CARNIVORE-*ISH*

125 Protein-Rich Recipes to
Boost Your Health & **Build Muscle**

Ashleigh VanHouten
& Beth Lipton

VICTORY BELT PUBLISHING
LAS VEGAS

First published in 2022 by Victory Belt Publishing, Inc.

ISBN-13: 978-1-628601-47-3

Cover design by Kat Lannom

Cover photo by Tatiana Briceag

Interior design by Kat Lannom and Charisse Reyes

Photos by Beth Lipton, Heather MacDonald, and Amy Zambonin

Illustrations by Allan Santos

Printed in Canada

TC 0122

CONTENTS

PREFACE

We bonded over butter.

Well, technically it was ghee. We met at a press event for a ghee company in New York City—both of us health writers, food enthusiasts, and constant learners looking to have new experiences, try new things, and meet new people in the relatively small world of ancestral health and nutrition. We hit it off right away, and as our understanding of and work in the world of healthy eating grew, so did our friendship. But yes, in the beginning, our connection boiled down to boiled-down butter.

One of the big things we've always had in common is that we both appreciate the value of animal-based food, which still, shockingly, seems a rarity in mainstream "health culture," especially as it relates to—and is marketed to—women. We feel strongly that the keys to deep, long-lasting health can be found in nature, in our bodies' innate wisdom, and in the wisdom that's been handed down through countless generations regarding what the human body craves at a cellular level. While the modern world affords us plenty of information, convenience, and entertainment, it obscures the truth around what our bodies and minds require to live a robust, happy, and healthy life. Unfortunately, there simply isn't much money to be made in a happy, healthy, self-sustaining society, so instead, an industry embodying diet culture, a sick-care medical system, and endless ineffective quick fixes leaves us misinformed, medicated, hungry, and frustrated. And the worst part is, we usually blame ourselves when we don't feel better or reach our goals.

We know this because we've been there; we've seen its effects. With a combined twenty-five-plus years in the health industry, we've seen—and tried—our share of diet and fitness plans, fads, biohacks, and experiments, only to keep coming back to what makes the most sense in our hearts and brains and bones: to move our bodies in ways that feel good; to nurture deep connections and relationships; to do work that is meaningful to us; to manage stress; to enjoy the sun and sleep deeply; and, at the center of it all, to eat a variety of nutrient-dense food that's as close to nature as we can get it. People are smart, but we're not smarter than nature; we haven't (and won't) create a "foodlike product" in a lab that will rival the pleasure and health that can be found in a perfectly cooked steak (maybe cooked in a little ghee).

If you are fed up with "wellness" or "diet" culture, you're not alone. It's normal to be overwhelmed by all of the conflicting information out there, and even to want to give up entirely. That's actually part of the sell; it's why we keep falling for quick fixes. We are here to tell you (women especially, since we're most often the target of this morality- and aesthetic-based health marketing) that you don't have to buy what social media or the latest influencer is selling. If it feels wrong to be told that the way humans have eaten throughout history is suddenly cruel, unhealthy, and unsustainable—well, that's because it *is* wrong.

Though there are those who truly believe it, the narrative demonizing animal protein is, for the most part, a marketing tactic. It is not grounded in fact, no matter what you might have seen in a Netflix "documentary." Cherry-picked science is not science. We'll get into that later.

We wanted to write a book based not on rules, or dogma, or fear, but based on a love of nutrient-dense animal foods—a celebration of nourishing food that is meant to be shared and savored. We want to show that eating a protein-forward diet is healthy, versatile, and delicious and that there are many ways to "eat whole foods." We want to show you that a healthy diet can be satisfying, even decadent—and these meals can also be simple and fun to prepare, even for the kitchen novice. Healthy eating is about how you feel just as much as what you eat; a stressed-out body won't digest food well. We want this book to be a tool to help you let go of the shame, guilt, or fear you might be feeling around animal protein and truly enjoy it on every level so you can find your path to true wellness.

Ultimately, we're just two friends who love to eat meat, and we want to share that love with you—with a little history, education, and humor thrown in. A meal is meant to be enjoyed and shared, and we hope this book helps you do just that.

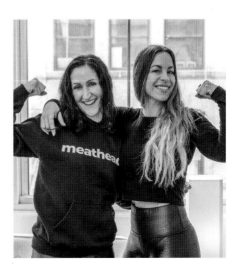

—Ashleigh and Beth

INTRODUCTION

We hope you'll find this book fun to use. We want it to be a resource to help you understand why an animal protein-forward diet can help you feel great and reach your body composition goals, a primer on how to do it deliciously without hassle, and a resource for tasty recipes to give you plenty of variety.

Here's a guide to the book to get you started:

- Explaining the carnivore diet and the carnivore-ish approach: It may seem like it's all beef all the time, but the carnivore diet actually can have a lot of variety. This section explains what this approach is, why people do it, and how you can use it in small doses as a tool. Carnivore-ish is not the same as the carnivore diet, so this section outlines the differences and the myriad advantages to a lots-of-meat-but-not-all-meat approach.

- Your carnivore-ish kitchen: This section will help you outfit your kitchen for success, both in terms of the tools and equipment you'll need and the ingredients you'll want to have on hand. There are some items in the book not listed here, but this section includes the ones you will need the most, for this book and for life beyond it.

- Get to know your proteins: We interviewed a host of experts to bring you this section, which gives you insider tips, busts myths, and corrects common mistakes about all kinds of animal proteins. Reading it will help you get the most bang for your buck and cook the way the pros do. We learned a ton from writing it, and we hope you get a lot from reading it.

- The recipes: Divided into chapters based on protein type, the entree recipes cover all times of day and every situation, from simple weeknight meals to show-stopping holiday celebrations, for all kinds of tastes. Beyond that are sides, sauces, and condiments designed to enhance and elevate the entrees. Then we have a chapter of appetizers and snacks and one of desserts and beverages, because life is too short to not have those. Some of the recipes in those chapters don't incorporate animal protein, but they complement animal protein well—though we sneaked it in there as often as possible, and in pretty creative ways, we think.

A few notes on the recipes:

- Recipes are guides, not laws. Often we point out ways to customize the recipes in this book. But you can do that anywhere you like, and we encourage you to do so (and to tag us on your creations if you post to social media). We bet it will come out great most of the time. And if it doesn't, laugh it off and try again another day. We all have our food fails; it's part of the fun and the learning experience. (Trust us, we had our share in the process of making this book.)

- We are loosey-goosey with seasoning, by design. We often instruct to season to taste with salt and pepper. The fact is, how much you need changes depending on the meat you're using, the type/brand of salt you're using, what else you're adding to your plate, and your individual taste. We encourage you to salt meat generously—but that may mean something different to us than it does to you. Again, please experiment: start with light seasoning and add more as you go. Over time, you'll develop a feel for how much you need for different applications.

- We don't call for grass-fed this or organic that in the recipes themselves. As you'll see in the first two chapters, we encourage you to shop for the highest-quality animal protein your budget allows. But if conventionally raised is what you have access to, that's OK. No one tells you not to eat vegetables if you can't afford all organic. Just because meat isn't 100 percent grass-fed doesn't mean it's devoid of health benefits.

- Carnivore reset/meal plans: We think a meat-based (and in some cases, strictly carnivore) temporary diet reset can be beneficial for many people, for a host of reasons. We explain those reasons here, as well as how exactly to go about a carnivore reset—and for fun, we put together some menus and meal plans based on the recipes in this book in case you'd like to throw a carnivore-ish brunch, holiday party, or picnic.

- Carnivore-ish on a budget: Animal protein can be quite pricey, and not everyone has unlimited funds to splurge on food all the time (we know we don't). This section gives you some solid strategies for procuring high-quality proteins no matter what your budget or where you live.

- Resources and recommended reading: Though this book is chock-full of information and recipes, there's always more to read and learn. In these two sections, we provide our research sources, favorite places for you to shop for meaty goods, and other information for you to nerd out on.

PART 1

GETTING *STARTED*

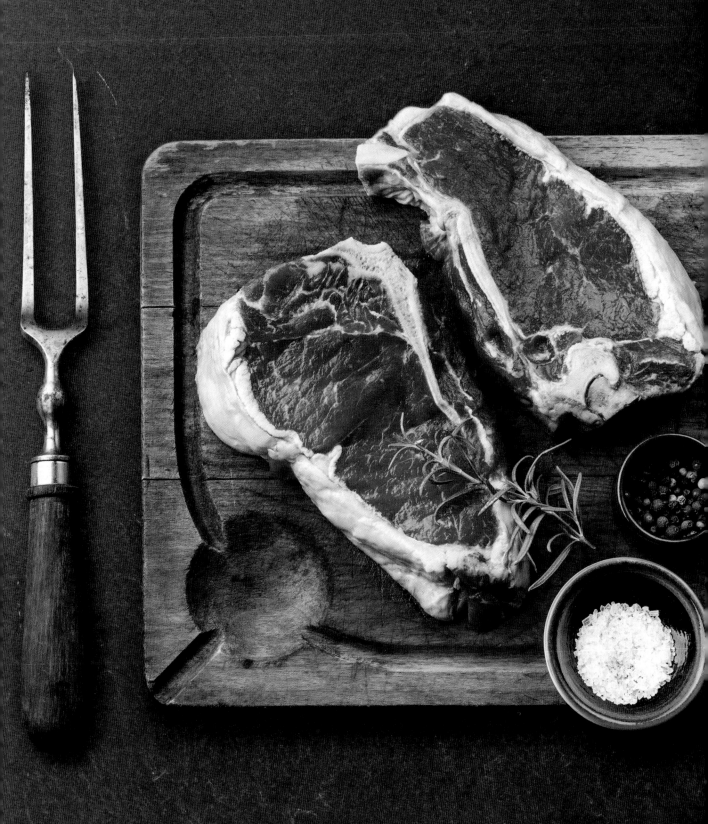

CHAPTER 1:

WHAT IS THE CARNIVORE DIET?

Most of you are probably familiar with the term *carnivore*—although it's usually attributed to fearsome animals, like sharks or some of the scarier dinosaurs. What it really means, though, is an animal that exclusively eats meat due to its physiology. Carnivores eat meat because that's the healthiest option for those animals to absorb nutrients, get energy, function properly, and thrive.

Simply put, a carnivore diet is one that incorporates only animal products. In this chapter, we explain what it means to be carnivore-ish, discuss how a carnivore approach can work as a temporary reset, and offer meal plan suggestions.

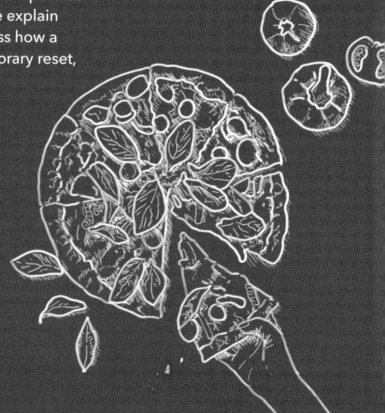

ARE HUMANS MEANT TO BE CARNIVORES?

Humans are omnivores; we are physiologically flexible and cunning enough to be opportunistic eaters. Our systems are set up to handle, digest, and use a wide array of plant and animal foods, and throughout history, humans from all over the planet have survived this way: by eating whatever was handy, available, and nourishing. Just look at how varied the traditional diets of humans all over the world are to this day, and you'll see what we mean.

In many cases, ancient humans relied on plant foraging (seeds, fruits, and tubers) to fill their bellies while they waited for the "good stuff"—the less frequent but much more nourishing and satisfying big meals comprised of an animal from the land or sea. While in the run of a day many of our ancestors would have spent time eating roots and seaweed, it was the less frequent fish, fowl, or large game catch that really ensured their survival.

In fact, evolutionary biologists and archaeologists have widely theorized that it was cooking and eating meat that made early hominids decidedly human, shrinking their stomachs and growing their brains dramatically over the course of human evolution. This is largely what separates us from our ape cousins: our relatively big brains consume about 20 percent of our bodies' overall energy at rest (despite making up about 2 percent of our body weight), which is twice that of other primates. A diet rich in meat affords us those nutrient-dense calories that led us to the top of the food chain, which, in turn, took us to the moon, onto the internet, and everywhere else. (Imagine how difficult it would be to create art and technology if we had to spend 80 percent of our waking hours eating leaves—like gorillas do—just to keep from starving.)

So, no, humans aren't technically carnivores. We're definitely not vegetarians, either. Though, of course, some of us choose to be carnivores and others, vegetarians. We're a complex mix, and where you fall on the spectrum depends on several factors: your ancestry, where you live, your unique goals or health challenges, and your personal preferences (or the preferences put on you by your culture or community).

OK, THEN WHAT DO YOU MEAN BY "CARNIVORE-*ISH*"?

With the rise in popularity of a strict carnivore diet—thanks in part to influential individuals like Dr. Shawn Baker, Joe Rogan, and Mikhaila Peterson, who subscribe to strict carnivore approaches with positive benefits—and the pervasive messaging about plant-based diets (more on that in a minute), we think it's time to take a step back, shut off all of the shouting voices, strip away the misinformation and marketing, and take a more instinctive, realistic look at how we eat.

"Carnivore-ish" is our cheeky way of saying that we value and emphasize animal protein for its nutrition and taste. But we're not here to demonize vegetables, fruit, spices, or desserts—you'll see them all over this book. The carnivore-ish approach keeps animal protein front and center while acknowledging that preferences and availability wax and wane: we may want to eat differently when we're training for something, whether it's summer or winter, or because we just happen to crave steak one day and eggs scrambled with vegetables the next. We're carnivore-ish because we know that diet is fluid and flexible and should be pleasurable, not punishing.

If we remove emotion and our general, modern discomfort with death, it's easy to see that animal protein is a crucial part of our evolution, function, and health, and that we thrive when we can enjoy healthy sources of animal protein. We're not here to tout one "best" way of eating. What we hope to show you, over the course of this book, is that animal protein is undeserving of the bad reputation it's received in the mainstream press and money-driven health industry. In fact, emphasizing it may be the hiding-in-plain-sight "secret" to the energy, good health, longevity, and, yes, body composition we all strive for.

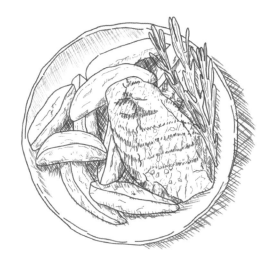

With our combined backgrounds in recipe development, cookbook writing, nutrition and food journalism, and various other work in the health and wellness industry, we understand how complex and dogmatic the world of healthy eating can be. What usually sells books, diet plans on social media, and products in the grocery store is a strict set of rules to follow and a tribe to join and identify with. The reason these don't work in the long term is that a successful approach to eating involves nuance, choice, and flexibility. We each need to find the diet that is nourishing, sustainable, and enjoyable for *us,* no matter what someone on the internet says is the right choice. This book is our answer to that—a tool we've created to help you find what works for you as the individual you are.

DEBUNKING 8 BIG MYTHS ABOUT EATING MEAT

My [sister, BFF, favorite influencer] says that plant-based is best.

Yeah, we know.

We're bombarded every day with messages that say eating animals is inherently cruel and unnatural; that it is negatively impacting the environment; that it will give us cancer or other terrible diseases. These claims are largely baseless and originate from special interest groups who are working with incomplete information, make money by keeping us fat and sick, or are trying to sell us expensive products. (No, we don't think your sister is evil or trying to hurt you; rather, it's the people she's getting her information from.)

The pressure to eat more (or only) plants is real, we get that. But again, if you zoom out, you'll see that much of the powerful messaging falls apart.

An argument can be made that a largely plant-based diet—one that is rich in variety and low in processed foods—may be healthier than the standard American diet (SAD). Many folks transitioning from the SAD to vegetarianism notice immediate health benefits. They assume it's the removal of meat that did the trick, when it most likely was getting rid of inflammatory foods and other processed junk.

The thing is, just because a plant-based diet is better than the toxin-filled SAD doesn't mean it's optimal. We seem to have the notion that if some of something (e.g., vegetables) is good, a lot is better, and the most extreme version (veganism) is the best. In reality, though, that's rarely true when it comes to health. Try giving up meat and going plant-based without eliminating junk foods; you'll likely see it wasn't the meat that was hurting you. (Please don't actually do this; we're just making a point here.)

Taking this a step further, some research has posited that a vegan diet is dangerous for pregnant women and children, and some places (like Belgium) have determined that feeding a child a vegan diet without significant monitoring and supplementation amounts to criminal negligence. In North America, women are frequently encouraged to eat a "wholesome, plant-based" diet, but then, for the sake of the baby's health, that advice is reversed when the woman becomes pregnant. If that doesn't speak to a systemic lack of care for women's health in favor of what's trendy and marketable, we don't know what does.

Red meat is bad for you.

There are so many other experts who have spent years researching this topic and can speak to it in a more in-depth way, so we'll cover it generally here and recommend that you learn more and read the works of Diana Rodgers, Weston A. Price, and others. The main point we want to get across is that human beings have been following our instincts and eating red meat for as long as we've been in existence, starting long before internet influencers began telling us what to do. In the span of human existence, only in the last handful of decades have we seen obesity, chronic disease, and diet-related illness skyrocket, and this is happening in conjunction with people eating less red meat and animal fat than ever before. They're replacing it with highly processed foods, trans fats, vegetable oils, and sugar (and combining that with less movement and sunshine and more chronic stress).

Red meat is an excellent source of protein and essential amino acids, as well as vitamins B_6 and B_{12} (the latter being an essential nutrient that is important for blood formation as well as brain and nervous system health, and that is derived almost exclusively from animal sources), phosphorus, zinc, iron (in heme form, which our bodies absorb much more readily than plant-based non-heme iron), and niacin. It's also rich in an antioxidant called glutathione, conjugated linoleic acid or CLA (a naturally occurring trans fat that has many health benefits when combined with a healthy diet), and cholesterol, another maligned compound that is actually crucial to many processes in the body, including brain function.

Many of the pervasive anti-meat narratives are unfortunate (and, in many cases, perhaps willful) misinterpretations of study data around human eating behavior. Many of these studies show a possible connection between meat eating and disease/mortality but no correlation, and they do not take into account limitations like individual self-reporting or the myriad other connections that could be made between combined lifestyle factors and health but were not highlighted. In other words, if a study participant eats fast food, smokes, drinks a lot, doesn't exercise, and is in poor health, many studies conclude it was the meat on the fast-food burger that caused the problem, not any of the other lifestyle factors. Much more recent and well-designed studies have disproved the outdated concept that red meat is directly linked to mortality and cancer, although this new information has taken some time to enter into the mainstream conversation—perhaps largely because it would upset the current consumer landscape that so many massive, influential corporations rely on.

It may be one of our most costly nutrition fallacies, in fact, that one of the more maligned and feared foods on the planet—red meat—is actually one of the most healthful and nutrient-dense. The micronutrients found in abundance in meat (and most bioavailable via meat, based on our physiology) are required for body function and, perhaps more importantly than ever, in decreasing the instances of depression. We're not here to tell you that eating steak will make you a happier person; we're simply suggesting that giving your body the fuel it needs can help establish a robust, resilient, and well-functioning body and mind, and that quality animal products are an optimal way to provide that fuel.

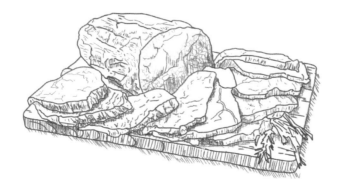

Eating meat is cruel.

It can be incredibly difficult to separate emotion from fact when it comes to topics of life, death, pain, and personal opinions of ethics and morality. But the more we attempt to look at these important topics from an objective, science-based approach rather than a personal, emotional one, the more apt we are to make sound decisions.

If you've ever watched a nature documentary, you know that life is harsh and death is inevitable. In our modern world, we've grown uncomfortable with the idea of death, but that doesn't make it go away. Life involves death. That doesn't mean animals shouldn't be raised ethically, cared for well, and slaughtered as humanely as possible. They absolutely should, and if it's important to you, you can choose to buy meat from animals that were raised that way. We do. But the idea that animals won't die if we don't eat them is patently false; in fact, many of them would suffer much more if killed by starvation or predators. If humans didn't exist and the rest of the animal kingdom ruled the world, do we think death would cease to exist? Our bodies nourish other bodies, as well as the soil and plants. Why are we so narcissistic as to think we are not a part of the natural circle of life?

When a person chooses a plant-based diet, they can't ensure that animals don't die in the process of making their food. Vegan diets are absolutely not blood-free; the razing of crops often requires the deaths of thousands of small rodents and other animals. According to farmer, registered dietitian, and *Sacred Cow* author Diana Rodgers, "Many animals lose their lives in the process of farming vegetables... Birds and butterflies are poisoned by chemicals, rabbits and mice are run over by tractors, and vast fields of monocropped vegetables displace native populations of animals that once lived on the land."[1] (Monocropping is the practice of cultivating a large single-plant crop like corn or wheat on the same land, year after year, without rotation, which results in soil depletion and erosion, among other detrimental environmental impacts. It provides higher yields—and higher earnings—for those planting the crops, but it's often harmful to the environment and the land. It involves overuse of pesticides, fertilizers, and water and contributes to declining biodiversity, pest issues, pesticide resistance, and other negative impacts.) You could argue that sustainable agriculture—in which animals are raised in a healthy, happy, and humane environment; they are killed painlessly; and their bodies are used for sustenance—is a much more useful and respectful way to honor their lives than mowing them down with a tractor to harvest monocrops while making no use of their bodies.

[1] Rodgers, D., "Sentience: Black & White? Good & Bad?," *Sustainable Dish* (blog), July 4, 2017, https://sustainabledish.com/sentience-black-white-good-bad/

We're not trying to get people who truly don't want to eat meat to do so. We are not in the business of pushing our beliefs on anyone, and we acknowledge that there is a wide range of healthy diet options for human beings depending on individual preferences and goals. But so many people are fighting their instincts to eat meat, battling their desire for it, based on arguments that simply aren't true. If you are open-minded enough to read this book and still decide that plant-based eating is for you, more power to you. We just want everyone to have the information required to make the best decisions possible.

Eating meat is unnatural.

The argument that eating meat is unnatural (that is, not something humans are meant to do) is categorically false and easy to disprove. Humans are physiologically omnivores and have received the majority of their nutrients and calories from meat since the beginning of human existence, across the globe. The stark fact of our physiology can't be disputed, despite many overtly false articles on the internet claiming humans are naturally herbivorous.

The evidence is right in front of our faces—*in* our faces, actually. Our teeth include flat, chewing molars (great for breaking down plants) as well as sharper incisors and canines, ideal for ripping meat.

Our system of digestion also reveals our nature. Our bodies lack cellulases, enzymes for breaking down vegetables, that many herbivores have, although we do have sucrases for digesting fruit and an abundance of proteases for breaking down animal protein. Human beings require vitamin B_{12} to thrive, which historically could come only from bacteria or animal sources. Our digestive tracts are longer than those of carnivorous animals like lions and wolves but shorter than those of herbivores like cows and sheep, making us capable of digesting fats and proteins as well as some (but not all) vegetable matter. Cows, which thrive on grazing grasses and other plant matter, have four stomachs—just think about what would happen to our digestion if we were suddenly forced to eat their diet. Instead, nature created a system where cows eat the grass and we eat them. Our closest evolutionary relatives, chimpanzees, are also omnivorous.

One argument we hear often is that just because we can kill and eat animals doesn't mean we should. While we would apply that reasoning to some things (just because you can eat an entire box of donuts in a sitting doesn't mean you should), it doesn't make sense here. To do so ignores the complex fabric of nature. We can kill animals and eat them, and, in fact, that is our place in the ecosystem.

Eliminating meat is the answer to climate change.

Again, there is an abundance of resources and information on this topic already out in the world, and it's actually a relatively complex one—understanding how carbon emissions and carbon sequestration and global warming all work—so we'll try to keep this as short and sweet as we can and encourage you to continue to do your own learning and research.

A common refrain is that our current farming practices make up a dizzying proportion of the climate-changing carbon emissions on our planet: more than all transportation emissions combined. Many of those working in sustainable agriculture argue that it's not animal farming as a whole that's to blame; it's unethical and unsustainable farming practices, and there are ways to raise animals that actually provide a carbon sink (meaning the soil will absorb and store carbon, reducing the amounts of carbon in the atmosphere), which is a benefit for our environment.

Grazing cows add microorganisms to the soil through their manure and stimulate grass growth through their movements, which encourages healthy pasture—pasture that is not appropriate for crop growth, meaning that grazing land for animals does not take away crop land for plants. (Some 70 percent of grazeable land is not appropriate for crops and could not be used for this purpose whether the animals were there or not.) This type of natural, cyclical interaction does not happen in a monoculture farming environment. While vast chemical-supported monocrops deplete the soil, sustainable agriculture supports soil health by replenishing nutrients through water, compost, and natural movement. Poor agricultural practices and continuous grazing contribute to soil erosion and nutrient depletion, while research shows that regenerative grazing practices (including moving cattle to different spaces to allow natural processes to occur and avoid overgrazing) can significantly improve soil carbon and soil health, and even can help restore brittle or dying land back to health.

There is so much more we could cover here, but the overall message is that it is unsustainable agricultural practices in both animal and plant farming that are harming our planet. Rather than vilifying animals (who have always existed and roamed the earth in a symbiotic way), we should aim to improve those agricultural practices to support a regenerative, health-promoting system. The idea that we can a) stop all humans from consuming meat; b) replace all grazing land with crops; and c) improve human health and the health of the planet by eating only plants simply isn't accurate or realistic.

People—especially women—are supposed to eat "light," low-fat, and plant-based.

The notion that women are supposed to eat "light" to maintain health is downright harmful on a number of levels. Not only is it unrealistic (this is why people who lose weight on traditional diets often gain it all back and even add more), but it also causes unnecessary suffering. Plus, we've attached morality (or a lack thereof) to our desire for nourishment. What does "light" even mean? We've seen vegan desserts and a vegetarian burrito or two that could never be described as light.

Some of the recipes in this book will seem indulgent at first glance. They're full of meat, full-fat dairy, eggs, butter, and other foods that we've been taught to think of as rich, decadent, or even "bad" in an "it tastes so good it must be bad" kind of way. Sadly, many of these foods fall under the category of guilty pleasures, stuff that people enjoy but feel bad about enjoying—another fallacy we're hoping to fix.

We believe that humans are attracted to these foods not because life is about a constant struggle between what we want and what's good for us but rather because nature is on our side, pushing us toward what we need. News flash: Sex feels good because we need to keep doing it to propagate the species. It's the same with food. These rich, indulgent foods are also nutrient-dense, and our bodies are designed to use them for fuel. We're supposed to want them because they help us to live well.

You may be thinking, "OK, but why do I crave sugar so much?" Well, maybe because you don't eat enough meat. Our ancient ancestors lived in cycles of feast and famine. If you had an unsuccessful hunt, you didn't order in; instead, you went without food. Filling up on meat wasn't gluttony; it was survival. And when they found some honey or a lot of fruit was in season, they ate it, because who knew when they'd find it again?

For most people, all of that is completely out the window now. You can get all manner of sweets anytime (you can't wait in line to check out at Office Depot without facing a wall of king-size Twizzlers, Milky Ways, and Skittles), and you've been sold this bill of goods about making meat a condiment while you pound "healthy" carbs all day. So you're left hungry and unsatisfied and riding the wave of needing sugar and having junk food thrust in your face all the time. Even if you eat a lower-carb diet, the pressure to incorporate more plant-based foods is real, and this constant pressure can take time and patience to unlearn.

We think you'll find that as you shift your eating habits to prioritize protein—specifically the protein that's richest in nutrients and the most bioavailable, *animal protein*—you will "need" sugar less. You will feel more satisfied in general, and your sugar cravings will abate.

Does that mean you'll never want a brownie again? Nope. You will. (We would worry if you didn't.) But you will "need" it less; the cravings won't rule you as much. And the best part: you'll be in much better shape, with the body composition you want and the metabolic flexibility that allows you to enjoy the hell out of that occasional brownie and then move on with your life.

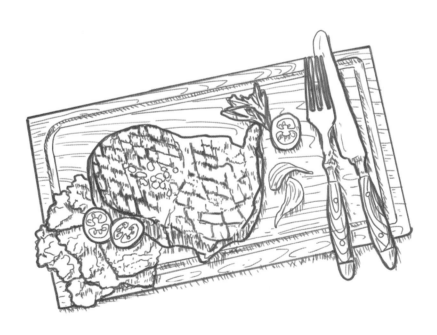

Women shouldn't eat too much protein.

Related to, but different from, the eating "light" issue, this may be one of the more frustrating arguments considering that much of the longstanding misinformation around women's nutrition and health is deeply entrenched in sexist notions of how women "should" look and behave. The massive fitness and health market targeted toward women has long prioritized mainstream concepts of beauty, attractiveness, and femininity over health, happiness, sustainability, and performance. The depth of fear-based marketing and pseudoscience involved in creating a culture whereby certain foods are more appropriate for certain genders is truly mind-boggling, if you stop to think about it. When was the last time you saw an advertisement of a laughing man eating low-fat yogurt, promising long-lasting happiness as a result of feeling lighter and looking thinner? It sounds outrageously silly, but women have to contend with this type of misogynistic marketing all day, every day.

By many accounts, women make up as much as 85 percent of the consumer market; they are buying more products and more of the food for their households, so it makes sense that most food marketing is geared toward a sense of "fixing women's problems," whether it's how they look, how much they weigh, or how they're feeding and supporting their families. (Ironically, many of these problems are created or perpetuated by companies that then conveniently offer the solutions—for a price. From fast-food chains offering ultra-processed "plant-based alternatives" and massive junk food conglomerates buying up pseudohealthy brands, the manipulation at play here is deeply layered.) As Diana Rodgers writes on her website:

I love working with women to teach them about the importance of eating meat, because in most cases, if you can help women understand good nutrition, you've fixed the whole household. Iron deficiency is the most common nutritional deficiency, with prevalence highest among young children and women of childbearing age, particularly pregnant women. We're not going to fix this with more salads. We need to let women know that it's OK to eat meat. Red meat has gotten such a bad reputation, but meat is an incredibly nutrient-dense food.[2]

[2] Rodgers, D., "Women and Meat," *Sustainable Dish* (blog), October 17, 2016, https://sustainabledish.com/women-and-meat/

The reality is, women and men are both human, with bone, muscle, and a digestive system, and the foods we require to support those systems are the same. (Do you think our hunter-gatherer or even preindustrial ancestors had special "women's foods"?) Due to women's unique hormonal makeup and fluctuating requirements during various stages of life (reproductive age versus menopause, for example), we may need to prioritize protein—and its important micronutrients like iron—even more than men. Women show an increased tendency toward sarcopenia (muscle wasting) and bone density loss as we age, meaning that we must prioritize a diet that minimizes and even reverses these issues. Muscle wasting, bone breakage, osteoporosis—many of the challenges we consider inevitable aspects of aging—are largely preventable, or at least drastically slowed, through a supportive, nourishing diet and movement plan. That means, yes, eating more animal protein and lifting heavier weights, two things we're expressly discouraged from doing by mainstream advertising. (There's a reason why the 3-pound dumbbells are usually pink.)

While many online resources point to the "minimum daily requirement for protein" landing at around 10 to 15 percent of total calories, or 0.8 gram of protein per kilogram of body weight, which equates to 50 to 60 grams of protein daily, we must remember that the minimum requirements for survival are not the same as the optimal amounts for robust health and long life.

Most of the world is not at risk of eating too much protein; in fact, the opposite problem is true, as our food culture leads us further down the path of sugar and processed carbohydrate consumption. It's worth noting that a significant body of research shows that overeating protein will not cause you to gain fat, whereas overeating fat and carbohydrates will. On the contrary, protein intake plays a pivotal role when it comes to weight loss, not only because it helps to build and maintain lean muscle, improves satiety, and costs your body more calories just to digest but also because it is not easily converted to body fat the way carbohydrates are.

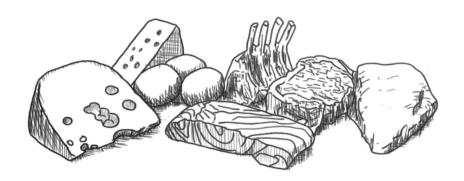

Plant protein is just as good as animal protein.

Most well-intentioned plant-based nutritionists we've come across will admit that in order for strict vegan eaters to optimize their nutrition and health, they have to supplement, sometimes significantly, to obtain ideal amounts of essential amino acids and some vitamins and minerals. While it's certainly possible to eat a meat-heavy diet and still be missing some key nutrients, omitting animal protein from your diet sets you up for a significant disadvantage nutritionally. Although supplements have their place and can be useful, our bodies absorb nutrients more optimally from easily digestible whole foods (and often best in the presence of fats), which is why this should always be the first option, with supplementation as more of a last resort.

Let's break down why animal protein is objectively a more complete source of nutrition than plant protein.

Protein is composed of amino acids; there are twenty amino acids that make up the human body. Nine of these are considered "essential" amino acids, in that our bodies require them and cannot make them, so we must obtain them from food sources. All animal proteins have all nine essential amino acids, whereas very few plants contain all nine, and you generally need to eat much larger amounts of those plant foods to absorb the optimal amounts of those necessary amino acids. For practicality and efficiency reasons, animal protein is a far superior source.

Specifically, animal protein is the richest source of leucine (a key essential amino acid responsible for triggering muscle growth and repair) and creatine (a protein molecule made from the essential acids arginine and methionine that is shown to support athletic performance and recovery), both of which are critically important when it comes to building lean muscle mass.

Even the complete plant proteins—including soy, hemp, and quinoa—contain protein and amino acids in such relatively low amounts that you'd have to eat much more of them to get the requisite nutrients, which is not practical from a digestion or caloric standpoint (we'd rather eat three ounces of beef than three full cups of quinoa). And if you aren't eating complete proteins from plant sources, the level of chemical alchemy needed to ensure you're getting the most from your diet is exhausting, time-consuming, and inefficient.

Animal versus Plant Proteins

3 OUNCES 80:20 BEEF

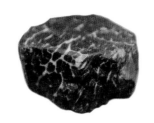

3 OUNCES QUINOA

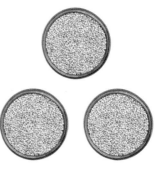

216	calories	102
17g	fat	1.6g
0g	carbs	18g
15g	protein	3.7g

3 OZ. WILD-CAUGHT SALMON

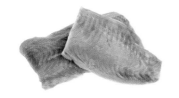

3 OZ. CHICKPEAS

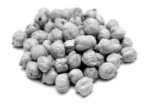

130	calories	135
4g	fat	2g
0g	carbs	23g
22g	protein	8g

HOW TO APPROACH A CARNIVORE RESET

As we've indicated, we don't think you have to adhere to a strict diet, or any kind of dietary dogma, to be healthy and nourished. Just because a specific plan worked for someone else—or even worked for you previously—doesn't mean you have to try it or stick to it forever. We are all individuals, with different challenges, goals, and preferences. That's what makes our health journeys fun, if also more complicated than we might want them to be.

Having said that, we also believe there is space for focused and *temporary* dietary "resets." These short periods of restriction can be a helpful tool for many reasons. Here are some circumstances in which a reset may be beneficial:

- As part of a monitored elimination-diet protocol to determine which foods may be causing inflammatory responses, digestive problems, or other issues in your body (followed by a period in which foods are mindfully reintroduced so you can monitor their effects)

- To remove processed foods, sugar, or vegetable oils from your diet

- To reset hunger and satiety signals after a period of bingeing or just eating too much suboptimal food (for example, after an indulgent vacation or the holidays)

- As a temporary fat loss tool

We recommend that you speak to a trusted health professional (hopefully one who is knowledgeable about nutrition and won't try to convince you that "animal fat is dangerous" and tofu and peanut butter are your best sources of protein) and use discretion whenever you undergo a dietary change.

In mainstream circles, these resets often look like juice fasts or seven- to thirty-day vegan challenges. Obviously, that isn't what we're talking about here; you already know why those approaches are both counterproductive and unhealthy. (The juice cleanses just kill us: you're essentially stripping out much of what's good from fruits and vegetables—fiber—and drinking only liquid sugar, and somehow this is what your body needs to "detox"? No.) Instead, we're talking about short carnivore resets. We've found these to be effective for addressing the previously listed issues, without the side effects that juice or vegan "cleanses" have, including a lack of nutrients and severe hunger.

Prolonged fasts—where you consume nothing but water for a period of days—are another approach. While this type of fasting can be a great tool for some people, we'd rather enjoy many of the same blood sugar-regulating and anti-inflammatory benefits while still eating satisfying animal protein, supporting our bodies' functions, and maintaining (or building) muscle.

For most of us, a three-, five-, or even seven-day "strict" carnivore approach can be sufficient to kick-start many of the goals we're looking to achieve: eliminate sugar cravings, regulate blood glucose, decrease bloating and inflammation, and even drop a pound or two. You may choose to keep these approaches going for longer—up to a month or more—and again we encourage you to pay attention to your body, get your bloodwork done so you have before-and-after metrics to study, and work with an experienced health professional.

Note: A reset may not be appropriate for someone with an eating disorder or a history of disordered eating. If this describes you, or you even suspect it might, please speak with a trusted mental health professional before restricting your diet.

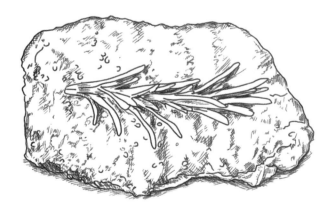

How to do a carnivore reset:

- Decide how long you're going to do it. Having a goal in mind is helpful. Though a carnivore reset is easier to do than other types of elimination diets because it's so satiating, there's still a mental hurdle around having any restrictions, and it can be somewhat inconvenient if you eat meals with others and have to explain what you're doing. Set your goal, mark your calendar, and get yourself mentally ready for the task.

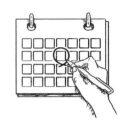

- Consume only animal products. We recommend a variety of meats from different sources, different cuts, and different preparations (three days of nothing but ground beef or steak can get boring). Prep your favorite ground meats, chicken thighs and hearts, shredded chicken, beef, pork, fish, shellfish, canned fish, eggs…you get the point. Use animal fats to prepare and cook these proteins: for example, tallow, schmaltz, butter, and ghee.

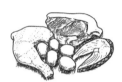

- Grab the salt. Use high-quality salt to season your food and ensure proper electrolyte balance and hydration. Salt helps the body absorb water, so don't be shy about salting your food— but no need to overdo it. Salt to taste.

- Season more…or don't. In terms of seasonings other than salt, it depends on your goals. If you're using a carnivore reset to determine whether you have any food sensitivities, you may want to skip spices, as some can have an inflammatory impact. But if you're just looking to ditch the sugar and cravings or feel better after a booze- and junk food–fueled vacation (we've been there), feel free to sprinkle in some of your favorites to keep things interesting, like cumin, garlic powder, paprika, and so on.

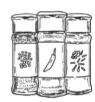

- Consume dairy at your discretion. You may include dairy such as cream, yogurt, and cheese if you want to and if you tolerate and digest it well. Keep it full fat and obviously no sugar added. Bonus points if you have access to raw dairy.

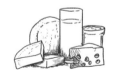

- Snack if you need to. Depending on your goals and comfort level, you can play with carnivore snacks like beef jerky, dehydrated cheese, and pork rinds. Mixing up flavors and textures will keep you from getting food fatigue.

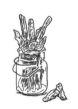

- Stay hydrated...with water. Make sure to drink plenty of water. If you are "detoxing" from highly processed foods, carbs, and alcohol, you may find yourself eliminating some bloat and stored water, and while meat has a high water content, it can be easy to become dehydrated. Water is your only beverage if you're going 100 percent carnivore; if you're giving yourself some leeway, coffee (black or with cream), tea, sparkling water, and no-sugar electrolyte beverages are fine to include. But, for the length of your reset, you'll need to skip the booze, kombucha, and other beverages (especially those with artificial sweeteners).

- Eat to satiety. We can't tell you exactly how many ounces of what or how often to eat; that's up to you to figure out. We encourage you to pay attention to your hunger and satiety signals and use them as your guide on how much (and even when) to eat and stop eating. Now, if you're someone who really needs some numbers to work with, think of it this way: try to stick as close to your maintenance calories as possible, but don't sweat it if you end up under that. You will not starve on an all-beef, chicken, and sardine diet for a few days, we promise. This will be an excellent exercise in listening to your body, slowing down your eating, and practicing mindfulness. Practice sitting down with your food and having no other distractions, taking a few deep breaths and smelling your food before eating it, setting your fork down between bites and chewing thoroughly, and really thinking about the nourishment you're putting into your body as you eat. In our experience, it is extremely difficult to overeat when meat is all you're eating. Steak frites, sure (because of the frites), but when it's just the steak, your body usually gives you pretty clear messages that you've had enough.

Common pitfalls to avoid:

- Carb or junk food loading in preparation and then going "cold turkey" (no pun intended). Get rid of the "last meal" thinking. This is a temporary reset, not the last time donuts will ever be available. Depending on your diet before you undertake a reset, you may experience some discomfort as your body adjusts to fewer carbohydrates and less sugar, alcohol, or other inputs than it is accustomed to. You may have heard of the "low-carb flu" that some people experience when cutting carbs or going keto, which can include 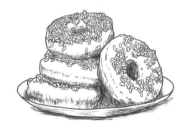 headaches, fatigue, irritability, and generally feeling crappy for a day or two as the body switches from exclusively burning sugar to burning both stored and exogenous fats. Don't make it harder on yourself by bingeing before you reset. All that does is set you up for a miserable experience. We recommend gradually reducing the amounts of whatever it is you'll be forgoing—whether it's caffeine, alcohol, sugar, or all of the above—in the days leading up to your reset to give your body its best chance to function optimally.

- Eating the same thing over and over. Life is both too short and too long to be bored with your food. We understand that not everyone loves spending time in the kitchen, and many simply don't have time to spend cooking. But eating the exact same thing over and over—even for just a few days—creates food fatigue, boredom, and increased likelihood of giving up, and it can even increase the chances of food intolerance. The best way to avoid all that is to have as much variety as possible in your carnivore reset (and in your diet in general). As we mentioned earlier, even a "meat-only" diet can provide near-endless combinations of tastes, flavors, and textures if you use a little imagination. Even if you have only ground beef for three days, you can prepare it in different ways—made into burgers or cheese-stuffed meatballs, folded into an omelet, slow-cooked in fat until it's crisp (check the Beef Confit recipe on page 100), and so on. But there's no reason to have only ground beef. Stock up on whichever kinds of meat, pork, poultry, eggs, fish, seafood, and game you like and make the reset fun and pleasurable. You're doing something good for yourself, and there's no reason it should feel like a punishment. We are firm believers in enjoying what you eat, and a little effort can go a long way.

- Going too strict for too long. Just because a week felt great doesn't mean a month is necessary. In our culture, we seem to think that if a little of something is good, then a lot is better, and the most extreme form is the "best." In fact, that's rarely the case when it comes to nutrition or health overall. Time and again, we've seen this "more is better" approach result in people crashing and burning—going too long without any carb sources while also training hard; mental exhaustion from being super-strict with your diet, which can impact your social and family time; being overly obsessed or preoccupied with your diet when it's not truly necessary; and the list goes on. Only you know how your choices are truly impacting your body and mind, so we can't tell you what kind of approach is appropriate for you, but we do know that when your dedication to a diet begins to negatively impact your physical and mental health, stress levels, and relationships, it's time to take a step back and reevaluate why you're doing it. A reset is meant to be just that; it isn't a long-term lifestyle.

- Not being mindful with reintroducing foods after the reset. We get it—it's been three, five, or seven days (or longer) since you've had anything but animal products, and you may be looking to dive headfirst into a pizza and a beer. But that can mean undoing all of the good that your reset did for your body and missing out on learning how some of your "normal" foods are impacting you. If you're doing an easy three-day reset to get back on track after a vacation, this shouldn't be an issue, but if you're going strict carnivore for a week or more to try to figure out which foods may be negatively impacting you, it's important that you add these foods back one at a time and wait at least a day (ideally two) after reintroducing a food before you add another one. Keep a journal of the foods you're adding back in, including the quantity you ate, what you ate it with, when you ate it, and how you felt immediately after, an hour or so after, the next day, and so on. Pay attention to your digestion, energy, mood, and sleep; depending on your goals or challenges, tracking your blood sugar may be appropriate as well. It sounds like a hassle, but this short-term investment can give you priceless information about what foods work for you and which ones might be holding you back. You've already committed to the work, so be patient and methodical with your data collection—it will pay off.

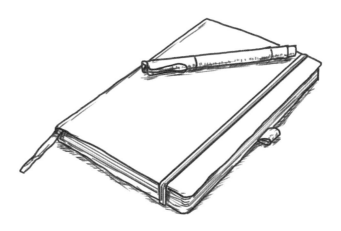

SAMPLE 3-DAY CARNIVORE RESET MEAL PLAN

Reminder: Serving sizes and actual meal breakdowns are up to your discretion. If you like to eat fewer larger meals or prefer to snack all day, that's up to you. Think of this as a guide to what a few days of carnivore eating can look like rather than a strict meal plan that you must stick to. Most of these recipes are, or can be made, strict carnivore by omitting non-animal-based ingredients.

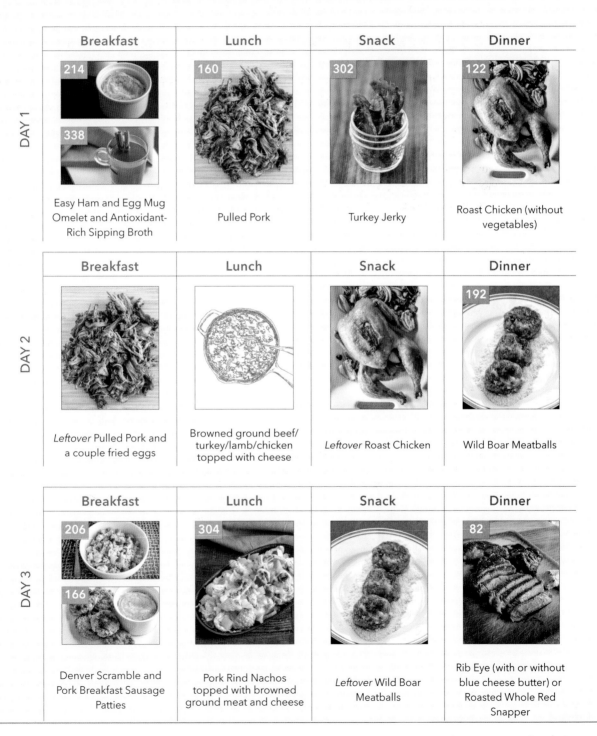

DAY 1

Breakfast	Lunch	Snack	Dinner
214 / 338	160	302	122
Easy Ham and Egg Mug Omelet and Antioxidant-Rich Sipping Broth	Pulled Pork	Turkey Jerky	Roast Chicken (without vegetables)

DAY 2

Breakfast	Lunch	Snack	Dinner
			192
Leftover Pulled Pork and a couple fried eggs	Browned ground beef/turkey/lamb/chicken topped with cheese	*Leftover* Roast Chicken	Wild Boar Meatballs

DAY 3

Breakfast	Lunch	Snack	Dinner
206 / 166	304		82
Denver Scramble and Pork Breakfast Sausage Patties	Pork Rind Nachos topped with browned ground meat and cheese	*Leftover* Wild Boar Meatballs	Rib Eye (with or without blue cheese butter) or Roasted Whole Red Snapper

CARNIVORE-ISH MENU IDEAS

Carnivore-ish Brunch

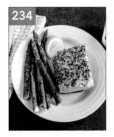

Everything Bagel Salmon

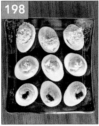

Deviled Eggs Three Ways

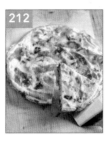

Caramelized Onion and Leek Frittata with Prosciutto

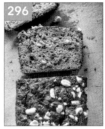

Elvis Banana Bread

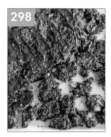

Dark Chocolate–Coconut Granola Clusters

Carnivore-Curious Dinner

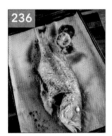

Roasted Whole Red Snapper

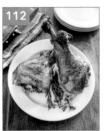

Turkey Legs Confit

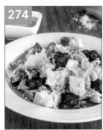

Caesar Salad with Pork Belly "Croutons"

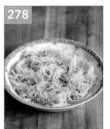

Garlicky Spaghetti Squash

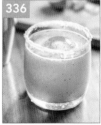

Spicy Toro Shot

High-Protein Picnic

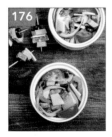

Italian Sub Salad

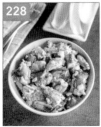

Lemon-Tarragon Lobster Salad

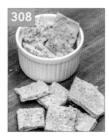

"Animal" Crackers

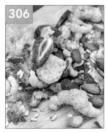

Forager Trail Mix

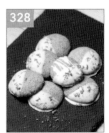

Orange White Chocolate-Dipped Duck Fat Sugar Cookies

Kid's Lunch

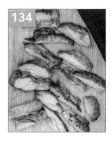
Spicy Air Fryer Chicken Thighs

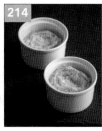
Easy Ham and Egg Mug Omelet

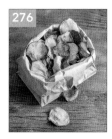
Air Fryer Mixed Sweet Potato Chips

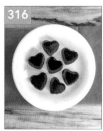
Fruit Jellies

Special-Event Spread

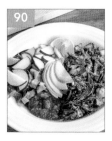
Chipotle Shredded Beef

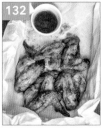
Hot Honey Chicken Wings

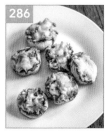
Stuffed Mushrooms

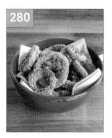
Pork Panko Onion Rings

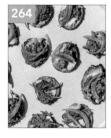
Tongue Sliders

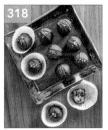
Secret-Ingredient Cookie Dough Truffles

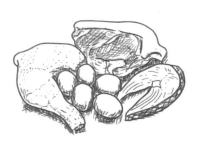

Dinner Party on a Budget

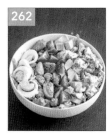
Grilled Chicken Heart Cobb Salad

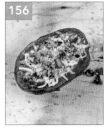
Loaded Sweet Potatoes

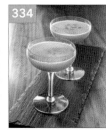
Blood Orange Gin Fizz

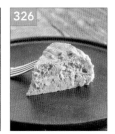
Japanese-Style Cheesecake

CHAPTER 2:

YOUR CARNIVORE-ISH KITCHEN

Here's the good news: a kitchen that's optimized for a carnivore-ish diet isn't all that different from a kitchen that's aimed at any approach to healthy eating. All you need are a few good tools and, of course, great ingredients. Here's what we recommend to make your carnivore-ish cooking as easy, fun, and delicious as possible.

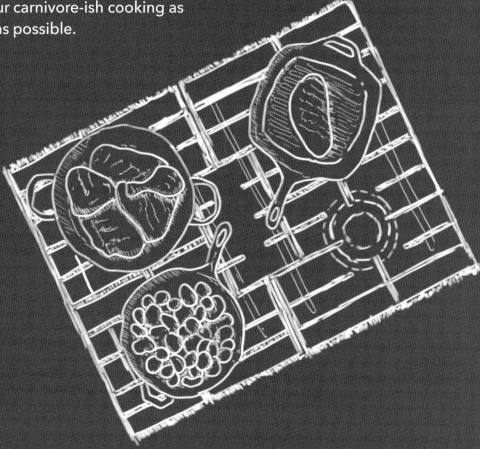

UTENSILS/COOKING EQUIPMENT

A well-outfitted kitchen isn't one that has every flashy gadget. Even if you don't live in a tiny New York City apartment like Beth does, avoiding clutter is key to stress-free, streamlined cooking. The following list highlights the essentials, with the occasional mention of some cool gadgets you may want if you're into that and have the space.

Knives

Knives are among the most important items in your kitchen, full stop. Though you can spend bundles of cash on knives and get a different one for just about every task, the truth is, you really need only three:

- **Chef's knife:** This is the knife you'll use most often. It's great for slicing and chopping, carving meat off of bones, and removing skin from fish. When in doubt, grab your chef's knife. They range in size and weight, though most people tend to gravitate toward an 8- to 10-inch chef's knife. If you are going to buy one, we recommend going to a store and holding the knives in your hand to find the one that is most comfortable.

- **Serrated knife:** This is the knife to use for slicing. It looks like a kitchen version of a saw, and that's essentially what it is. It's best used for foods with thick surfaces and softer interiors, like bread (in fact, it's sometimes called a bread knife). It's also great for slicing produce that is soft in the center but has a firm skin, like melon and eggplant. There's some debate over whether it's OK to use a serrated knife to carve roasts. We don't use it for that task, but if you do and you have success with it, there's no reason to change.

- **Paring knife:** This smaller knife has a shorter blade and is essential for more delicate jobs that require precision, like julienning and peeling. It's also useful if you're going to make a small cut in the center of a piece of fish to check for doneness.

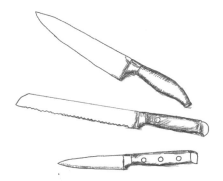

Depending on how much and what type of cooking you do, you may also want to invest in a slicing knife, which is long and thin like a serrated knife but with a straight edge. It's useful for slicing meat such as roasts and steaks, along with poultry and fish. Cooks who don't like the drag of a serrated blade on meat usually prefer a slicing knife. You can go all-out and get a cleaver and a boning knife, but these tools aren't necessary for the average cook.

PRO TIP: CARING FOR YOUR KNIVES

You don't need fancy, expensive knives—what you do need is sharp ones. Sharp knives make every job easier and neater, and they're safer to use. As such, get yourself a sharpening stone and a blade honer. How frequently you sharpen your knives depends on how often you use them; generally, every few months is OK. Honing is not the same as sharpening. (When you see chefs on TV running their knives over a long metal tube with a flourish, they are honing, not sharpening.) Sharpening actually removes metal from the blade to create a fresh edge. Honing realigns the center of the blade, which does help with sharpness but isn't the same as sharpening.

If you have access to professional sharpening via a kitchen supply store or department store, it's worthwhile to get your knives sharpened by a pro at least once a year.

Lastly, be sure to thoroughly clean and dry your knives by hand after each use. Never put them in the dishwasher. Store them in a wooden block or mount them on a magnetic strip, whichever suits your space. Don't let them rattle around in a drawer; this can damage them and is unsafe for you.

Cutting Boards

People have strong opinions about wood versus plastic; we're agnostic. We have both and use them for different applications. Plastic cutting boards are great for raw protein and smelly foods, like onions and garlic, because you can put the boards in the dishwasher to sanitize them and remove the odor. Wooden ones are more attractive and sometimes can double as serving vessels (for a charcuterie plate, for example), and arguably they can be easier on your knives. It's a good idea to have at least two so you can use one for raw items and another for things like fresh vegetables. Don't put your wooden cutting boards in the dishwasher; they'll warp. Instead, use very hot water, dish soap, and a brush or sponge. Be sure to clean both sides of the board whether you cut on the surface or not, because there could be bacteria on the counter and/or something may have dripped onto the other side.

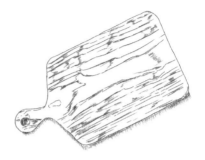

Instant-Read Thermometer

This essential tool can mean the difference between consistent success in cooking meat and…well, the opposite. By checking the internal temperature of meat, poultry, and fish (and other things, like custards), you can tell whether they're cooked to a safe temperature (as in poultry) and to the right level of doneness (as in a medium-rare steak), with no guessing. There are a lot of options out there. Beth wrote a story for a magazine where she tested six popular ones to find the best, so we'll save you the trouble: we like the ThermoWorks Thermapen ONE best overall, and the best one on a budget is the Kizen Instant Read Meat Thermometer.

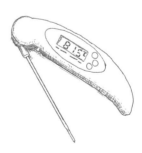

Peeler

If you have one of those flimsy metal peelers that you bought at a supermarket, toss it and get yourself a good one. (You can tell yours is crappy if peeling a carrot is difficult in any way.) You can buy a good one for less than $10, and it's so worth it. Whether you get a regular peeler or a Y-shaped one depends on your preference. Make sure the blade is sharp and the handle is comfortable.

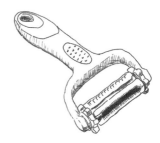

COOL GADGET:

> *Serrated peeler. This tool is great for peeling thin-skinned foods like tomatoes and peaches. If you do that a lot, get one. It will save you from having to blanch the items to remove the skins.*

Whisk

There are many different whisk shapes available, but we find the traditional teardrop or balloon shape does the trick. One is plenty; an 11-inch whisk can handle most jobs. But if you feel like it, having a few in different sizes can come in handy. We especially like having a 7-inch whisk, which is great for re-emulsifying dressings, blending a few eggs, whisking collagen into coffee, and other small jobs. You can buy a set with 11-, 9-, and 7-inch whisks at a kitchen store.

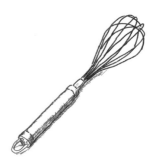

Spatulas

You need two kinds: the standard type, also known as a pancake turner and traditionally made of metal and used for flipping foods, and a silicone spatula, used for so many things, such as stirring, mixing, folding, and scraping every bit of batter from a bowl. To avoid scratching your pans, we suggest you get both types with silicone heads, which are heat resistant. Rubber-topped spatulas can melt into your food.

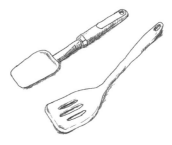

Fish spatula. This is a cousin to the pancake turner, with a longer, more flexible, slotted plane, usually made of stainless steel, sometimes with silicone on the edge for use in nonstick pans. The edge is asymmetrical and the head is longer and thinner than that of a pancake turner. This spatula is great for flipping fish because the design allows you to get under a delicate fillet more easily. You can also use it for burgers, eggs, and crepes.

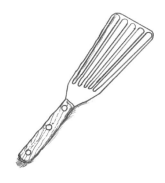

Tongs

This is an incredibly useful and versatile tool, and it's one we reach for all the time. Use tongs to flip steaks, toss and serve salad, keep the food moving in a stir-fry or sauté, stir vegetables in a roasting pan, transfer a whole chicken to a cutting board or platter, remove hard-cooked eggs from a steamer basket, and reach things on high shelves (if you're short like us). We like the ones with silicone tips because they won't scratch nonstick and cast-iron pans.

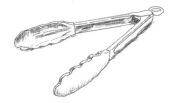

Wooden Spoons

These are useful for stirring and breaking up ground meat as it cooks. They're easier on skillets and pans than metal spoons, too. One that's around 11 or 12 inches long is sufficient, but again, you can buy a set with 12-, 10-, and 8-inch spoons for very little money, and you're likely to use all three. A longer-handled spoon is useful for cooking items in a high-sided pan or Dutch oven, whereas a shorter-handled one is good for stirring food in a smaller skillet (and if you cook with kids, they may find a smaller one easier to manage).

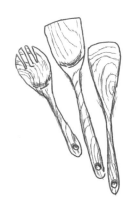

Zester/Grater

A rasp-style zester (such as a Microplane) is fantastic for zesting citrus as well as finely grating hard cheeses, garlic, ginger, and even chocolate. One is plenty.

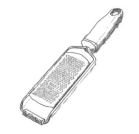

Rimmed Baking Sheets

We use rimmed baking sheets (aka sheet pans) for everything, from cookies to roasts. (Don't confuse these with cookie sheets, which are the flat ones with no rims.) Definitely get rimmed ones; the flat ones are basically only good for things you don't need to stir, like cookies. You also can't use the flat ones for anything that will create liquid or fat during cooking, like bacon. One exception to our near-complete preference for the rimmed baking sheet is when we need to slide something on parchment paper onto a baking sheet; that step goes more smoothly on a cookie sheet. But even in that instance, you can still use a rimmed baking sheet.

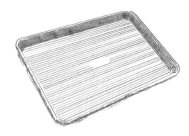

A standard size is 18 inches by 13 inches. This size is known in the professional cooking world as a half-sheet pan, but this is the size that fits in most home ovens (a full sheet is designed for commercial kitchens). We prefer plain aluminum to nonstick pans because they're much more versatile—you shouldn't broil on nonstick pans, for example—and they're easy to clean. As you may be cooking different elements of a dish at the same time, or portions that require more than one pan, we find it useful to have at least two rimmed baking sheets.

COOL GADGET:

> *Silicone baking mat.* You can use this in place of parchment paper to line baking sheets for some applications. It can save you money and is a nice option sustainability-wise.

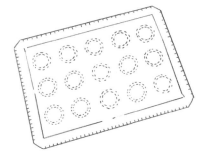

Roasting Pan

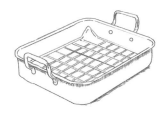

Get a large one with a rack—this pan is great for, well, roasting. Items like whole birds and larger cuts of meat go in the rack so the meat cooks more evenly and there's space for the drippings to collect below, either to make the base for gravy or to flavor vegetables (or both). You can also braise in roasting pans. They are made to withstand high heat, and the high sides trap in heat, so they're a better option for roasting than baking pans or rimmed baking sheets. Bonus: You can place a roasting pan on the stove and make your gravy in it.

Enameled Dutch Oven

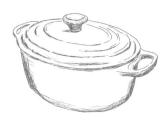

This is a large, deep, heavy pot with a tight-fitting lid, made from cast iron covered in a layer of enamel. Dutch ovens can be pricey, but you can often find a good one for less than $100 if you shop strategically (think factory outlet stores and holiday sales). We recommend a 5- to 7-quart enameled Dutch oven. That is enough volume for all of the recipes in this book and likely most of the recipes you'll encounter elsewhere. Also, cast-iron pots are heavy, but with this size, you can transfer it from stove to oven and oven to table, even full of food, without too much struggle. Some say enameled is less sturdy because the coating can chip; we haven't had this problem ourselves in many years of Dutch oven cooking, and enameled is much easier to clean.

We love our Dutch ovens for braising, making soups and stews, and more. They conduct heat really well, they're stovetop- and oven-safe, and they're usually attractive enough that you can even serve out of them. They're also sturdy and built to last, so they're a good investment. We like oval ones; they give you the most surface area to work with, so searing meat requires fewer batches.

Saucepans

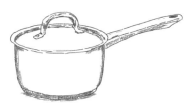

You need at least one medium saucepan (2 to 3 quarts), but if you have the space and budget, it's worth having a smaller one (about 1 quart) and a larger one (4 quarts) as well. We use all three sizes in the recipes in this book. A good saucepan will feel sturdy and have a well-fitting lid and a handle that doesn't get crazy hot.

Skillets

Having a few skillets in different sizes is useful: at least one small one (6 to 8 inches), one medium (around 10 inches), and one large (12 inches or larger). In general, we prefer heavy-bottomed stainless-steel skillets. They're the most versatile, they can withstand high heat, and most are oven-safe (check the manual to make sure yours is). It's nice to have at least one large and one medium nonstick skillet for things like eggs and crepes, but it is not the pan to use for stir-frying or searing meat because most nonstick coatings are not made to withstand high heat.

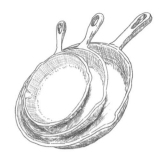

We also recommend having at least one well-seasoned cast-iron skillet. What other equipment do you know of that actually improves over time? As you use it, your cast iron will get more and more nonstick and well seasoned. Cast-iron skillets hold heat very well, so when you have gotten your pan really hot for searing a steak, the temperature doesn't drop as dramatically after you put the steak in the pan as it does in other types of skillets. That's why meat sears so beautifully in cast iron. Plus, it adds a teeny bit of iron to your food when you cook in it. If you're intimidated by cast-iron pots and pans, don't be—they're easier to clean and maintain than you think, and nowadays most new ones come preseasoned.

We call for medium and large cast-iron skillets in this book, meaning 8 inches and 10 inches, respectively. If you have both sizes, great—but if you have just one that's 9 to 10 inches, that size will work well for all of the recipes in this book. In general, you want a skillet that's large enough to accommodate a large steak or a generous amount of food, but cast iron is heavy, so you don't want one that's so large you can't handle it comfortably.

Springform Pan

This is a baking pan with a base and sides that lock on but can be removed. It's useful for items that can't be turned out onto a rack, such as cheesecake (that's what we use it for in this book) and ice cream cake. It also can be used for quiche. You remove the sides and slide the cake off the base onto a serving dish or cut and serve it right off the base. We use a 9-inch springform pan in this book. We find that to be the most convenient size because many recipes are developed for it.

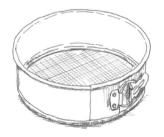

If you are using a springform pan to bake something that needs to go into a water bath, such as a cheesecake, be sure to wrap the base and locked sides in a double layer of foil to prevent water from seeping in.

Cooling Racks

A wire cooling rack is essential for cooling foods because it allows air to circulate underneath the rack. You can also use it in a rimmed baking sheet to keep foods like onion rings (page 280) and waffles warm in the oven when you want them to stay crisp. We recommend having at least two cooling racks.

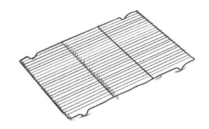

Loaf Pans

We recommend loaf pans made from light-colored sturdy aluminized steel. These yield consistent, evenly baked items. Avoid glass pans; you'll find that the sides of the food brown too much before the center is cooked, which is obviously not desirable.

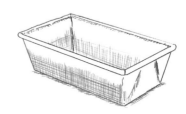

In general, we don't love nonstick baking pans. The darker ones have the same problem as glass pans. Plus, you can't use cooking spray on them because it can ruin the nonstick coating. This is all just too fussy for us. Use a light-colored metal pan, line it with parchment paper, and you get even cooking and easy cleanup. For the recipes in this book, you'll need an 8 by 4-inch loaf pan and a 9 by 5-inch pan.

Pie Plate

A plain glass 9-inch pie plate is the most versatile, and we find that it bakes the most evenly out of all of the pie plates we've tried. You can get a deep-dish one, too, though it isn't essential. If you have a metal pie plate, that's also fine to use. Metal conducts heat better than glass, so your crust is likely to brown faster than in a glass dish. If you have a metal pie plate, consider reducing the oven temperature by 25°F.

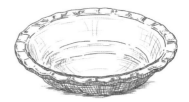

Baking Dishes/Pans

It's useful to have at least two sizes: a rectangular one that's 9 inches by 13 inches (for casseroles) and a smaller 8-inch square one (hello, brownies). Aluminum, ceramic, or sturdy glass, like Pyrex, all work well, though the timing may be somewhat different depending on what you use. Cook times for glass and ceramic are a bit longer because those materials take longer to heat up than metal. We don't recommend silicone because we find foods don't brown as well in pans made from that material and find the flexibility of those pans awkward.

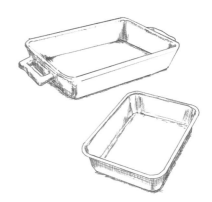

Parchment Paper

We like the precut sheets that come in half sheet pan size (because we're lazy...or efficient?). But a whole roll that you cut into sheets works just fine, too. We use parchment paper to line pans to prevent sticking and for easy cleanup. Only use parchment at temperatures below 450°F and never under the broiler; higher temperatures and proximity to a broiler could cause the paper to catch fire.

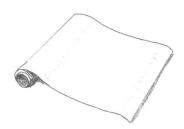

Measuring Cups

Be sure to have a set of dry measuring cups and at least one liquid measuring cup. Trying to measure dry ingredients in a liquid measuring cup or liquids in a dry measuring cup is such a pain and not as accurate. For dry measuring, metal cups are sturdier and tend to last longer, and we think they look nicer. For a liquid measure, make sure you have one that goes as low as ¼ cup. You may find it useful to have a smaller liquid measure, say 1 cup, and a larger one that goes up to 4 cups.

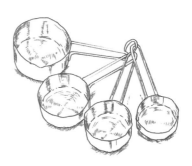

Measuring Spoons

Get yourself at least one set of these; again, we find metal to be superior to plastic. You need ¼, ½, and 1 teaspoon and 1 tablespoon. Some sets have ⅛ and even 1/16 teaspoon, and some have ½ tablespoon. Those are nice to have but not necessary. Pro tip: If you have more than one set, take them off the rings, put them in a mug, and leave them on your counter; no more hunting through drawers trying to find that ¼ teaspoon.

COOL GADGET:

> *Along with traditional round spoons, you can now find rectangular measuring spoons. These are great for fitting into jars with small openings, like some spice jars.*

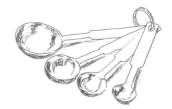

Kitchen Scale

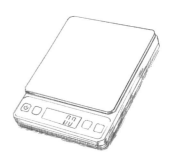

This tool falls under the "cool gadget" category in that you don't absolutely have to have one but we strongly recommend it, especially if you're going to bake often. Weighing dry ingredients is faster and easier than spooning them into cups and leveling them off, and you will get more consistent results. Plus, you can use your scale to make sure foods like burger patties and meatballs are evenly portioned for more accurate cooking. You can buy a good scale for less than $50, and it doesn't take up much space. We predict that once you get it, you'll wonder how you did without it. Make sure you get one that has both metric and imperial measurements (that is, grams and ounces).

We use both types of measurements in this book. Sometimes we list the weights of ingredients in ounces and pounds (as with meat), and other times in grams (as with baking ingredients). We do so because this is generally how we shop. In the U.S., the weights for meats are given in ounces and pounds, whereas the weights of ingredients such as almond flour are usually listed on the package in grams. We followed that pattern to make it as simple as possible to buy ingredients and execute the recipes.

APPLIANCES

Air Fryer

We admit to being slow adopters of these relatively new appliances—but once we each got one, we found ourselves using them a lot and really enjoying them. Air fryers don't actually fry; they have strong fans that blow hot air around, cooking food quickly and crisping up items like chicken wings without a lot of oil. It's easy to use an air fryer: preheat the fryer, place the food in a single layer on the fryer's perforated tray, set the timer, and cook, usually turning the food over at least once during cooking.

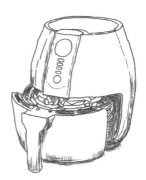

A few things to know about preheating an air fryer: They don't all operate the same way. Some air fryers have a preheat setting that goes for a set amount of time and a certain temperature; with others, you set it to preheat and give a temperature and specify an amount of time. Unlike ovens, some air fryers turn off after they've finished preheating, and you have to set the temperature and time again to cook. In the recipes in this book that call for an air fryer, we give a temperature and a time of 5 minutes for preheating, but feel free to adjust that if your model works another way (check the instruction manual if you aren't sure). If yours turns off after the preheating time is over, be sure your food is ready to cook before you preheat.

For a family of three or four, a 6-quart size will cover most of your needs. If your air fryer is a smaller model (3 quarts or less), you will likely need to cook the recipes in additional batches, which will increase the overall cooking time; if yours is larger, you may be able to cook the recipes in fewer batches and reduce the cooking time.

If you don't have an air fryer and you're not inclined to buy one, you can still make nearly all of the recipes in this book. Wherever possible, we have offered alternative cooking methods for the air fryer recipes.

Food Processor

Making quick work of chopping and dicing is what food processors are best known for, though they're also useful for making dips, nut butters, spreads like pesto, and more—plus, they often have attachments that allow you to shred and slice. Food processors are different from blenders in that they are better for drier mixtures, whereas blenders can accommodate more liquid (food processors leak when filled with too much liquid). We highly recommend investing in one if you don't already have one. 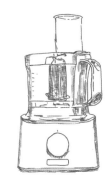 They come in sizes ranging from 3 to 14 cups; an 8- to 10-cup model will get the job done in most kitchens and accommodate the recipes in this book. If space and budget allow, consider also getting a small food processor (3 or 4 cups), either a stand-alone model or one that comes as an attachment to an immersion blender (see below). These smaller models work great for blending dressings and sauces when the quantity is too small for a full-size processor or blender.

Blender

There are bar blenders and high-powered blenders; you don't need both, but having one or the other is handy for pureeing soups as well as blending sauces, dressings, smoothies, frozen drinks, and more. With a high-powered blender (such as a Vitamix), you can mix hot or cold liquids with the lid on; with a bar blender, it's important to remove the center of the lid and place a kitchen towel on top when blending hot liquids to 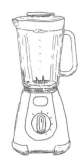 allow steam to escape (failure to do so can cause pressure to build up and the lid to fly off, so you end up scraping hot soup off the ceiling). High-powered blenders are more powerful than bar blenders but tend to be pricier; you can do perfectly well with a bar blender if that's what your budget allows.

Immersion Blender

An immersion blender is a nice-to-have if not crucial piece of kitchen equipment. Also known as a stick or hand blender, this gadget allows you to puree right in a pot or saucepan—no need to transfer the mixture to a separate blender. An immersion blender is easy to pull out of a cabinet and doesn't require much space, so it can be useful in a small kitchen. Plus, it works on both hot and cold mixtures. You can buy a model that's just an immersion blender or get one that has attachments, such as a whisk (handy for whipping cream or egg whites) and a mini food processor.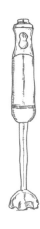

Slow Cooker

This countertop device is very popular because you can toss ingredients in, set it, and leave it, coming home at the end of the day to a ready-to-eat meal with minimal effort. A slow cooker is also really useful for making homemade bone broth, and it allows you to prepare an additional dish when your stove and oven are occupied, as in holiday meals. Slow cookers come in a wide range of sizes, from 1½ to 2 quarts (good for warming dips) all the way up to large 10-quart models. We find a 6-quart slow cooker to be the most versatile; along with a good batch of broth, you can make chili or pulled pork in a cooker that size. The recipes in this book were developed using a 6-quart slow cooker.

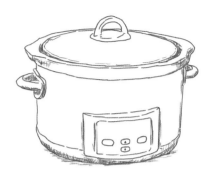

THE PANTRY

We're calling this the pantry, but it incorporates the fridge and freezer, too. Here are some basics, fresh and dry, to keep on hand.

Cooking Fats

We use a variety of cooking fats for different applications. It may seem like a hassle to stock an array of fats, but doing so is an easy way to elevate your cooking and will net you more success.

- **Avocado oil:** This is our favorite oil for high-heat cooking. It has a high smoke point, around 520°F, so you can use it for every kind of cooking application. It's also neutrally flavored.

- **Butter:** The saying "everything's better with butter" is true. We like to use unsalted butter so we can control the seasoning. Look for brands made from grass-fed cream. Butter can burn easily, so be careful when cooking with it (though gently letting it brown to a golden color with a nutty fragrance is divine).

- **Coconut oil:** This rich, luscious fat has received so much bad press because of its saturated fat content; don't believe it. Unrefined coconut oil is used widely in many cultures and does not cause heart disease. It's fantastic for curries, in baking, and in any dish where you don't mind a bit of coconut flavor. It has a smoke point of about 350°F, so if you're going to cook with it on the stovetop, it's best used for moderate-heat sautéing.

  Refined coconut oil, which has a higher smoke point and no coconut taste, is widely available, but we recommend sticking to unrefined oils. To refine the oil, many manufacturers put it through chemical processing, and we figure it's better not to bother with it and choose a different oil.

- **Duck fat/beef tallow:** Duck fat has a rich, smoky flavor that works perfectly for things like fried potatoes; it's also surprisingly good in baking. Beef tallow is more neutral but also rich and delicious as a cooking fat. Duck fat's smoke point is around 370°F and tallow's is closer to 400°F, so they're both useful in many applications, and the richness they impart makes them worth adding to your pantry.

  These animal fats are very traditional and have been used by human beings for centuries, yet they can be hard to find in stores nowadays. (They've been replaced by a sea of highly processed vegetable oils, which is criminal—those oils are highly inflammatory and terrible for you.) You may spot animal fats in high-end grocery and health-food stores like Whole Foods, or you can order them online. Epic is a brand that sells all of these fats, and they're very good. Alternatively, you can ask for them at your butcher shop. You can often get animal fats in farm stores and at farmers markets as well; see "How to Be Carnivore-ish on a Budget" (page 73) for more info on shopping.

- **Ghee:** This is butter with the milk solids removed, so it can withstand much higher temperatures than butter without burning; its smoke point is around 480°F. Because the milk solids are removed, ghee is safe for people with lactose intolerance, though not recommended for anyone with a dairy allergy. Ghee is delicious, great for gut health, and so versatile—plus, it doesn't require refrigeration.

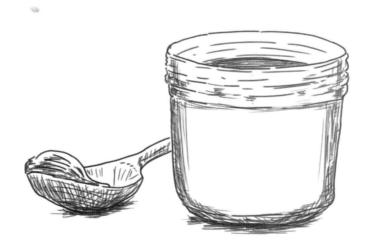

- **Extra-virgin olive oil:** No doubt you already know how healthy olive oil is. It has a relatively low smoke point, around 325°F. You can cook with it, but it's best for dishes cooked over low to moderate heat; it's not the oil to use for high-heat methods like stir-frying or searing. Olive oil is also great for baking, imparting a slightly savory flavor. (You don't have to worry about the smoke point for baking because the oil is mixed with other ingredients.) Use olive oil in dressings and sauces, and feel free to drizzle it on foods after cooking to add flavor and healthy fat.

  Pro tip: You can usually tell if olive oil is of high quality and fresh if you get a peppery kick at the back of your throat when you taste it.

- **Toasted sesame oil:** Technically, toasted sesame oil is not a cooking fat; it's a finishing oil. Drizzle it on after cooking to give Asian-inspired dishes like stir-fries a rich flavor, or blend it into dressings or sauces.

- **Cooking spray:** This is handy for lightly greasing baking dishes, skillets, and air fryer baskets and for evenly misting fat over food before cooking. Look for cooking spray made from olive, avocado, or coconut oil (though coconut oil spray usually has a coconut flavor, so factor that in when you're shopping); avoid any spray made from vegetable oils, which are inflammatory to the body. Also, check the label to make sure your cooking spray is free of propellants; these additives are not good for you, and they're unnecessary.

  Note: Cooking spray is not recommended for nonstick cookware, as it can damage the nonstick coating.

PRO TIP: SAVE YOUR BACON FAT

Whenever you cook bacon, transfer the rendered fat to a cup and keep it by the stove. Use it to cook stir-fries, eggs—really anything that could use a little smokiness. It's great in baking, too, in place of some of the butter. You can store bacon fat in the fridge if you won't use it quickly, but we find that when it's right there by the stove, we tend to use it up.

Aromatics, Fresh Herbs, and Spices

There's a reason why you see these items in just about every recipe, everywhere: they're essential to creating dishes with truly pleasing, satisfying flavor. Plus, they happen to be full of nutrients.

Aromatics

Think of these ingredients as the building blocks of dishes, infusing them with flavor and, yes, aroma. Although they aren't usually the main event in a dish, you'd miss them if they weren't there.

- **Garlic:** We like to have both fresh garlic and garlic powder on hand, as they're useful for different things. Buy whole heads of garlic, or do what Beth does and cheat by buying a bag of whole peeled cloves. A medium-sized clove will yield about 1 teaspoon of minced garlic; in this book, we give you the number of cloves and the yield, so you know how much you need no matter what size cloves you have. When cooking with fresh garlic, watch it carefully; if you let it burn, it will taste bitter.

- **Ginger:** As with garlic, we like to keep both fresh and powdered ginger on hand. While the powdered stuff is great for baking, there's no substitute for fresh ginger in stir-fries, curries, dressings, soups, and other dishes. Often you see large knobs of ginger in the store; go ahead and buy one, even if you need only a bit. Toss the rest in a resealable bag and freeze it. You can peel and chop the frozen ginger and then toss it into a dish; you don't even need to defrost it first.

  The easiest way to peel ginger is with the side of a spoon. Just run the edge of the spoon over the side of the knob of ginger, and the delicate skin will come right off. If your ginger is frozen, cut off the peel with a sharp paring knife.

  The recipes in this book call for the amount of minced or grated ginger you need; it's hard to tell you the size of the piece needed for each recipe because ginger pieces vary widely in diameter. For reference, a 1-inch piece that's about the width of your index finger will yield a generous tablespoon of minced ginger.

- **Shallots:** We love these elegant, tender, sweet members of the onion family. They add flavor and depth to dishes but are milder than onions. (Don't get us wrong, we love onions. But sometimes you want a subtler taste.)

Fresh Herbs

Fresh herbs impart a bright flavor and aroma as well as a pop of color to a dish, and they make beautiful garnishes. They fall into two categories: soft and hard (or woody). Make them last by wrapping them in a damp paper towel and placing them in a plastic bag in the crisper drawer. Basil, the one exception, should be treated like flowers: stick it in a cup of water and keep at room temperature.

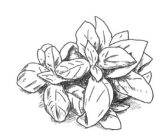

Here are some herbs that we use often.

Soft herbs:

- **Basil:** A classic in salads and, of course, as the base for a traditional pesto. Thai basil, which often has purple stems and narrower leaves, has more of an anise flavor to it. We love both types. Thai basil isn't nearly as common in stores. If you buy it, use it quickly because it usually spoils in a couple of days. Chop it up and add it to larb or other lettuce wraps (like the ones on page 126), toss it into salads, or stir it into curries. It's sturdier than Italian basil, so it holds up well in cooking.

- **Cilantro:** This herb is highly controversial. If you don't like it (many who don't like it say it tastes like soap), it may be because you have a variation in your olfactory receptor genes that causes you to pick up the soapy taste in certain compounds within the herb. If that's the case—or if you simply don't care for cilantro—leave it out or swap in parsley.

- **Dill:** With its bright flavor, dill adds great freshness to dishes. Be careful not to overdo it; too much dill will overpower the flavor of a dish. If you have fennel fronds on hand, they can sometimes stand in for dill if you don't mind the tinge of licorice flavor.

- **Mint:** Mint adds a coolness and a distinctive flavor to dishes. Similar to dill, it can be overpowering if you use too much.

- **Parsley:** We prefer flat-leaf parsley for cooking because it has a brighter, bolder flavor than curly parsley. Plus, it's easier to wash. If curly is all you have on hand, it's OK to use.

- **Tarragon:** Highly aromatic tarragon has a distinctive flavor similar to licorice, so it can be polarizing. We love its bold, fresh taste, but keep in mind that it's easy to overdo it, so be cautious with it. Tarragon is especially good with mild-tasting proteins like shellfish, eggs, and chicken.

Hard/woody herbs:

- **Rosemary:** This herb's distinctive flavor and aroma go beautifully in savory dishes—plus, rosemary makes a lovely addition to shortbread cookies.

- **Sage:** Pungent and earthy, this herb packs a punch, so a little goes a long way. Sage is fantastic in homemade sausage patties and as a seasoning for roast chicken or hearty vegetables like winter squash. Pro tip: Fry whole sage leaves in butter until crisp for a fancy garnish.

- **Thyme:** Use whole sprigs of this delicate herb to stuff a chicken cavity, to flavor roasted vegetables, or on top of fish. Try adding a sprig of thyme to lemonade, too.

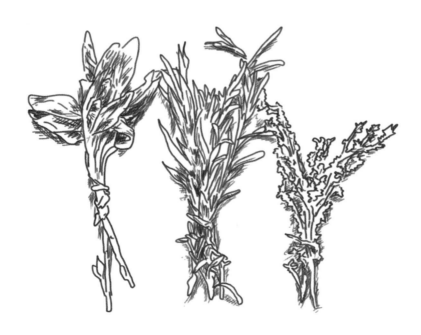

Spices

Variety is...well, the spice of life, right? Even if you tend to eat the same foods over and over, spices can help change up the flavor profile so you don't get bored. Plus, spices have numerous health benefits. So they make food taste better, and they up the nutrition—thanks, Nature.

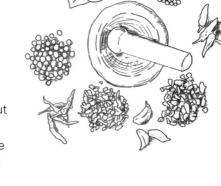

The following are the spices we use most often, but this is by no means a comprehensive or "must-have" list. Keep the ones you like on hand; if you're not sure where to start, begin with blends like chili powder, curry powder, herbs de Provence, Italian seasoning, and za'atar. Blends give you layers of seasoning without having to buy a lot of spices or guess at proportions.

Regarding black pepper, rather than purchase it preground, we prefer to grind it on the fly, so we use a pepper grinder and black peppercorns. Freshly ground pepper has a more pronounced flavor than preground; plus, most grinders are adjustable, so you can make your pepper more or less coarse depending on the application.

Here's what's always in our spice racks:

- Black peppercorns
- Cayenne pepper
- Celery seed, ground
- Chili powder
- Chipotle powder
- Cinnamon, ground and sticks
- Coriander, ground
- Cumin, ground
- Curry powder

- Dried bay leaves
- Dried oregano leaves
- Dried thyme leaves
- Everything bagel seasoning
- Garlic powder
- Ginger powder
- Hot paprika
- Mustard powder

- Onion powder
- Red pepper flakes
- Rubbed sage
- Smoked paprika
- Sweet paprika
- Turmeric powder
- Za'atar

PAPRIKA

This bright spice adds color and flavor to several of the recipes in this book. Although all paprika is made from dried peppers, there are differences among the types:

- **Sweet paprika:** In the U.S., this is the most common of the three, and the type your grandmother would have sprinkled on deviled eggs. Note that jars may be labeled "sweet paprika" but more often than not will be labeled simply "paprika." The trick is, it isn't sweet per se, just mild in flavor. It's a little bit fruity with a slightly bitter edge.

- **Hot paprika:** This spicy Hungarian variety is great for adding a complex heat to dishes. You can swap it for sweet paprika if you want a hotter dish, or you can use it in place of red pepper flakes or cayenne pepper, though the flavor is a bit different.

- **Smoked paprika:** This Spanish variety, made from either sweet or hot peppers that are dried and smoked, adds depth and richness. It's delicious in spice rubs. Keep in mind that a little goes a long way. It is also called pimenton.

Salt

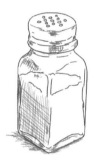

Most of the recipes in this book were developed using fine sea salt. Our favorite is Redmond Real Salt; it has great flavor and plenty of minerals. You can use any type you like; just make sure that it's an unrefined mineral salt. Iodized table salts are highly processed and have the minerals stripped out. Salt was widely fortified with iodine beginning in the 1920s to combat goiter, but chances are if you eat eggs and seafood regularly, you're getting plenty of iodine and don't need it in your salt.

You'll see flaky sea salt in a few recipes. These larger flakes add a lovely hit of salty crunch when sprinkled on at the end of cooking a dish. They work beautifully in savory and sweet applications (on a steak or on cookies, for example). Maldon is a well-known brand that's easy to find and very good.

We also use kosher salt for wet brining. Brining requires a lot of salt, most of which doesn't end up in the food; kosher salt is coarse, so you can use less of it to make the water salty. This is more efficient and more economical than using up a lot of fine sea salt in a brine. You can use kosher salt for salting the water if you're cooking potatoes or pasta, too. We like having a box of kosher salt in the kitchen for scrubbing cast-iron skillets, too.

Milk and Yogurt

You can use dairy or nondairy milks, creams, and yogurt depending on your preference. If you go with nondairy, make sure you choose something that's similar in flavor and thickness to its dairy counterpart. For example, canned coconut milk is thick and rich, like cream; rice milk is thin and sweet, like skim milk; and almond milk is somewhere in the middle. If you use nondairy milk, check the label to be sure it doesn't have added sweeteners or flavorings such as vanilla.

Pro tip: Frequently the "original" flavor of a nondairy milk is sweetened, so look for "unsweetened" on the label. Avoid milks with potentially problematic additives like carrageenan. Many contain stabilizers like guar gum; these are OK as long as you tolerate them well.

Flours

All of the recipes in this book are free of refined flours and gluten. We use the following flours instead:

- **Almond flour:** This is simply finely ground almonds. We prefer blanched almond flour, which has the skins removed, because it yields lighter, less dense results.

- **Arrowroot powder:** This is a powdery starch that's similar to cornstarch but grain-free. You can use it to thicken sauces and in baking in combination with almond and other flours to lighten the texture.

- **Cassava flour:** The most similar to all-purpose of all of the grain-free flours, cassava flour is great to start with if you're new to grain-free baking. It has a neutral flavor and behaves similarly to wheat flour—though it's more absorbent than all-purpose, so you may not be able to substitute it at a 1:1 ratio. We recommend weighing baking ingredients for the best results, and this is especially true for cassava flour. A little too much can ruin the end result.

- **Coconut flour:** Made from dried coconut meat, this flour is highly absorbent; very little goes a long way. A recipe may call for only 1 or 2 tablespoons of coconut flour and what seems like a lot of liquid. Don't be alarmed. Note that almond flour and coconut flour are not interchangeable.

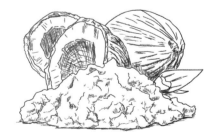

- **Oat flour:** Though most of the recipes in this book are free of grains, we make an exception for oat flour, which is made by finely grinding rolled oats. Like oats, oat flour is slightly sweet, with a mild flavor, and it adds bulk and body to snacks and baked goods.

- **Premixed Paleo or gluten-free flour blends:** In general, we find that a mix of grain-free flours works best for a light texture and an even crumb. Luckily, nowadays you can get these mixes premade. We like Bob's Red Mill Paleo Baking Flour, which is a grain-free blend of almond, arrowroot, coconut, and tapioca. For an easy swap for all-purpose flour, a gluten-free blend is handy (note that these mixes are not grain-free). Bob's Red Mill comes to the rescue again; its Gluten Free 1-to-1 Baking Flour, a blend of rice flours and potato starch, works beautifully.

  Premade blends can be a convenient (if sometimes pricier) option that takes the guesswork out of choosing the right replacement flour or attempting to mix flours yourself to achieve the ideal consistency. Just note that while a gluten-free flour mix can generally be used in place of all-purpose flour, a Paleo flour mix usually can't. If you want a Paleo version of a recipe, we recommend finding one that is designed to be Paleo rather than trying to convert one that calls for regular flour.

Canned Goods

We keep the following canned items on hand:

- Coconut milk and coconut cream (*Note:* We always use unsweetened full-fat coconut milk and cream; we find it yields the best texture.)

- Diced tomatoes (preferably fire-roasted)

- Fish (sardines, tuna, wild-caught salmon)

- Olives (green such as Castelvetrano, kalamata, and ripe black olives)

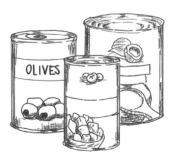

Anchovies

Anchovies are such a gift. They're salty and briny, and they provide fantastic flavor—plus, they're deeply nutritious, rich in omega-3 fats, calcium, vitamin K, and protein. Anchovies are also sustainable and low in mercury. Whether you buy tinned or jarred depends on your personal preference and what's readily available, but be sure to buy them packed in olive oil, not vegetable oil. When you sauté them, they essentially dissolve, leaving behind a rich salty flavor.

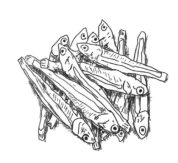

Canned Chipotle Peppers in Adobo

Chipotles are smoked jalapeños, and adobo sauce is a thick, rich sauce traditionally made from a variety of dried chilies. You'll find canned chipotles in adobo in most supermarkets. As with regular jalapeño peppers, the heat is in the seeds and ribs, so remove them if you like your food milder.

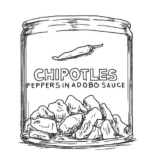

If you open a can and use only one or two chilies, you can freeze the rest. Place one chili and some of the sauce in each well of an ice cube tray. When frozen, pop them out and put them in a resealable bag to store in the freezer. (This will stain the ice cube tray, so you may want to have a dedicated tray.)

Tomato Paste

You'll always find this paste, made from tomatoes that have been cooked down and concentrated and then strained to remove the seeds and skin, in our fridges. It adds brightness, acidity, and deep umami to dishes, especially when you cook it in some fat and let it caramelize a bit. We prefer the tubes to cans or jars; we find the tubes easier to use since most recipes call for only a tablespoon or two. Once you open a can, you have to deal with storing the rest, and the jars often have openings that are too small for a tablespoon measure.

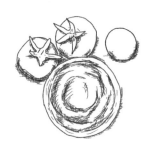

If you have extra canned tomato paste and no immediate need for it, you can freeze it in an ice cube tray, then pop out the frozen cubes and keep them frozen in a resealable bag. As with chipotle peppers in adobo, this will stain and likely flavor your ice cube tray, so keep a tray just for this purpose if you're going to do it.

Condiments and Flavoring Agents

These pantry items can be sprinkled or spooned onto dishes on their own to add flavor or be used as ingredients in sauces and dressings. We love to have a variety of condiments and flavoring agents on hand to enhance all kinds of dishes.

Coconut Aminos

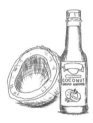

Made from coconut tree sap, coconut aminos is a great replacement for soy sauce. It's sweeter and far less salty than soy sauce, so season foods accordingly. In addition to being used in Asian-inspired dishes, it can add a subtle sweetness and umami taste to dressings and sauces.

Harissa

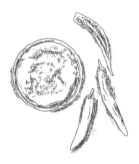

This spicy Middle Eastern/North African chili paste is worth keeping in your refrigerator, especially if you like spicy food. Harissa is usually made from a blend of chili peppers, garlic, olive oil, and sometimes spices like cumin and/or coriander. It's so versatile: use it to flavor marinades, soups, sauces, dips, or rice, or use it on its own as a condiment. Spoon some harissa on top of feta cheese and drizzle it with olive oil, and you have an instant appetizer. You'll find harissa in jars and tubes; choose whichever packaging you prefer.

Hot Sauces

Not everyone loves hot sauce; feel free to ignore this bit if heat isn't your thing. Here are the hot sauces we use most often:

- Buyo
- Cholula
- Frank's RedHot
- Pickapeppa Sauce
- Sriracha sauce

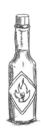

Mirin

Mirin is an Asian rice wine that's great for cooking. It's similar to sake, but milder and slightly sweeter. It's great in dressings, sauces, and marinades.

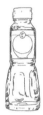

Vinegars

Having a few of these types of vinegar can come in handy. You can change up a dressing or sauce just by swapping in a different vinegar. Here are a few types we love:

- Apple cider vinegar (Look for a raw one that still contains the "mother"; it will have a cloudy appearance. As creepy as that sounds, the mother is just strands of protein that contain enzymes and beneficial bacteria.)
- Balsamic vinegar
- Distilled white vinegar
- Rice vinegar (We use unseasoned to avoid added sugar.)
- Sherry vinegar
- White wine vinegar

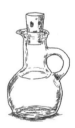

Nuts, Seeds, and Nut and Seed Butters

We like to have a variety of nuts and seeds on hand for snacking, baking, and cooking applications such as adding to a breading for fish or chicken. Nut and seed butters are essential in baked goods and sauces and for spreading on apple slices (or, let's face it, licking off a spoon). If you buy roasted nuts or seeds, make sure they're dry-roasted; others are usually cooked in vegetable oils such as sunflower or canola, which are highly inflammatory. When shopping for nut or seed butters, choose ones that are unsweetened and free of stabilizers like palm oil. Buying unsalted allows you to control the seasoning, but that isn't always possible. If only salted nut or seed butter is available, taste it before cooking with it so you have an idea of how much salt it is adding to your recipe. Whether you choose crunchy or smooth depends on how you're using it and your preference.

Here's what we usually have on hand:

- Almonds, sliced and whole

- Pecans

- Walnuts

- Hemp hearts (aka hulled hemp seeds)

- Sesame seeds, black and/or white, raw and toasted

- Shelled sunflower seeds, raw as well as dry-roasted and salted

- Almond butter

- Cashew butter

- Tahini and/or sunflower seed butter (both are nut-free)

- Unsweetened shredded coconut (Did you know that coconut is not technically a nut? Botanically, it can be classified as a fruit or a seed.)

Sweeteners

Treats are a must for both of us, though we try not to go overboard. One way to make treats that aren't a disaster for your health is to use sweeteners that are natural and as unrefined as possible. That isn't carte blanche to go crazy with sweets; sorry, sugar is still sugar. But for those occasional treats, and for adding sweetness to balance sauces and dressings, here are our favorites:

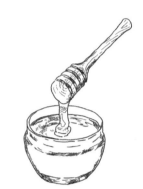

- Coconut sugar

- Maple syrup (Ashleigh is Canadian, so obviously.)

- Molasses

- Monk fruit

- Raw honey (Always buy it unpasteurized so the enzymes are left intact.)

- Stevia

Miscellaneous

Here are some other items that we keep on hand:

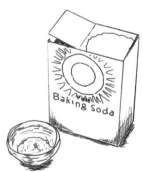

- **Baking powder and baking soda:** Both are chemical leaveners, and they are not interchangeable. Use whichever one a recipe calls for.

- **Pork panko:** Made from crushed pork rinds, these are a fantastic swap for breadcrumbs. You can make them yourself simply by grinding pork rinds in a food processor until they form fine, flaky crumbs. You'll need a 2.5-ounce bag to yield a generous cup of panko. We prefer to buy the panko premade; it saves a step, and we find it more consistent than making it ourselves. Our favorite brand is Bacon's Heir; it's the finest and has the most consistent texture and subtlest flavor.

- **Vanilla extract:** Get the pure stuff, never imitation, which doesn't taste nearly as good.

GET TO KNOW YOUR PROTEINS

One of the things we love most about cooking is that there's always more to learn. A different technique, a new combination of flavors—even the most experienced chefs in the world regularly seek out more and better ways to do things.

Even if you've been cooking proteins forever, we are confident that you'll find useful information here. We talked to experts in beef and pork, seafood, poultry and eggs, game, and offal, all of whom were incredibly generous in sharing their wisdom.

Beef and Pork

Experts:

- Ryan Farr, founder of San Francisco's 4505 Meats, an artisan whole-animal meat company devoted to sustainable practices; owner of 4505 Burgers and BBQ restaurant; and author of *Whole Beast Butchery: The Complete Visual Guide to Beef, Lamb, and Pork*

- Mike Salguero, founder and CEO of ButcherBox

What you need to know:

- **Pat meat dry.** Salguero says many people are afraid to handle meat, so they take it out of the packaging and put it right in the pan. But it's important to pat meat dry before cooking. This gives you more contact between the meat and the pan (or grill), and less liquid means less steam, which gives you a better sear.

- **Temper, temper.** Let the meat stand at room temperature before cooking it rather than slapping it on a grill or into a skillet straight out of the fridge. This allows for more even cooking. Following this recommendation, you'll find that we often call for removing red meat (including game) from the refrigerator at least 30 minutes before cooking to allow it to temper.

- **Don't be shy with salt.** If you use a quality mineral salt (see the information about salt on page 56), it is not bad for your health, and seasoning generously is key to flavorful meat. Along with adding salty flavor, salt amplifies foods' own flavor, so your steak will taste meatier and more savory thanks to salt. Farr recommends salting before tempering and then adding other seasonings right before cooking. If you forget, don't worry; you can season right before cooking and still get delicious meat, as long as you use enough salt.

- **Embrace heat.** Make sure your grill or pan is hot enough before you start cooking. If the grill or pan isn't hot enough, the meat is more likely to stick. Plus, you need high heat to get a good, deep sear on the surface. That sear will give the meat a pleasing crust as well as a rich, savory, caramelized flavor. On the stovetop, give your skillet a few minutes at high heat, then add a little oil. The oil should shimmer; that's an indication that it's hot enough. (Don't let your oil smoke—that note shows up in recipes often, but oil that smokes is breaking down, which will affect its flavor and cause it to release harmful compounds that can adversely affect your health. If your oil starts to smoke, remove the pan from the heat, let it cool, wipe it out, and start over.) For a grill, it's hot enough if you can't keep your hand above the grate for more than a second or two.

- **Pork should not be considered white meat.** Years ago, pork was marketed as "the other white meat," but if you cook pork until it's white, it tends to be dry and tough. Cook pork until it's still slightly pink in the center, and use a meat thermometer for accuracy; the internal temperature should be 145°F.

- **Let meat rest before eating it.** Allow meat to rest on a cutting board for at least 5 minutes after it's finished cooking. This allows the juices to be redistributed within the fibers of the meat. If you start to cut into it and it steams or juices run out, you're cutting it too soon. This will leave you with dry meat, says Farr.

- **Slice meat the right way.** Sometimes recipes instruct you slice meat against "the grain." This refers to how the muscle fibers line up. The grain is easier to see in some cuts (ropy steaks like flank) than in others (leaner cuts such as tenderloin); it's also easier to see before the meat is cooked. You want to cut across the grain rather than along it. Cutting against the grain shortens the fibers, which makes the meat more tender and easier to chew. Note that in some cuts, such as rib eye, the grains move in different directions in different sections of the steak. Cut the steak into pieces where the grains line up and then slice each piece against the grain.

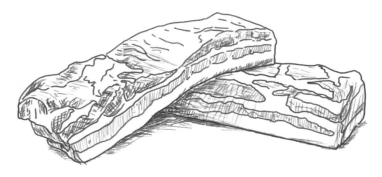

QUESTIONS TO ASK YOUR BUTCHER

- **Be specific.** Have a basic idea of your parameters—such as cooking method and amount of time you have—before going to the butcher. Then, instead of asking questions like, "What's good today?" or "What's the best way to cook lamb?" give them information like, "I have two hours to prepare, I'm cooking for four people, and I'd like to grill. Are lamb chops a good choice?" Most butchers will be happy to share, and with some basic info, they can guide you much more effectively.

- **Ask about sourcing.** As you know, a well-raised animal that's fed its natural diet and allowed to move and graze is healthier and happier, as well as being better for us and the planet. With that in mind, it's perfectly fine to ask your butcher where the meat you're buying came from, how it was raised, what it was fed, and if there are any other animal welfare claims, Salguero says. (If you buy from a source that sells only regeneratively raised meats, you can skip this step.) Even if 100 percent pastured and grass-fed everything isn't in your budget, there are different levels of animal care, so get as much information as you can.

- **Ways to be adventurous.** If you tend to buy the same cuts all the time, it's worth asking your butcher for different ones. (If you want grass-fed meat but find it too pricey, ask your butcher about more economical cuts, such as chuck.) We love rib eye as much as anyone, but coulotte (also known as picanaha) is also luscious and super flavorful. Tell your butcher what you usually enjoy and ask for suggestions.

Seafood

Expert:

- John Addis, owner of Fish Tales (a Brooklyn fishmonger); contestant on *Throwdown with Bobby Flay*

What you need to know:

- **Shop local.** If you have a local fishmonger, it's worth shopping there, even if it's a little out of your way. You're likely to get fresher fish and a wider array of choices than you'll find at a supermarket.

- **Fish should not smell fishy.** A lack of fishy smell is one indication of freshness. Feel free to ask your fishmonger to let you smell the fish you're interested in buying. Ask the fishmonger about the origins of the fish and when it came in.

- **Expand your palate.** If you always go for one or two types of fish, try something different. Tell your fishmonger what you usually buy and ask for recommendations. Inquire about the flavors and textures of different fish. Your fishmonger can tell you what's best that day and offer suggestions for how to cook it.

- **Mollusks should be closed.** If you're buying clams or mussels, look closely to make sure all of the ones you're getting are closed (or close quickly when tapped) and the shells are intact.

- **Fattier fish stand up better to freezing.** When frozen fish is thawed, moisture is drawn out of the fish. The fat in fatty fish such as black cod and wild salmon keeps the fish moist after thawing. When shopping for frozen fish, choose fattier types for the best texture. Stick to fresh for leaner fish such as sole and flounder, if possible.

- **Go beyond the eyes.** If you're buying whole fish, clear eyes are one indication of freshness. But a better one is a burgundy-hued and moist-looking gill plate (ask your fishmonger to gently open it so you can inspect it). If ice touches the eye, the eye will cloud over, so you might think the fish isn't fresh. When in doubt, check the gill plate.

- **Monday's fish may or may not be fresh.** Conventional "wisdom" is that the fish in the store on Monday is carried over from the weekend and is not fresh. Depending on where you live, that isn't necessarily true. Ask your fishmonger when the fish came in.

- **Fish doesn't have to be expensive.** There are flavorful, delicious fish that are very economical because there's abundant supply. Bluefish, mackerel, dorade, and porgy are a few types that are less pricey.

- **Don't overcook fish.** Depending on the type of fish, rare or medium-rare is fine, or cook it just until the fish flakes. Overcooked fish, like other proteins, tends to be dry and tough.

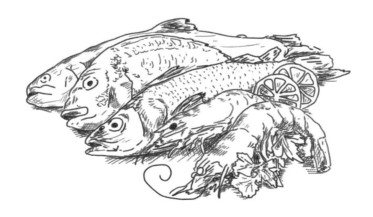

Chicken and Eggs

Experts:

- Jennifer Gregg, vice president of operations, Vital Farms

- Jess Coslow, livestock manager in charge of the poultry program, Stone Barns Center for Food and Agriculture

What you need to know:

- **Chickens are not vegetarians.** Be suspicious when you see "vegetarian fed" on a label. The best diet for chickens, which will yield the healthiest chicken and eggs, is a varied one that includes the grass, bugs, grubs, and worms they eat on pasture as well as grains, Coslow says.

- **Seek out better birds.** If you have access to pasture-raised chicken, it's worth buying. The meat is usually more flavorful and richer in iron and vitamins E and D. Plus, it tends to have more omega-3 fats than birds that aren't raised on pasture. Pastured chickens aren't always readily available in supermarkets; you'll often find them in butcher shops and farmers markets. Eggs from pastured hens are also richer in omega-3 fats and vitamins E and A. So, although pastured chicken and eggs cost more and getting them sometimes means taking an extra step, they're worth the effort and added cost.

- **Talk to your purveyor.** Ask your butcher or farmers market seller about the chickens: how they're raised, what they're fed, any cooking tips, etc. If you always cook boneless, skinless breasts, and you want to branch out into skin-on thighs or even a whole bird (which we strongly encourage), your purveyor may have good recipes and/or cooking tips for you.

- **Don't rinse chicken.** The direction to rinse chicken shows up in recipes sometimes (not in this book, of course), but it isn't necessary; in fact, it does the opposite of what it's meant to do. The idea behind it is to rinse away bacteria, but cooking to the right temperature kills any pathogens. Meanwhile, when you rinse chicken, you're splashing water all over the sink, countertop, your hands, and/or your kitchen towels, and that opens up the danger of cross-contamination. Instead, simply pat chicken dry thoroughly with paper towels.

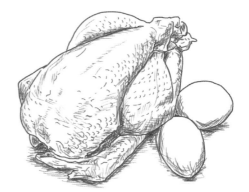

- **Brine your chicken.** We utilize both dry brine (for skin-on chicken) and wet brine (for skinless meat) methods in this book. Both work beautifully to infuse flavor and crisp the skin.

- **Know your egg labels.** Pastured eggs are the gold standard, but if they aren't available or they don't fit within your budget, here's Gregg's ranking of most to least desirable (though it's worth mentioning that even the lowest eggs on this list are still a healthy protein source): Certified Humane (the facility has met stringent third-party animal welfare standards), free range (the birds are able to leave the barn), cage free (the birds are not kept in small cages), and finally conventionally raised. If you don't see pastured but organic eggs are available, that label indicates not only that the birds' feed was free of synthetic pesticides and GMOs but also that they had access to the outdoors year-round (weather permitting).

- **Eggshell color doesn't matter.** Brown eggs are not more "natural," and white eggs have not been bleached or otherwise treated; the shell color doesn't indicate anything about the nutritional profile of the egg. The factor that determines the color of an egg's shell is the hen's earlobe. Yes, you read that right. Her earlobe. Some breeds include ISA Brown (brown eggs), Araucana (blue eggs), and Hy Line White (white eggs).

- **Double yolks are safe to eat.** A double yolk indicates that the egg was laid by a younger chicken. Younger chickens' reproductive systems haven't fully leveled off yet (not unlike how young people's menstrual cycles can take a while to become regular), so they are more likely to lay eggs with double yolks, Gregg says. If you get a carton and all of the eggs have double yolks, they were probably gathered from a young flock. We can't speak to whether it's good luck or not (though we like to think it is).

- **A blood spot in an egg is perfectly safe.** If you see a red blood spot on an egg, most likely the hen got scared and a blood vessel popped in the egg. You can remove it or scramble it in; it's safe to eat.

- **In the U.S., you need to refrigerate your eggs.** Beth's in-laws live in Mexico, and they keep eggs out on the counter; this is also a common practice in Europe. But it's not safe to do in the U.S., Gregg says. Eggshells are porous. During the process of laying an egg, the hen puts a protective coating on it, known as the "bloom." In the U.S., facilities are required to wash eggs. Doing so removes the bloom, exposing the porous shells, so refrigeration is necessary to keep pathogens out. To keep them fresh the longest, store eggs in the fridge at the back of a shelf, not on the door; the temperature fluctuates the most in the door.

Game

Experts:

- Ariane Daguin, founder of D'Artagnan

- Bri Van Scotter, author of *Complete Wild Game Cookbook*

What you need to know:

- **Game animals have seasons.** Because game animals are subject to varying experiences based on the season, the meat is different depending on when it's harvested. If a wild mallard duck is harvested in the spring, for example, the meat is very tender because it's young and food is abundant. In the winter, the bird is older and it's had to work harder to find food, so the meat may be firmer, more savory, and less sweet. (*Note:* Game animals and birds that are farm-raised, such as bison and some venison, may have fewer fluctuations.)

- **The meat is different.** Game animals tend to be leaner than domesticated ones. And many have eaten a variety of food, unlike domesticated animals, which tend to eat a more regulated diet. The meat is often darker than that of domestic animals because game animals tend to move a lot more and undergo more stress, from predators and from the need to find food.

- **Game birds vary a lot.** The fat level on game birds is a big differentiator among them and subsequently affects how you may choose to cook them and how much additional fat you use. Whereas ducks and geese have a lot of fat, pheasant and quail are extremely lean.

- **Cook game carefully.** Even domesticated game is going to be leaner than conventional meat, so it will cook faster and can dry out easily. Daguin recommends searing most game meats in a very hot pan to seal in the juices and leave the meat on the rarer side. With duck and goose, Van Scotter recommends rendering the fat from the bird and using it to cook the meat. Score the skin, cook it low and slow to render the fat, and then turn up the heat to sear the meat. With a leaner bird, she adds, be generous with cooking fat and baste often and/or wrap it in fat or bacon while it cooks. Without that added fat, lean wild game birds can dry out and get tough.

- **Start with something accessible.** If you've never cooked or even eaten game before, start with something somewhat similar to what you're used to. Daguin recommends quail because it's very mild. From there, you can try duck or squab (find our duck recipes on pages 114, 120, and 142); both are birds, so they'll feel familiar to handle, but the meat resembles steak and is best at medium-rare, so it's also familiar in that way. Plus, duck is rich and juicy but doesn't have a strong gamey flavor, so it's generally crowd-pleasing. Another option is to start with ground meat. Look in the freezer section or ask your butcher if they carry ground bison, elk, venison, or other game.

- **Some of the beef and pork rules apply.** Temper game, season it generously, and let it rest after cooking, just as you would with domesticated meat.

Offal

Expert:

- Ashleigh VanHouten, author of *It Takes Guts* (and co-author of this book)

What you need to know:

- **Offal means organs and more.** Offal includes all of the edible bits of an animal other than the traditional cuts of muscle meat: organs (e.g., liver, heart, kidney, sweetbreads, and tripe), blood, marrow, tendons, and pieces like tongue. Offal has been enjoyed by human beings since there were human beings on this planet.

- **It gives you the best bang for your buck, nutrient-wise.** Organ meats and offal are the most nutrient-dense parts of animals, boasting higher concentrations of all of the vitamins, minerals, and nutrients that make muscle meat healthy—and usually at a lower cost. The collagen, marrow, and gelatin found in bones (and bone broth), for example, are full of amino acids (the building blocks of all of our body's structures) as well as vitamins and minerals that support bone and tissue growth and fight inflammation. Heart is an organ that's also a muscle, so it has that beefy texture that most of us are used to, and is high in the powerful antioxidant CoQ10 as well as B_{12}, iron, and protein. Each animal heart has a flavor unique to the animal, but all are delicious (see our recipe for grilled beef heart on page 254).

- **It is far more versatile and accessible than you think.** While most people's minds immediately go to liver and onions when they think of organ meats, there is a vast and delicious world beyond that familiar dish. We generally recommend starting with heart (chicken, duck, or lamb) if you're squeamish about texture and strong taste. Heart is nutrient-dense but has a much more familiar taste and texture and is easy to prepare in a number of ways. We also suggest infusing foods you already love with extra nutrients by "hiding" organ meats in your favorite dishes: for example, having your butcher grind up a 4:1 ratio of ground beef to ground organs and making burgers, meatballs, and sausages; or adding collagen or desiccated liver to your baking.

- **Try them first.** If you're curious about organ meats and offal but intimidated by the idea of cooking them and not convinced you'll like them, head to a local restaurant and order some sweetbreads, tacos de lengua (classic Mexican tongue tacos), pho (Vietnamese soup with organs and tripe), or modongo (Puerto Rican stew with tripe). Finding the flavors and preparations you like best will help you know where to start when you're ready to cook with offal.

- **Source the best you can get.** As with any other animal protein (or food product), you want to source the freshest, highest-quality cuts you can, ideally from local farms. If you're lucky enough to have a farmers market or butcher shop nearby, make friends with the purveyors and get to know their meat—where it comes from and how it's raised, fed, slaughtered, and processed. Most professionals will be more than happy to share the details.

- **Make time for prep.** Generally, prep will include cutting away any hard fat, gristle, or membrane and, in some cases, soaking in cold salted water to further remove any impurities. Some recipes call for liver or kidney to be soaked in lemon juice or milk to tone down the flavor, but we don't think this is generally necessary. (Liver is going to taste like liver regardless.)

- **Have no fear.** There's a misconception that organ meats are inherently more dangerous to eat than other animal protein. But if you source high-quality meat and follow the proper protocol for prepping, cooking, and storing these cuts, there is no evidence that they are riskier to eat than any other part of the animal.

- **Start smaller.** You can go fancy or simple with organ meats, just like any other ingredient. Though there certainly is no shortage of next-level preparations out there, you don't have to make them. You can whip up a delicious chicken liver pâté in fifteen minutes; mix some liver into ground beef and make the simple burgers you're used to; or pan-fry chicken hearts and toss them into a salad in less time than it takes to fry a few eggs.

- **There is nothing "extreme" or "out there" about organ meats.** Throughout history and today, millions of people enjoy true nose-to-tail eating for its culinary pleasures and health benefits. We understand that these foods might seem strange if you didn't grow up eating them. But these are just other parts of the same animals you enjoy eating, and one way to respect them and to be mindful of sustainability is to utilize the whole animal. We encourage you to keep in mind that just because something is new or unfamiliar to you doesn't make it bad. In this case, opening your mind to organ meats can introduce you to a whole new world of nutrient-dense, tasty food and improved health.

HOW TO BE CARNIVORE-ISH ON A BUDGET

Animal protein can be expensive, there's no question. It can also be really cheap—but cheap animal protein is often not the most optimal food. So what can you do if you have a regular income and can't afford 100 percent grass-fed rib eye and wild-caught salmon three meals a day?

Fortunately, there's a lot you can do. There are myriad ways to save on high-quality animal proteins and strategies for what to do when even the less-expensive stuff costs too much (or it isn't available to you).

Good news right off the bat: the more high-quality protein you're eating, the less appetite you'll have for junk food. That alone can save you a ton of cash. It may seem like just a bag of chips here or a liter of soda there—and these foodlike substances do tend to be far cheaper than more optimal foods—but these small, nutritionally empty purchases add up; you may not even realize how much you're spending on those items. Simply crowding them out with healthier food—like meat—can go a long way toward keeping you within your budget. Beth had a coaching client a few years ago who balked at the "expensive stuff" on a shopping list Beth recommended, but with all of the junk food off the menu, she found her grocery bills were actually lower. And the client felt and looked better. Win-win.

Aside from the money you'll save on not buying junk, here are some strategies for saving money on animal protein.

Buy it online

Online sources for protein have proliferated over the last few years, which is great for you because you can pick and choose. Some are subscription services, where you get a box every couple of weeks or every month, depending on the service and how often you want delivery. Most have varying sizes so you can order depending on your needs. Some offer custom boxes you build yourself, or you can let the provider select for you. With other companies, there's no subscription; you just order à la carte as needed.

Many of these companies offer more than beef; you can get seafood, pork, poultry, game meats like bison and elk, organ meats, bone broth, and more.

Here are some of our favorite online providers. Depending on where you live, there may be services near you that work with local farms.

- ButcherBox
  www.butcherbox.com

- Crowd Cow
  www.crowdcow.com

- D'Artagnan
  www.dartagnan.com

- Porter Road
  porterroad.com

- US Wellness Meats
  grasslandbeef.com

- Walden Local Meat (Northeastern U.S.)
  waldenlocalmeat.com

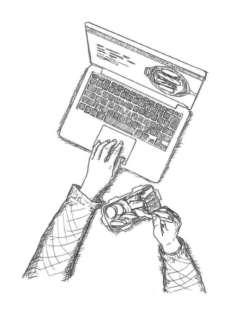

We recommend at least trying out the option to let the company choose for you, if it's offered. (Some let you set a few parameters so you won't end up with a box full of things you don't want.) That element of surprise can be really fun if you let yourself go with it. Plus, it may force you to learn how to cook a cut of meat you haven't worked with before, and you're likely to discover some new favorites.

Shop the farmers market and farm stores

Maybe you're already getting your produce at a local farmers market—if so, great. Farmers markets can also be a fantastic source for locally and often sustainably raised proteins. Get to the market early so you have the most variety to choose from. If you live in a coastal area, you may find fish; other markets will have poultry, beef, lamb, eggs, milk, cheese, and sometimes organ meats and bone broth. Some even have freshly caught game.

If you live in or near a rural area, close to farms, you may have access to a farm store, which can be a gold mine for great foods at a lower cost. Produce certainly, but farm stores can be excellent sources for fresh or frozen meat, small-batch cheeses and charcuterie, bone broth, organs, and more. Because there's no middleman, the prices are often surprisingly reasonable.

Buy less popular or traditionally cheaper items

Boneless, skinless chicken breasts, sirloin and rib-eye steaks, boneless center-cut pork chops, wild-caught salmon—all of these are crowd-pleasers. But because these familiar cuts are so popular, demand is high, which leads to high prices.

If you're on a budget, a simple way to save is to buy the other stuff. Bone-in, skin-on chicken thighs, lamb shoulder chops instead of tiny rib chops, mackerel or porgy instead of salmon—there's a whole world of cheaper proteins that taste just as good as (if not better than) the pricier ones. Visit the "Get to Know Your Proteins" section (see pages 64 to 72) to find out what the experts recommend in terms of lesser-known choices, as well as some of ours.

You can also focus more of your dollars on well-known cuts that are traditionally cheaper. Whole chickens, pork ribs, pork shoulder, ground meats and poultry, flatter beef cuts (such as hanger or skirt steak), brisket, shanks—there are so many cuts of meat that are full of flavor and good nutrition and are easier on the wallet.

The recipes in this book utilize many different cuts partially for this reason: most of us don't want to have to mortgage the house to put dinner on the table. So, although we do offer some special-occasion meals, we have tried to show you that you can make something awesome out of many different parts of many different animals.

Shop sales, and stock up

Proteins spoil, so, as they get closer to their expiration date, sellers will lower the prices to unload them. This is a great opportunity to stock up. Buy it and freeze it, or cook it and eat it for a few days, or cook a lot and freeze some. For example, you can take several pounds of ground beef, cook it seasoned with just salt and pepper, measure out how much you would need for individual meals, and freeze it in batches. Not only do you save on the cost of the meat, but future you gets some streamlined meals, which makes you less likely to spend money on takeout on a night when you're especially busy or tired.

Buy shelf-stable proteins

There was a time when shelf-stable protein basically meant canned tuna or tinned sardines, but these days, there are many great options. Even tuna has had a renaissance; you can get multiple species, packed in oil or water, in pouches with seasonings added, or fillets jarred in olive oil. There's also canned wild salmon, yellowtail, mackerel, cod, oysters, and shrimp. Plus, you can get canned cooked chicken breast. Not all shelf-stable proteins are created equal; we generally avoid the ones that contain a lot of preservatives and fillers, like canned sausage.

Spam presents a challenge. There's some concern among experts that sodium nitrate, the preservative in Spam and many other lunch meats, may be harmful; others say it doesn't pose a risk. Spam has become a part of the cuisine in some cultures; we respect that and as such will not list it in the "don't eat this" column. (It's also pretty tasty.) What we will say is that it's fine to eat Spam occasionally, but perhaps not as frequently as other shelf-stable proteins.

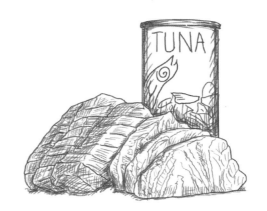

Buy conventional strategically

If grass-fed/pastured meat just isn't going to work for your budget, aim to buy leaner cuts. Research suggests that toxins from pollutants and pesticides are fat-soluble, so they collect in the fatty parts of the meat. By sticking to leaner cuts, you avoid the fat, so you lessen your exposure to the toxins.

This is not us encouraging you to avoid fat in general—hopefully by now you know that we are pro-healthy fat. When you buy those leaner cuts, cook them in a healthy fat like avocado oil or ghee, and/or drizzle on a sauce or add a slice of compound butter. That way, you'll reap the benefits of the fat-soluble nutrients in the meat while minimizing your exposure to potential toxins.

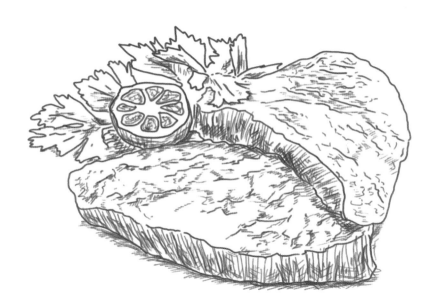

PART 2

THE
RECIPES

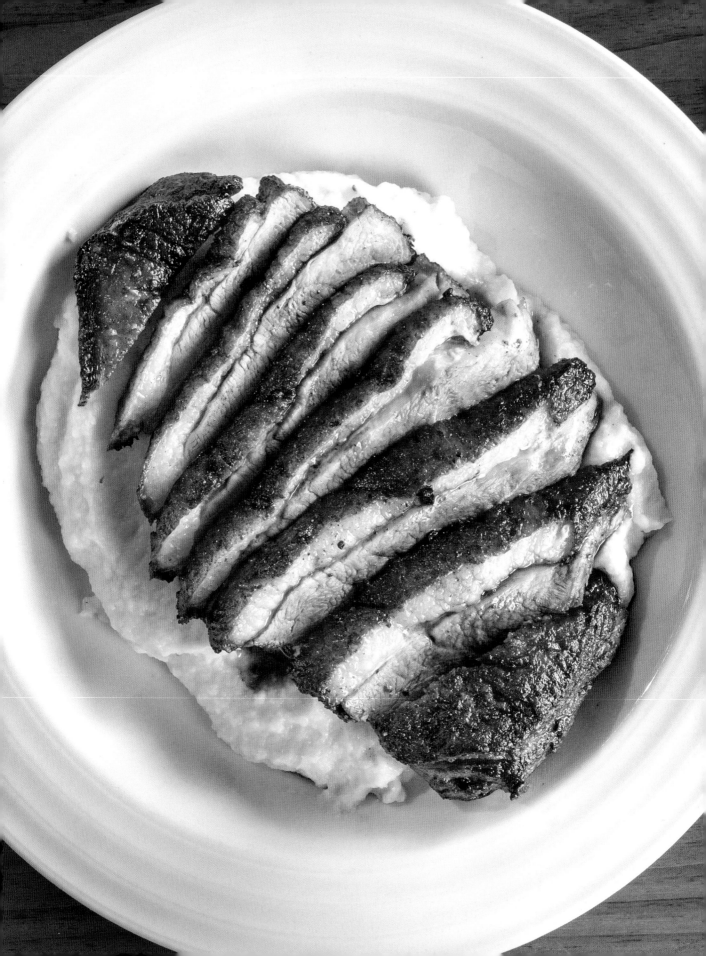

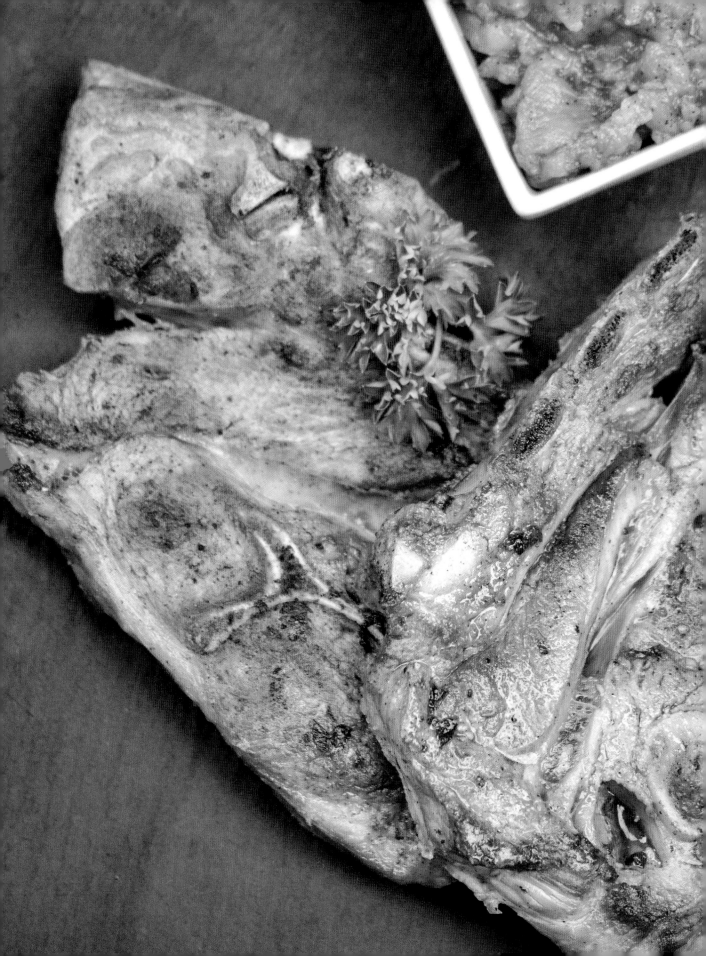

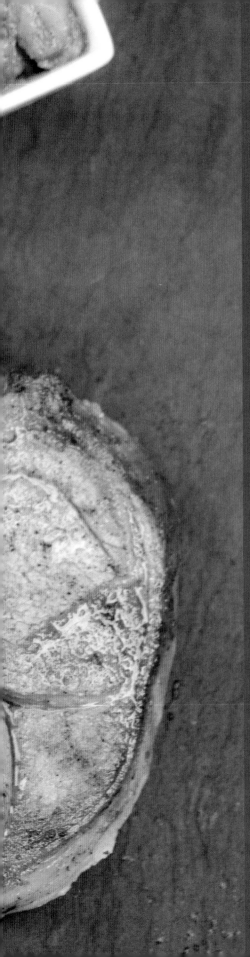

CHAPTER 3:

BEEF, LAMB & GOAT

RIB EYE WITH BLUE CHEESE BUTTER

SERVES: 4 | **PREP TIME:** 15 minutes, plus 30 minutes to chill butter |
COOK TIME: 10 minutes

A good rib eye is a thing of beauty. Since it's a fattier cut, it's glorious on its own, simply seasoned with salt and pepper, no sauce or topping needed. But adding the blue cheese butter—it's so easy, requiring just a bowl, a fork, and a few very simple ingredients—really elevates it. The keys to success here: get your skillet screaming hot for a good sear on the steak, and be generous with the salt.

4 tablespoons (2 ounces) unsalted butter, at room temperature

3 tablespoons crumbled blue cheese (about 1½ ounces)

½ teaspoon chopped fresh thyme

¼ teaspoon garlic powder

Fine sea salt and freshly ground black pepper

1½ pounds boneless rib-eye steak (preferably grass-fed), 1 inch thick

1 tablespoon avocado oil

1. In a medium bowl, mash together the butter, blue cheese, thyme, and garlic powder until combined. Season to taste with salt and pepper. Roll into a log, wrap, and refrigerate for at least 30 minutes. (You can make the butter up to 2 days ahead; keep it covered and refrigerated.)

2. Let the steak stand at room temperature for 30 minutes before cooking. Preheat a large cast-iron skillet over medium-high heat until very hot. Pat the steak thoroughly dry and season it generously with salt and pepper. Swirl the avocado oil in the pan, then add the steak. Cook until well seared on both sides and cooked to medium-rare (an instant-read thermometer stuck into the thickest part should read 130°F), flipping a few times, 8 to 10 minutes total, or slightly longer if your steak is more than 1 inch thick.

3. Transfer the steak to a cutting board, cover loosely with foil, and let rest for 5 to 10 minutes. Cut the blue cheese butter into thin slices. Slice the steak against the grain, top each portion with a few slices of the butter, and serve.

> **NOTES:**
>
> *You're likely to have leftover butter. Use it on another steak or on burgers, eggs, or chicken.*
>
> *The grain on rib eyes often goes in different directions. Separate the pieces that have different grains and slice each piece individually. It's more important to slice against the grain than it is to have longer slices.*

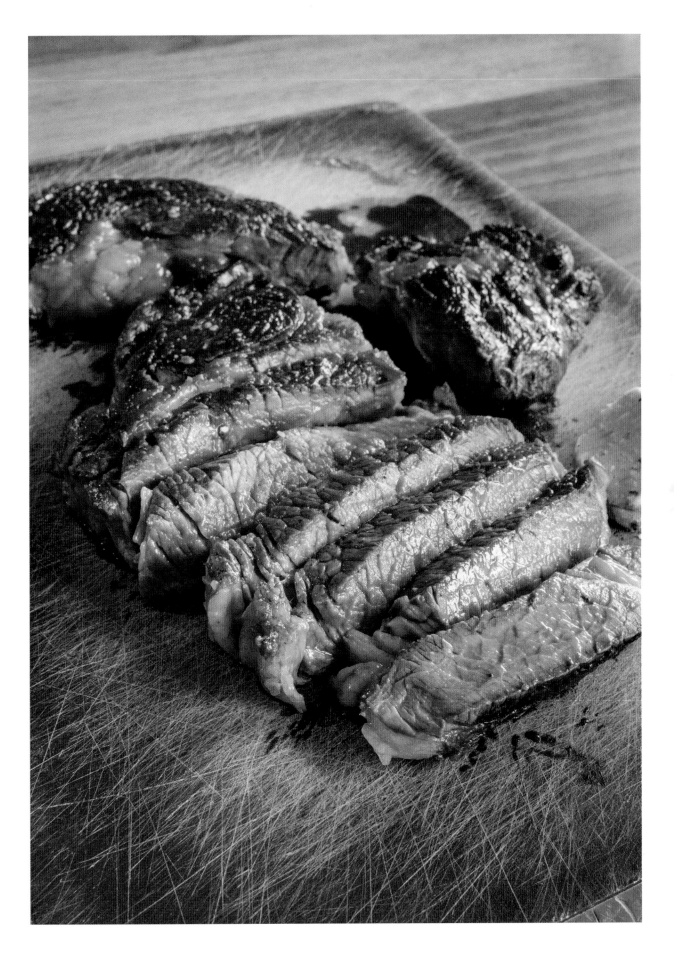

CHEESEBURGER SALAD

SERVES: 4 | **PREP TIME:** 15 minutes | **COOK TIME:** 20 minutes

Ground beef, special sauce, lettuce, cheese, pickles, onions: there's so much going on in this protein-forward salad, inspired by a certain famous fast-food burger, that you'll never miss the sesame seed bun. Look for fermented pickles in the refrigerated section of the supermarket to get the gut health benefits.

DRESSING *(MAKES ⅔ CUP):*

⅓ cup avocado oil mayonnaise

3 tablespoons unsweetened ketchup

1 teaspoon dill pickle brine

1 teaspoon coconut aminos

¼ teaspoon hot sauce (optional)

Fine sea salt and freshly ground black pepper, to taste

SALAD:

1 tablespoon ghee or avocado oil

1 small onion, chopped (about 1 cup)

Fine sea salt

1½ pounds ground beef

Freshly ground black pepper

1 medium head romaine, chopped (about 3 cups)

1 cup halved cherry or grape tomatoes

1 medium whole dill pickle, chopped (about ¾ cup)

¾ cup shredded cheddar cheese (about 3 ounces)

1. Make the dressing: Whisk all of the ingredients in a small bowl until well combined. (You can make the dressing up to 2 days ahead; keep it covered and refrigerated. Whisk before using.)

2. Make the salad: Warm the ghee in a large skillet over medium heat. Add the onion, sprinkle with salt, and cook, stirring occasionally, until very tender and lightly caramelized, about 10 minutes. Transfer to a bowl. Add the ground beef to the skillet, season with salt and pepper, and cook, stirring and breaking up the meat, until cooked through and browned in spots, about 10 minutes.

3. While the meat is cooking, place the lettuce, tomatoes, pickle, and cooked onion in a large bowl. Add 3 to 4 tablespoons of the dressing; gently toss, adding more dressing if desired. Add the meat and cheese; toss again. Divide the salad among four bowls and serve, passing the remaining dressing on the side.

NOTE:

If you're not serving all four portions at once, toss only what you're going to serve with dressing; store the remaining salad and dressing in separate covered containers in the fridge. The salad will keep for up to 2 days, the dressing for up to 4 days.

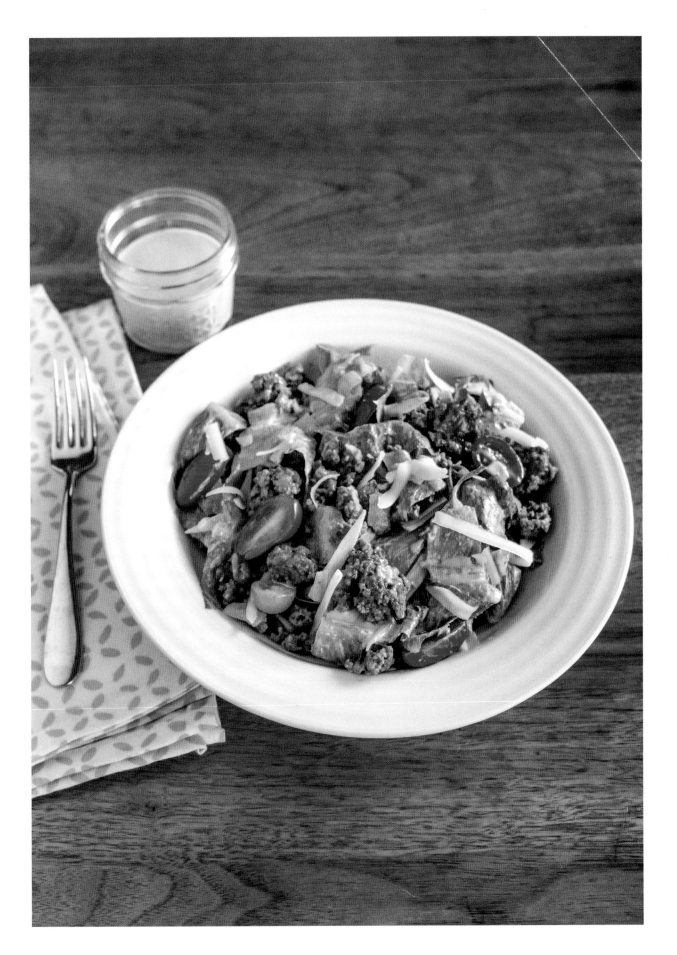

ZA'ATAR LAMB SHOULDER CHOPS

SERVES: 4 | **PREP TIME:** 10 minutes, plus 30 minutes to marinate | **COOK TIME:** 10 minutes

Shoulder chops are among our favorite cuts of lamb. They're rich and flavorful, easy to cook, and economical, especially compared to the sexier rib chops (we love those, too, of course). Though these chops are often braised, they work really well with a quick pan-sear. Za'atar, a Middle Eastern spice mix, is a simple, stress-free way to dress them up.

4 bone-in lamb shoulder blade chops, ¾ to 1 inch thick (about 2¼ pounds)

3 tablespoons avocado oil, divided

1 tablespoon za'atar

Fine sea salt and freshly ground black pepper

Tzatziki, homemade (page 352) or store-bought, for serving (optional)

1. Pat the lamb chops dry and rub them all over with 2 tablespoons of the avocado oil; sprinkle with the za'atar. Place on a large plate and let stand at room temperature for 30 minutes.

2. Preheat a large cast-iron skillet over medium-high heat until very hot. Season the chops generously with salt and pepper. Swirl the remaining 1 tablespoon of oil in the skillet, add the chops, and cook until well seared on both sides and an instant-read thermometer stuck into the thickest part away from the bone reads 130°F, 3 to 5 minutes per side, depending on thickness. Transfer to a cutting board, cover loosely with foil, and let rest for 5 minutes before serving. Serve with tzatziki, if desired.

NOTE:

Cook the chops in batches if necessary. It's better to do that than to overcrowd the pan, which will prevent the chops from cooking properly. Keep the first batch warm under foil as you cook the second batch.

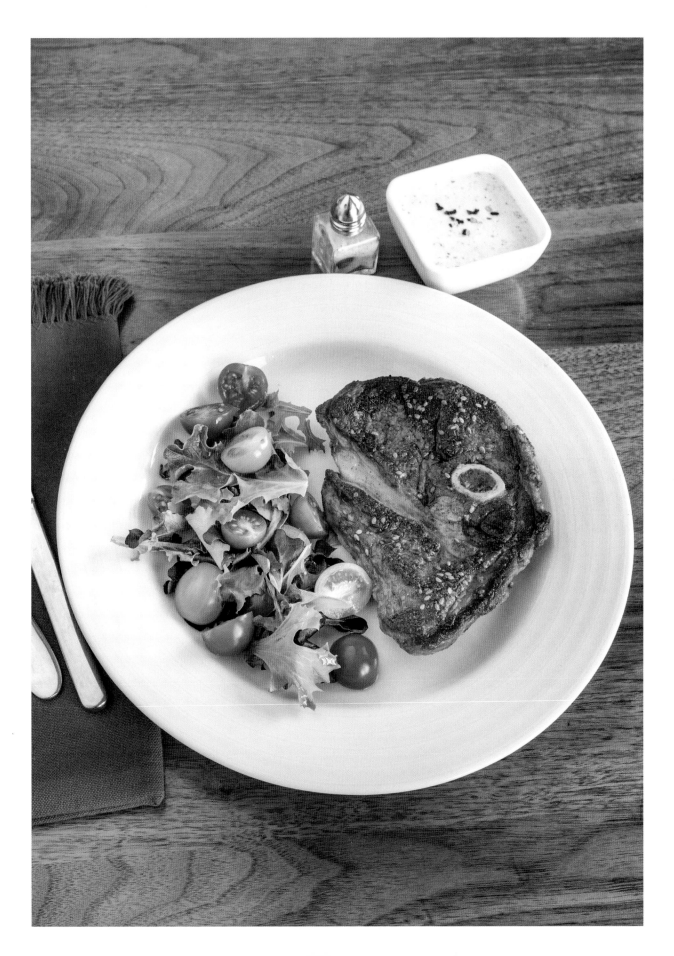

LAMB KEFTA

SERVES: 3 to 4 | **PREP TIME:** 5 minutes, plus 30 minutes to chill | **COOK TIME:** 10 minutes

If you're getting bored of eating the same ground beef dishes over and over again, subbing in lamb, adding some unique spices, and even shaping your meat into a slightly different form are all simple ways to ratchet up the flavor and keep things interesting. These Persian-style sausages, often called *kofta,* are deeply flavorful and juicy and taste fantastic with Tzatziki (page 352) or Garlic and Dill Yogurt Dip (page 354). A drizzle of tahini, thinned with water if needed, or a spoonful of hummus are good serving options, too. Traditionally, kefta are skewered and grilled, but we've opted to save a step and simply pan-fry them.

3 tablespoons minced white onions

2 tablespoons minced fresh flat-leaf parsley

2 tablespoons minced fresh mint

3 cloves garlic, minced (about 1 tablespoon)

1 teaspoon ground coriander

1 teaspoon fine sea salt

½ teaspoon freshly ground black pepper

¼ teaspoon ground cinnamon

1 pound ground lamb

2 tablespoons (1 ounce) unsalted butter

1. Toss the minced onions, parsley, mint, garlic, coriander, salt, pepper, and cinnamon together in a medium bowl. Add the ground lamb and mix with your hands until combined. Cover the bowl and refrigerate for 30 minutes.

2. Divide the meat mixture into 6 equal portions. Using your hands, form the mixture into oblong sausagelike shapes, 3 to 4 inches long and 2 inches thick.

3. Melt the butter in a large skillet over medium heat. Add the sausages to the skillet and cook until deep brown on one side, 4 to 5 minutes. Flip carefully with tongs and continue cooking until the meat is cooked through, 3 to 4 minutes longer. Serve hot.

NOTE:

> Though kefta are most often formed into oblong shapes, there are no hard-and-fast rules. You can form the meat mixture into patties or meatballs if you prefer. You can also swap out the ground lamb for ground beef if you like.

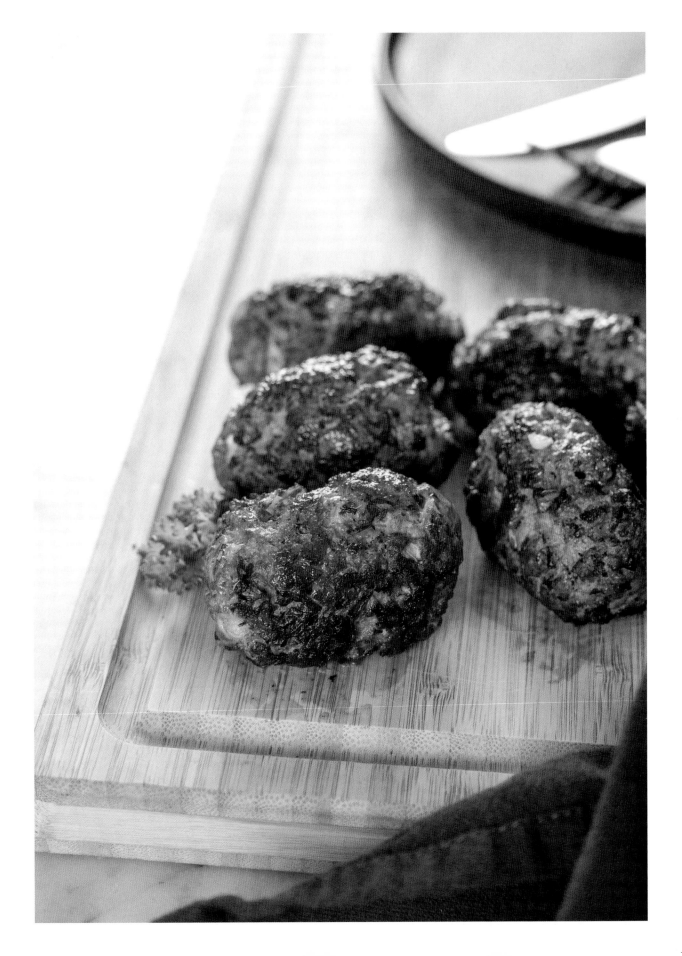

CHIPOTLE SHREDDED BEEF

MAKES: About 6½ cups (4 to 6 servings) | **PREP TIME:** 20 minutes |
COOK TIME: 3 hours 15 minutes

A big pot of shredded beef is a great way to feed a crowd for a Super Bowl party—or you can just make it on a Sunday and eat it over several days. This beef is loaded with flavor, with a touch of heat from the chipotles. Try it in tacos, on a salad, or in an omelet.

3 canned chipotle peppers in adobo sauce, seeded, plus 1 tablespoon sauce from the can

¼ cup fresh orange juice (from 1 small orange)

3 tablespoons fresh lime juice

2 teaspoons dried oregano leaves

1 teaspoon ground cumin

¼ teaspoon ground cinnamon

1 tablespoon avocado oil, plus more as needed

1 (3-pound) boneless beef chuck roast, trimmed of excess fat and cut into 2-inch chunks

Fine sea salt and freshly ground black pepper

1 small onion, chopped (about 1 cup)

4 cloves garlic, minced (about 1⅓ tablespoons)

½ cup chicken bone broth

1 dried bay leaf

1. Preheat the oven to 275°F.

2. In a blender or small food processor, blend the chipotles, adobo sauce, orange juice, lime juice, oregano, cumin, and cinnamon until smooth.

3. Warm the avocado oil in a Dutch oven over medium-high heat. Pat the beef chunks dry; season with salt and pepper. Brown the beef on all sides, 5 to 7 minutes. (Work in batches to avoid overcrowding the pan, if needed. Add more oil between batches.) Transfer the cooked beef to a bowl.

4. Lower the heat to medium. Add the onion to the pot; season lightly with salt. Cook, stirring, until the onion is tender, 3 to 4 minutes. Add the garlic; sauté until fragrant, about 1 minute. Return the beef to the pot along with any juices that collected in the bowl. Stir in the chipotle mixture, broth, and bay leaf; bring to a simmer.

5. Cover the pot and transfer to the oven. Cook until the meat is very tender and shreds easily, about 3 hours. Remove and discard the bay leaf. Shred the meat and serve. Let any leftovers cool, then cover and store in the fridge for up to 4 days.

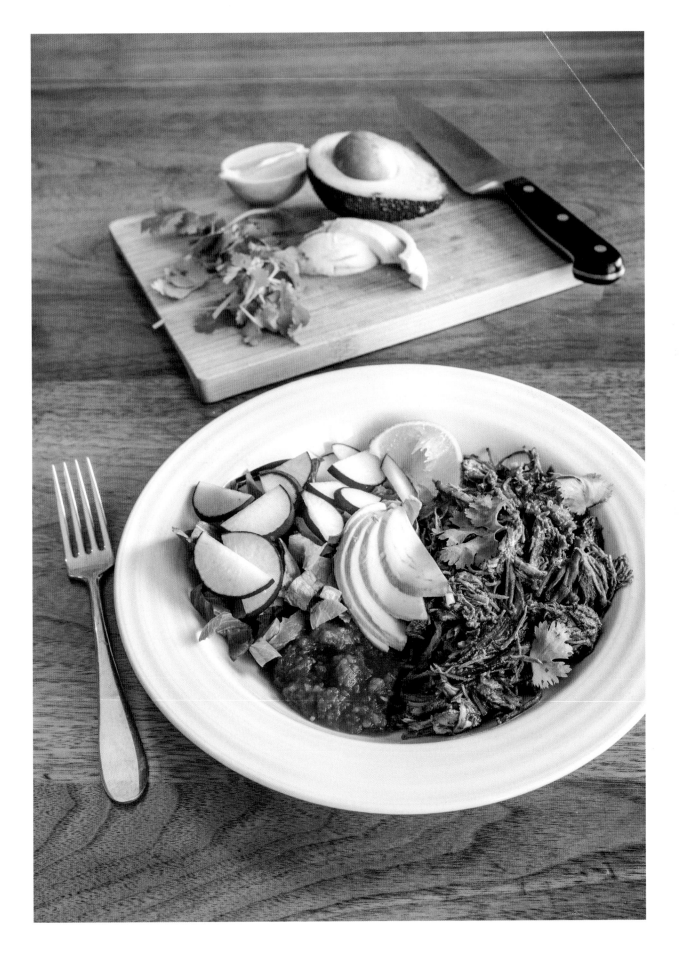

SUPER MEATY CHILI

MAKES: About 9 cups (4 to 6 servings) | **PREP TIME:** 25 minutes |
COOK TIME: 55 minutes

In Texas, they don't add beans to chili—and though this isn't quite a traditional Texas recipe, we wholeheartedly agree that the meat should be the star. If you prefer it spicier, leave the seeds in the jalapeño and/ or the chipotle. Enjoy the chili in a bowl with your favorite toppings, or spoon it over hot dogs. The sweet potato chips on page 276 would go great on the side.

2 tablespoons bacon fat or avocado oil, divided

2 pounds ground beef

Fine sea salt and freshly ground black pepper

1 large onion, chopped (about 2 cups)

1 large or 2 small jalapeño peppers, seeds and ribs removed, minced (about ⅓ cup)

3 medium carrots, chopped (about 1¼ cups)

1 medium rib celery, chopped (about ½ cup)

6 cloves garlic, minced (about 2 tablespoons)

2 canned chipotle peppers in adobo sauce, seeded and minced (about 2 tablespoons), plus 2 tablespoons sauce from the can

1 tablespoon dried oregano leaves

2 teaspoons chili powder

1½ teaspoons ground cumin

1 (15-ounce) can fire-roasted diced tomatoes

2 tablespoons tomato paste

1½ cups chicken or beef bone broth

TOPPINGS (OPTIONAL):

Sour cream

Thinly sliced radishes

Chopped avocado

Shredded cheddar or Jack cheese

Fresh cilantro

1. Melt 1 tablespoon of the bacon fat in a Dutch oven over medium heat. Add the ground beef, season well with salt and pepper, and cook, stirring and breaking up the meat, until well browned, 7 to 10 minutes. Use a slotted spoon to transfer the meat to a bowl. (If there's a lot of liquid in the pot, pour it off.)

2. Add the remaining 1 tablespoon of fat to the pot. Add the onion, jalapeño, carrots, and celery; season well with salt and cook, stirring, until the vegetables are tender, 8 to 10 minutes. Stir in the garlic, chipotles, adobo sauce, oregano, chili powder, and cumin; sauté until fragrant, 1 to 2 minutes.

3. Return the meat and any accumulated juices to the pot. Stir in the tomatoes, tomato paste, and broth. Raise the heat to medium-high and bring just to a boil, stirring. Reduce the heat to low, partially cover, and simmer for 30 minutes to allow the flavors to meld. Taste and season with salt and pepper.

4. Serve hot with toppings, or let cool, cover, and refrigerate to serve later. The chili will keep, covered and refrigerated, for up to 4 days.

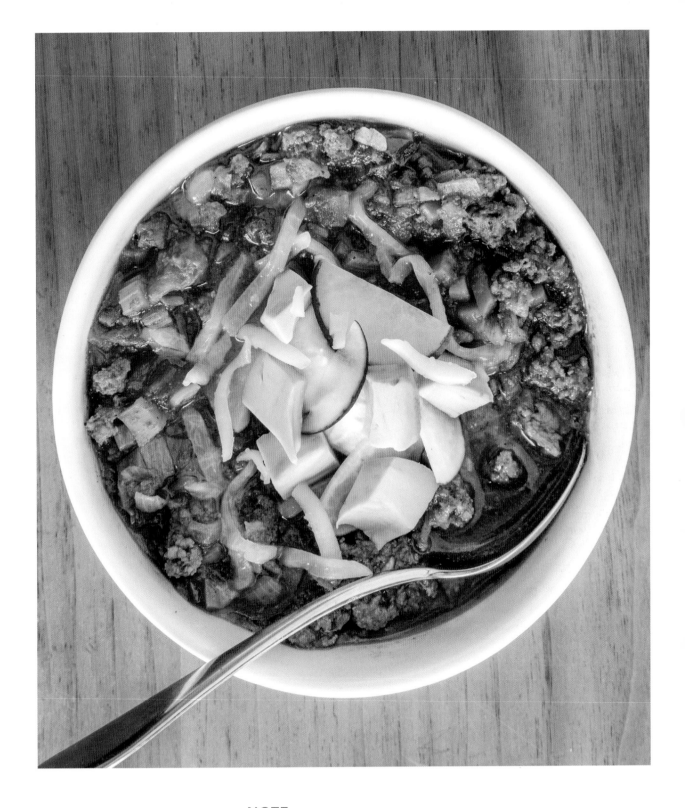

NOTE:

Chili tastes even better after it's had a chance to develop. If you have time, make it the day before you intend to serve it. Rewarm it gently on the stove.

CARNE ASADA

SERVES: 4 | **PREP TIME:** 10 minutes, plus 1 hour to marinate |
COOK TIME: 10 minutes

Technically, *carne asada* means "grilled meat," yet we cook this flavorful
marinated skirt steak in a cast-iron skillet. The thing is, we love this
steak so much, we don't want to have to wait for grilling season to eat
it. If you do want to grill it, go right ahead: just place it over high heat
for 3 to 5 minutes per side.

1½ pounds skirt steak,
patted dry

½ cup fresh orange juice (from
1 large orange)

¼ cup fresh lime juice (from
2 medium limes)

3 tablespoons coconut aminos

2 tablespoons avocado oil,
divided

Fine sea salt and freshly
ground black pepper

TACO FIXINGS (OPTIONAL):

Guacamole

Salsa

Warm grain-free or corn
tortillas

Fresh cilantro

Sour cream

1.   Cut the steak into a few pieces so that it fits into a large cast-
iron skillet. In a large bowl, combine the orange and lime juices,
coconut aminos, 1 tablespoon of the avocado oil, ½ teaspoon of
salt, and ¼ teaspoon of pepper. Add the steak to the bowl and turn
it to coat all of the pieces with the marinade. Cover and refrigerate
for 30 minutes, then put it on the counter and let it come to room
temperature, about 30 minutes longer.

2.   Remove the steak from the marinade; discard the marinade.
Preheat a large cast-iron skillet over medium-high heat until very
hot. Pat the steak dry and season with salt and pepper.

3.   Swirl the remaining 1 tablespoon of oil in the skillet, then add
the steak. Cook, turning once, until the steak is seared on both
sides and cooked to medium-rare, 3 to 5 minutes per side (an
instant-read thermometer stuck into the thickest part should read
125°F). Transfer to a cutting board; cover loosely with foil to keep
warm and let rest for at least 5 minutes. If serving tacos, have all of
your fixings on the table. Slice the steak thinly against the grain and
serve.

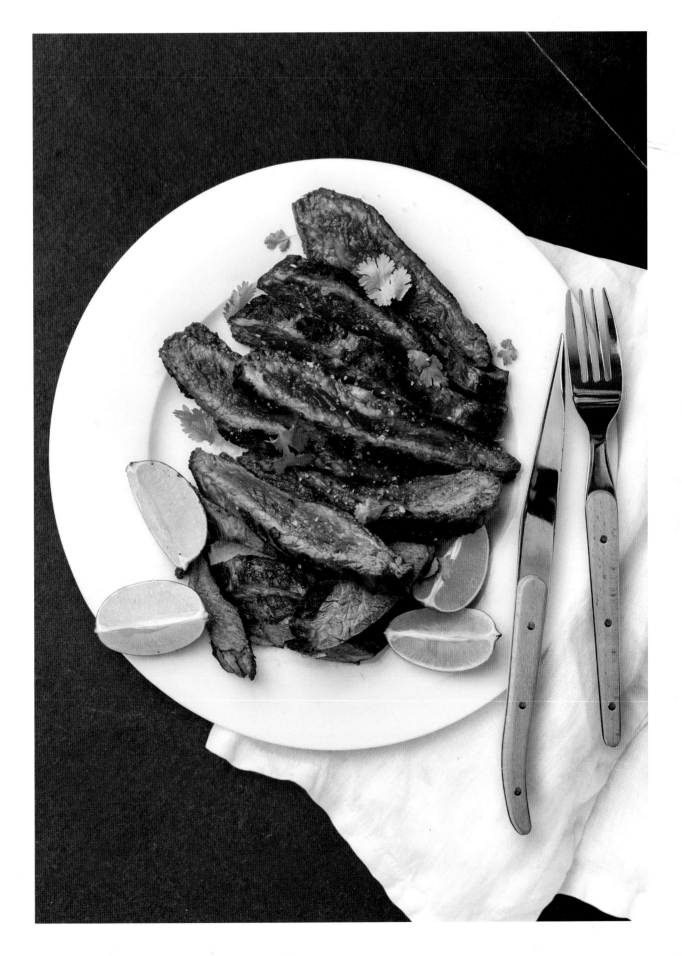

BEEF TENDERLOIN ROAST WITH BOURBON PAN SAUCE

SERVES: 6 | **PREP TIME:** 20 minutes, plus 30 to 60 minutes of standing time |
COOK TIME: 1 hour

A center-cut beef tenderloin, also known as Châteaubriand, is a
beautiful (and pricey) cut; it feels worthy of a special occasion. It's
super lean, so a sauce really elevates it; you also can serve it with slices
of compound butter (see pages 348 to 351). This one is cooked using a
reverse-sear method; instead of searing it in a hot skillet and finishing
it in the oven, you cook it low and slow in the oven until it reaches just
below the right temperature for medium-rare, then finish it in a skillet.
This makes it much easier to get a beautiful sear and a perfectly cooked
interior—just what you want with a showstopping roast like this.

ROAST:

1 (24- to 28-ounce) center-cut
beef tenderloin roast

Fine sea salt and freshly
ground black pepper

1 tablespoon melted ghee

1 tablespoon avocado oil

SAUCE:

2 medium shallots, minced
(about ⅔ cup)

2 cloves garlic, grated (about
2 teaspoons)

½ cup bourbon

1 cup beef or chicken bone
broth

2 tablespoons heavy cream,
at room temperature

2 tablespoons (1 ounce) cold
unsalted butter, cut into pieces

Fine sea salt and freshly
ground black pepper

1. Pat the roast dry and season it liberally with salt and pepper. Let
stand at room temperature for at least 30 minutes or up to 1 hour.
Pat dry again and season with additional salt and pepper.

2. Preheat the oven to 300°F. Fit a rimmed baking sheet with a
cooling rack. Brush the roast with the ghee, sprinkle with salt, and
tie up with kitchen twine at 1- to 1½-inch intervals. Trim any excess
twine. Place the roast on the rack-lined baking sheet and roast
until an instant-read thermometer stuck into the thickest part reads
125°F, 40 to 50 minutes, turning the roast over halfway through.

3. Preheat a large cast-iron skillet over high heat. Add the avocado
oil and swirl in the skillet. Place the roast in the pan and cook,
turning with tongs, until seared on all sides, 2 to 3 minutes. Transfer
to a cutting board, cover loosely with foil, and let rest for 15 minutes.

4. Meanwhile, make the sauce: Lower the heat under the skillet
to medium. Add the shallots and sauté until tender, 1 to 2 minutes.
Add the garlic; sauté until fragrant, about 1 minute. Pour in the
bourbon and stir to scrape up any browned bits from the bottom of
the pan. Boil until reduced by half, 1 to 2 minutes. Pour in the broth
and cream and cook, stirring occasionally, until reduced by half, 2
to 3 minutes. Remove the pan from the heat and whisk in the butter
a few pieces at a time until all of the butter is incorporated and the
sauce is thickened and silky. Taste and season with salt and pepper.

5. Slice the roast and serve with the pan sauce.

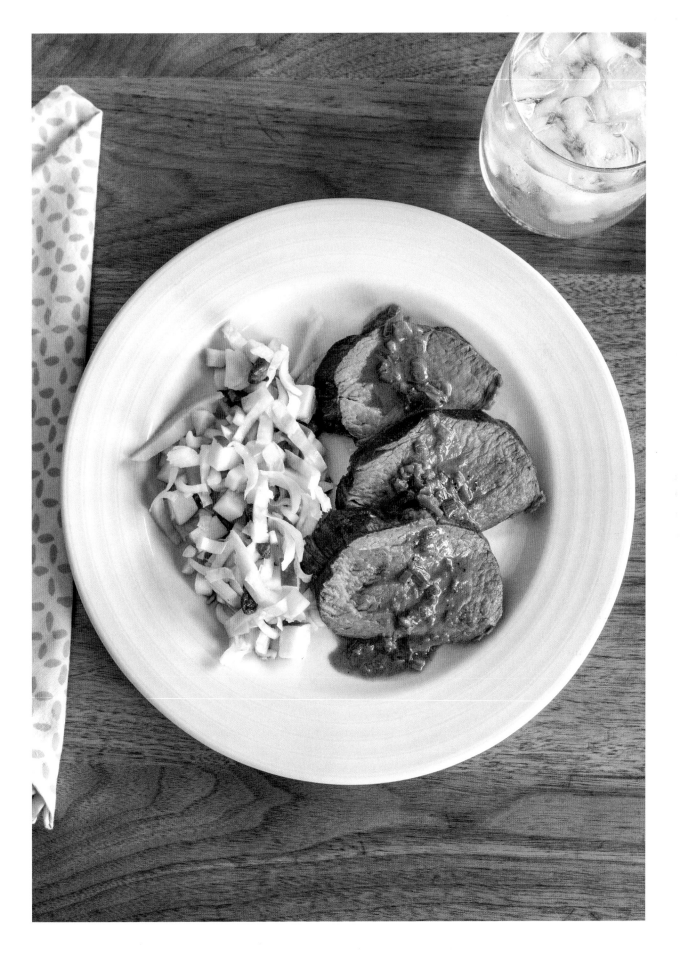

KOREAN-STYLE GROUND BEEF

SERVES: 4 | **PREP TIME:** 10 minutes | **COOK TIME:** 25 minutes

We love Korean food; in fact, the first time our husbands met each other was over an epic Korean meal in New York City. This Korean-inspired dish is bursting with flavor, though it's remarkably simple and unfussy to make. We like it over rice, with kimchi on the side, but it also works beautifully in lettuce wraps. If you have any left over, rewarm it the next day and enjoy it with a runny fried egg on top.

1 tablespoon avocado oil

1½ pounds ground beef

Fine sea salt

5 cloves garlic, minced (about 1⅔ tablespoons)

2 tablespoons minced fresh ginger

3 scallions, sliced on a diagonal (about ⅓ cup); reserve sliced dark green parts for garnish

⅓ cup coconut sugar

½ cup coconut aminos

½ teaspoon red pepper flakes

Freshly ground black pepper

1 tablespoon toasted sesame oil

Sesame seeds, for garnish (optional)

Cooked white rice, Cauliflower Rice (That Doesn't Suck) (page 268), or Bibb lettuce leaves, for serving

1. Warm the avocado oil in a large skillet over medium-high heat. Add the ground beef, season with salt, and cook, stirring and breaking up the meat, until nearly cooked through, 7 to 9 minutes. (If there's a lot of liquid in the skillet, pour off all but about ¼ cup.) Add the garlic, ginger, and sliced white and light green parts of the scallions; cook, stirring, until tender and fragrant, about 1 minute.

2. Stir in the sugar, coconut aminos, and red pepper flakes; season with black pepper. Stir until all of the ingredients are incorporated. Spread out the mixture in the skillet and cook undisturbed until the sauce thickens, 2 to 3 minutes. Stir and allow to cook for another 2 minutes. Repeat until the meat is well coated and browned and the sauce clings to the meat, once or twice more. Remove the pan from the heat, drizzle with the sesame oil, taste, and season with additional salt and pepper, if needed.

3. Spoon the rice into four shallow bowls, or place a few lettuce leaves in each bowl. Top with the beef mixture and sprinkle with the sliced scallion greens and sesame seeds, if desired. Serve hot.

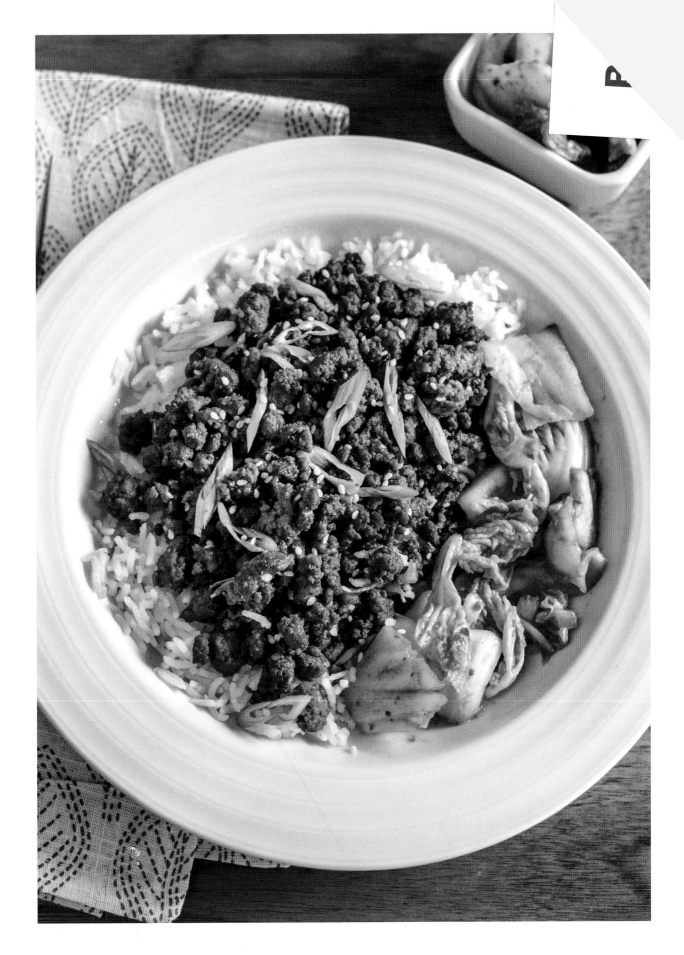

BEEF CONFIT

SERVES: 4 | **PREP TIME:** 2 minutes | **COOK TIME:** 1 hour

This simple but decadent recipe, inspired by *awarma,* a Lebanese lamb dish, is excellent with over-easy eggs, added to salads, or atop your favorite grain, like the simple couscous pictured here. To reheat, simply place the meat in a pan or skillet over medium heat for a few minutes, stirring occasionally, until the fat melts and the beef is warmed through.

1 pound beef tallow

1 pound ground beef

1 tablespoon fine sea salt

½ teaspoon ground cinnamon

¼ teaspoon ground cardamom

¼ teaspoon ground cloves

1. In a large cast-iron skillet, melt the tallow over low heat. Add the ground beef and cook, stirring occasionally, until the beef caramelizes and turns deep brown, about 50 minutes. Stir in the salt, cinnamon, cardamom, and cloves and cook until the beef starts to develop a hint of a caramelized crust, about 10 minutes longer.

2. Serve immediately or let cool to room temperature (about 10 minutes) and store in an airtight glass jar. It will keep in the fridge for up to a week.

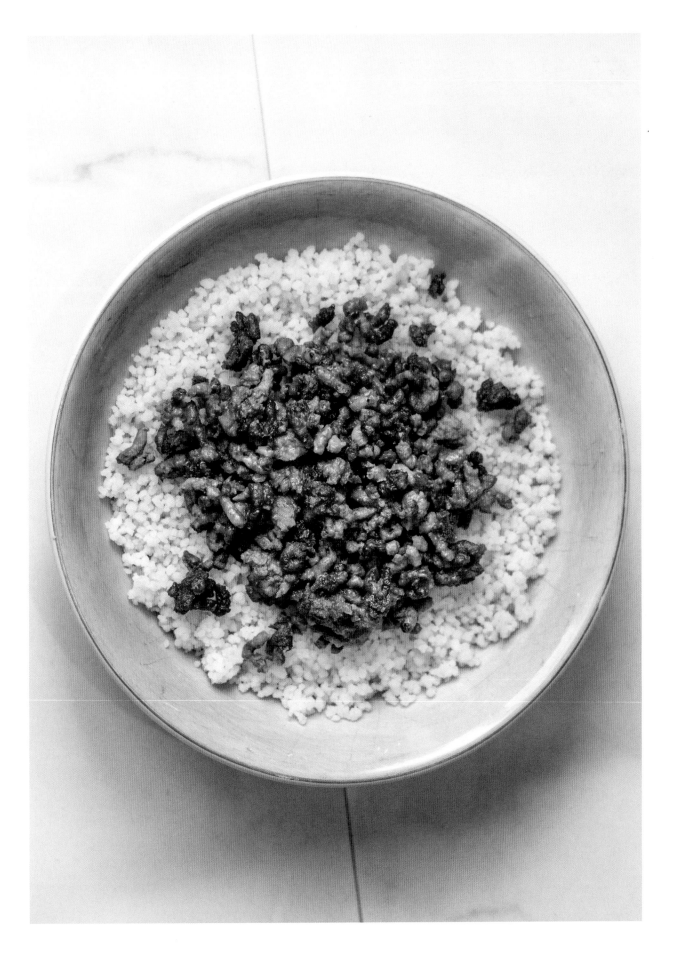

GARLIC-HERB LAMB CHOPS
WITH **APPLESAUCE**

SERVES: 4 | **PREP TIME:** 15 minutes, plus 1 hour to marinate | **COOK TIME:** 35 minutes

Applesauce is usually paired with pork chops, but here we sub in flavorful lamb loin chops. It's a fast, easy meal that's unfussy enough for a weeknight but still feels special. Mashed potatoes or cauliflower rice (see our recipe on page 268) would make a nice side dish.

LAMB CHOPS:

4 bone-in lamb loin chops, about 1 inch thick (about 1½ pounds)

2 tablespoons extra-virgin olive oil, divided

6 cloves garlic, crushed to a paste or minced

½ teaspoon freshly ground black pepper

1 tablespoon minced flat-leaf fresh parsley

1 tablespoon fine sea salt

2 tablespoons (1 ounce) unsalted butter

APPLESAUCE:

6 medium apples, peeled, cored, and chopped (we recommend Fuji or McIntosh)

2 tablespoons coconut sugar (optional)

½ teaspoon ground cinnamon

1. Put the lamb chops in a shallow dish.

2. In a small bowl, stir together the olive oil, garlic, pepper, and parsley. Rub the mixture over the chops. Cover and refrigerate for at least 1 hour or up to 12 hours.

3. Make the applesauce: Combine the apples, ⅓ cup water, sugar (if using), and cinnamon in a medium saucepan and bring to a boil over medium-high heat. Reduce the heat to low, cover, and simmer until the apples are very tender, 15 to 20 minutes. Remove the lid and simmer until thickened, about 5 minutes longer. Mash the apples with a potato masher or fork for a chunky consistency or puree with an immersion blender for a smooth consistency. Set aside or, if you prefer it cold, let cool, cover, and refrigerate.

4. Remove the chops from the fridge and season with the salt. Let sit on the counter for about 10 minutes to temper.

5. Preheat a large skillet over medium-high heat. Melt the butter in the pan, then add the chops and cook until they are medium-rare, 4 to 5 minutes per side (an instant-read thermometer stuck into the thickest part away from the bone should read 135°F). Transfer the chops to a platter, tent with foil, and let rest for 5 minutes. Serve the chops with the applesauce on the side.

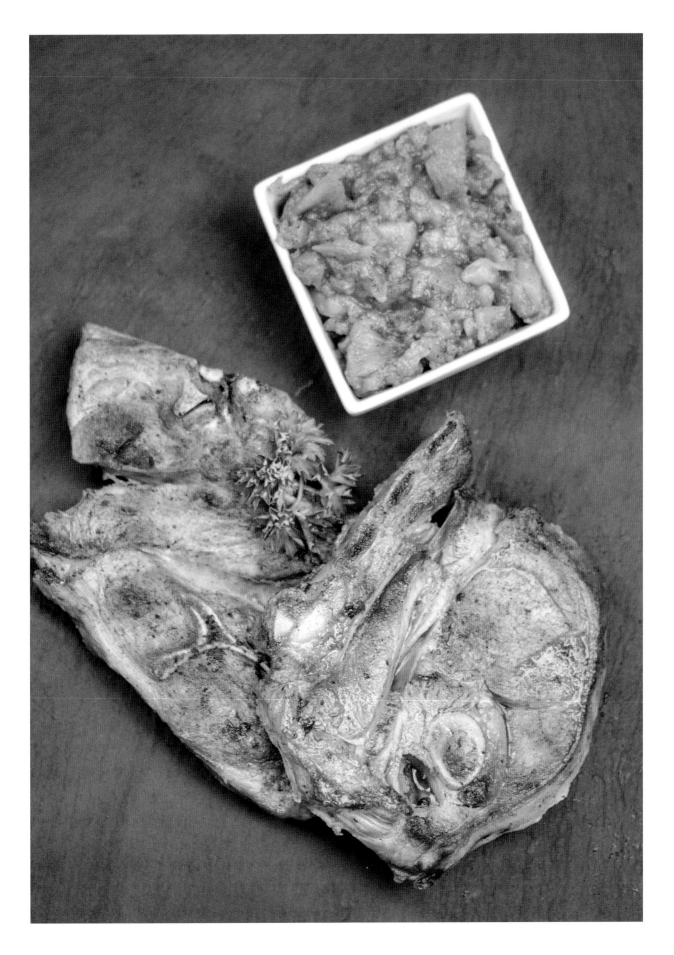

STUFFED CABBAGE ROLLS

SERVES: 6 | **PREP TIME:** 25 minutes | **COOK TIME:** 85 minutes

Consider this recipe another genius way to wrap meat in vegetables to get the best of both worlds. After years of buying and enjoying cabbage rolls, we took the plunge into making them ourselves and were pleasantly surprised; they're easier to make than they look.

1 head green cabbage

1 pound lean ground beef (90% lean)

1 cup cooked white rice or Cauliflower Rice (That Doesn't Suck) (page 268)

½ small white onion, finely chopped (about ½ cup)

3 cloves garlic, minced (about 1 tablespoon)

2 cups tomato sauce, divided

3 tablespoons chopped fresh flat-leaf parsley

1 large egg

1 teaspoon fine sea salt

½ teaspoon freshly ground black pepper

1. Bring a large pot two-thirds filled with water to a boil. Immerse the cabbage head in the boiling water. Cook until the cabbage leaves are pliable, 3 to 5 minutes. Peel off 6 to 8 large leaves (depending on the size of the leaves).

2. Preheat the oven to 350°F.

3. Put the ground beef, rice, onion, garlic, ½ cup of the tomato sauce, the parsley, egg, salt, and pepper in a large bowl. Lightly moisten your hands and use them to gently but thoroughly mix the ingredients until combined.

4. Lay each cabbage leaf on a flat surface. Use a paring knife to cut a V-shaped notch to remove the thick stem at the base of each leaf.

5. Divide the meat mixture into 6 to 8 equal-sized balls, according to the number of cabbage leaves, and shape each into a log. Place each meat log in the center of a cabbage leaf. Roll the leaf around the meat mixture, tucking the top of the leaf in first to close the top and doing the same to the bottom after rolling. Repeat with the remaining meat mixture and cabbage leaves.

6. Coat a 9 by 13-inch glass baking dish with cooking spray or avocado oil. Spread half of the remaining tomato sauce in the bottom of the dish. Place the cabbage rolls in the dish. Top with the remaining sauce.

7. Cover the dish with foil. Bake until the cabbage is tender and the filling is cooked through, 60 to 80 minutes. Serve hot.

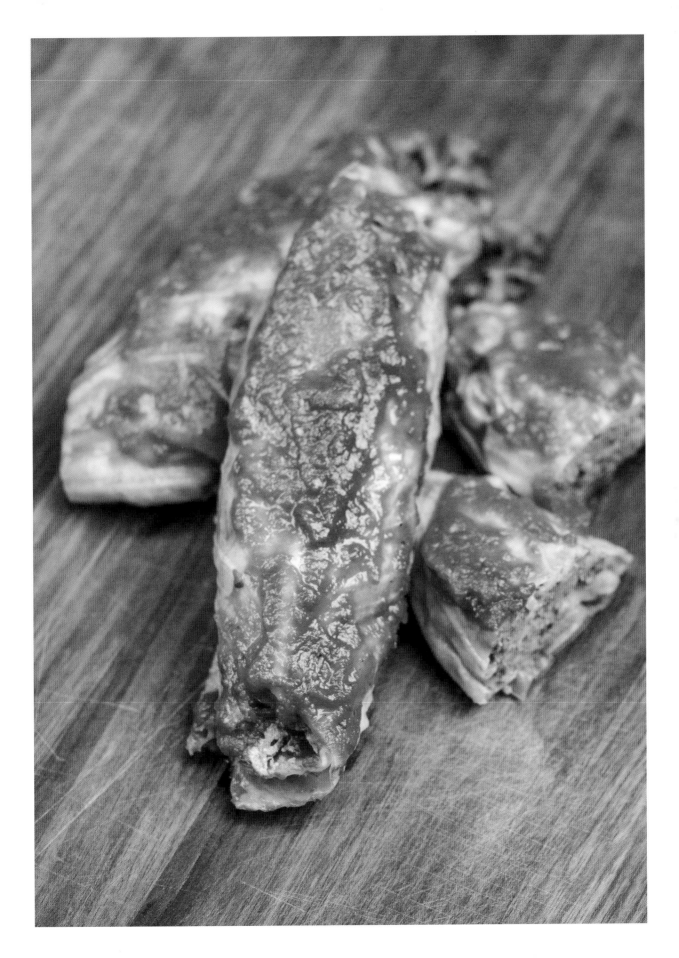

SPICE-RUBBED GOAT RIBS

SERVES: 4 | **PREP TIME:** 5 minutes, plus 1 hour to marinate | **COOK TIME:** 3½ hours

This combination of spices is reminiscent of a Jamaican rub, minus the addition of Scotch bonnet peppers for heat. Our version works well with the unique sweetness of goat meat, which is accentuated by a touch of molasses. Make this dish to impress your rib-loving friends who are looking for something delicious, but a little different.

SPICE RUB:

2 teaspoons ground allspice

1 teaspoon freshly ground black pepper

1 teaspoon fine sea salt

1 teaspoon garlic powder

½ teaspoon ground cinnamon

¼ teaspoon ground cardamom

¼ teaspoon ground nutmeg

1 rack goat ribs (about 2 pounds) (see Notes)

2 tablespoons molasses

Grated zest of 1 lemon

1. Combine the seasonings for the spice rub in a small bowl. Place the rack of ribs in a large glass container, rub the rack all over with the spice mix, then pour the molasses and lemon zest over the top. Cover and refrigerate for at least 1 hour or up to overnight.

2. Preheat the oven to 325°F; put the container with the ribs on the counter while the oven preheats.

3. Transfer the ribs to a 9 by 13-inch glass baking dish. Add ½ inch of water to the dish to keep the meat moist during roasting. Cover the dish with foil and roast until the meat begins to pull away from the bones, 3 to 3½ hours. Remove from the oven and let rest for
10 minutes, then remove the foil, cut between the bones to separate the ribs, and serve.

NOTES:

Sourcing goat ribs isn't as easy as buying your typical steak or even pork ribs. If you have a local butcher shop, you may be able to order them there. Another option is to seek out a halal butcher or Caribbean butcher in your area, if there is one. If there are no local options, see page 364 for a list of online purveyors.

Goat ribs, like other types, have a silvery membrane on the underside. Removing it is optional, but we recommend it. Carefully slice one side of the membrane with a paring knife, then pull it off with your fingers.

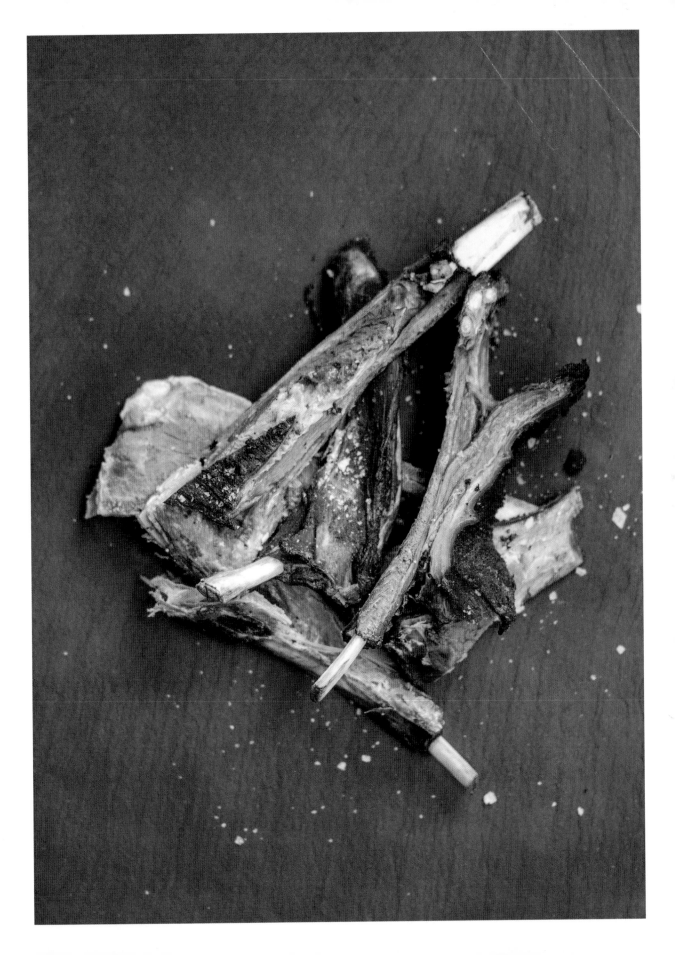

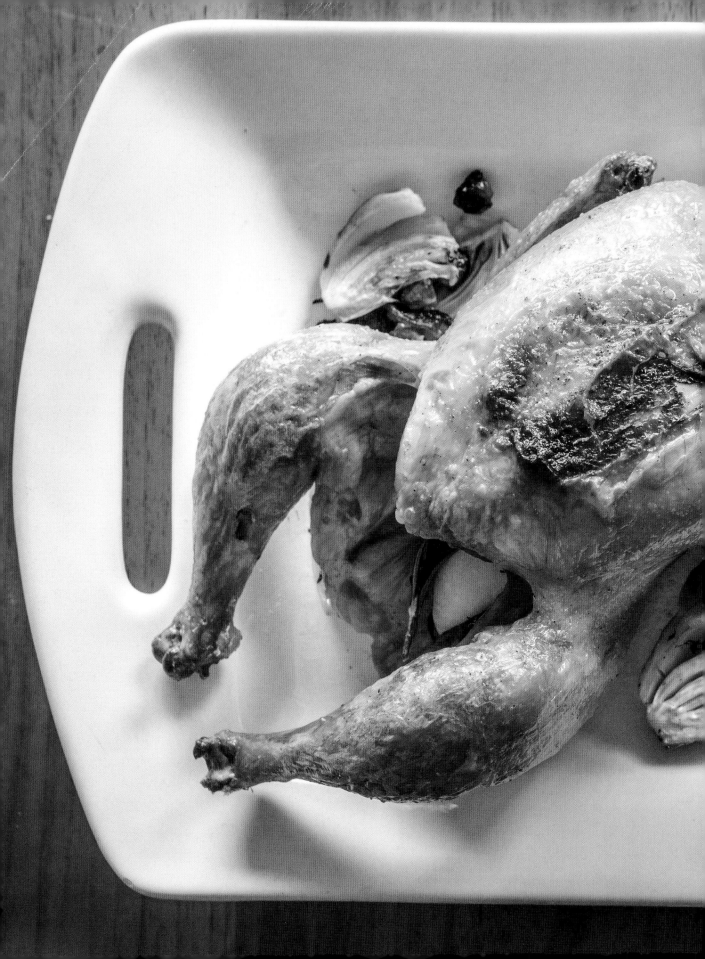

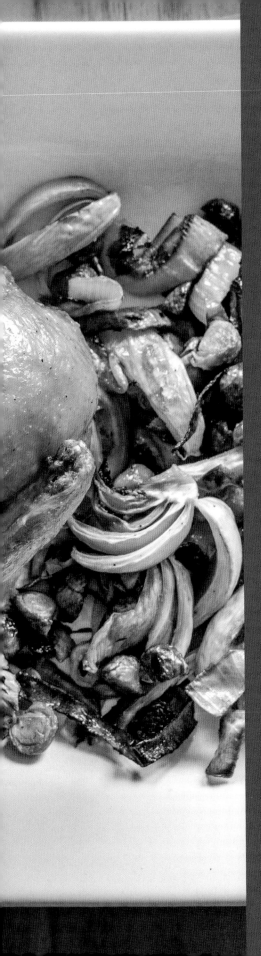

CHAPTER 4:

POULTRY

CHICKEN PICCATA

SERVES: 4 | **PREP TIME:** 20 minutes | **COOK TIME:** 16 minutes

Thin chicken cutlets make this classic dish come together quickly. If they aren't available, you can slice two regular chicken breasts in half horizontally, then place them between sheets of plastic wrap or parchment or waxed paper and pound to ¼-inch thickness with a meat mallet or rolling pin.

½ cup blanched almond flour

2 tablespoons arrowroot powder

1 pound thin chicken breast cutlets (about ¼ inch thick), patted dry

Fine sea salt and freshly ground black pepper

4 tablespoons (2 ounces) unsalted butter

2 tablespoons extra-virgin olive oil

¼ cup dry white wine

¼ cup chicken bone broth

3 tablespoons fresh lemon juice

3 tablespoons drained capers

1 to 2 tablespoons chopped fresh flat-leaf parsley

1. In a shallow bowl, combine the almond flour and arrowroot. Season the chicken cutlets generously with salt and pepper. Dredge in the almond flour mixture, shaking off the excess.

2. Melt the butter with the olive oil in a large skillet over medium-high heat. Add the chicken and cook until golden on one side, 3 to 4 minutes. Flip and cook until golden on the other side, about 3 minutes longer. Transfer to a plate. (*Note:* Do not overcrowd the skillet. Work in batches if needed, adding 1 tablespoon each additional butter and oil between batches.)

3. Pour the wine into the skillet; stir to scrape up any browned bits. Boil until the mixture is reduced by half, about 1 minute. Add the broth, lemon juice, and capers. Cook, stirring, until the sauce begins to thicken, 1 to 2 minutes.

4. Lower the heat to medium-low. Return the chicken to the pan along with any juices that have collected on the plate. Turn the chicken to coat it with the sauce and simmer to rewarm the chicken, 4 to 5 minutes. Taste the sauce and season with salt and pepper, if needed.

5. Divide the chicken among four plates. Spoon the sauce over the chicken, sprinkle with the parsley, and serve.

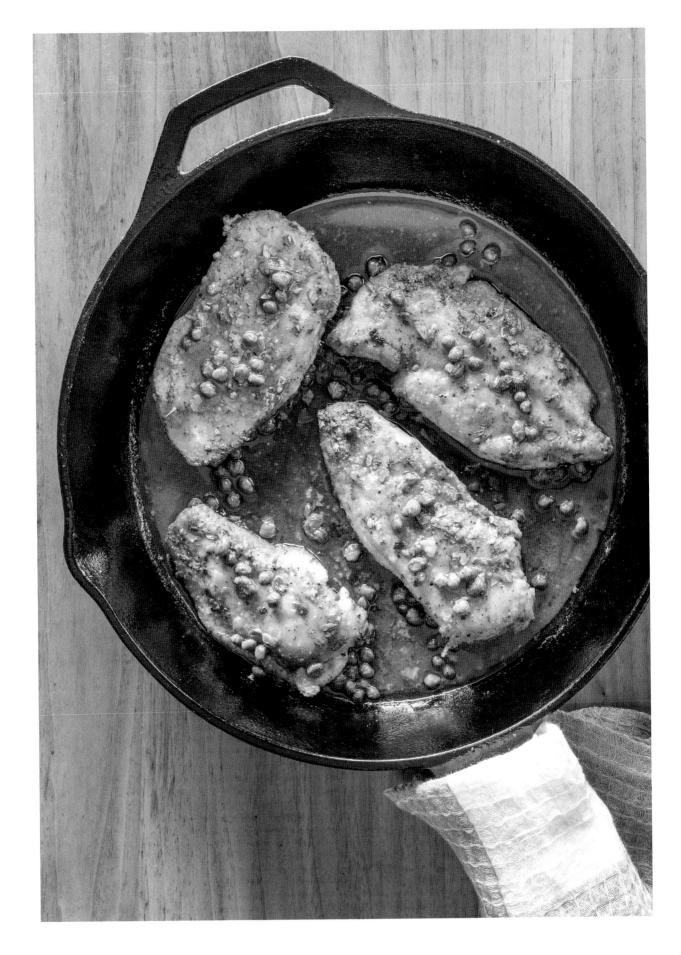

TURKEY LEGS CONFIT

SERVES: 4 to 6 | **PREP TIME:** 10 minutes | **COOK TIME:** 3 hours 20 minutes

When you think of confit, duck probably comes to mind. But confit—originally a preserving method and now just used because the result tastes so freaking good—works for all kinds of things. We love to confit turkey legs because turkey can be, let's face it, kind of pedestrian and not all that exciting. After it's been slow-cooked at a low temperature in a boatload of fat, however, it's luscious and feels really special.

1 (11-ounce) jar duck fat, divided

4 turkey legs (4 to 5 pounds), patted dry

Fine sea salt and freshly ground black pepper

10 cloves garlic, peeled and smashed with the side of a knife

1 medium sweet onion, such as Vidalia, chopped (about 1½ cups)

1 lemon, scrubbed and dried

4 sprigs fresh thyme

2 sprigs fresh rosemary

1 dried bay leaf

3 to 4 cups melted bacon fat or extra-virgin olive oil or avocado oil, or as needed

1. Preheat the oven to 300°F.

2. Warm ¼ cup of the duck fat in a Dutch oven over medium-high heat. (Warm the remaining duck fat in a small saucepan over low heat.) Season the turkey legs generously with salt and pepper. Cook the turkey, turning the legs a few times, until browned all over, 9 to 11 minutes total. (Do not overcrowd the pot; work in batches if needed.) Transfer the turkey to a platter. Add the garlic and onion to the pot, sprinkle lightly with salt, and cook, stirring occasionally, until the onion softens and the mixture is fragrant, 2 to 3 minutes.

3. Meanwhile, use a vegetable peeler to peel 3 long strips of zest from the lemon, taking care to get only the yellow part and avoid the white pith. Add the strips to the Dutch oven along with the thyme, rosemary, and bay leaf. Return the turkey legs to the pot. Pour in the remaining duck fat and enough bacon fat and/or oil to nearly cover the turkey legs. Cook over medium-high heat until the fat barely simmers (do not let it boil), 2 to 4 minutes.

4. Remove from the heat, cover the pot, and place in the oven. Cook until the meat is very tender and falling off the bone, 2½ to 3 hours, turning the legs over halfway through. Remove the turkey from the fat, shred the meat, if desired, and serve.

NOTES:

You can strain the cooking fat and use it to fry vegetables or potatoes, or place it in a jar, cover, refrigerate, and use it for cooking; it's good for up to a month. It will be flavored by the herbs and may be salty, so factor that in when deciding how to use it. It's delicious for simple things like scrambled eggs.

Leftovers can be covered and refrigerated for up to 3 days.

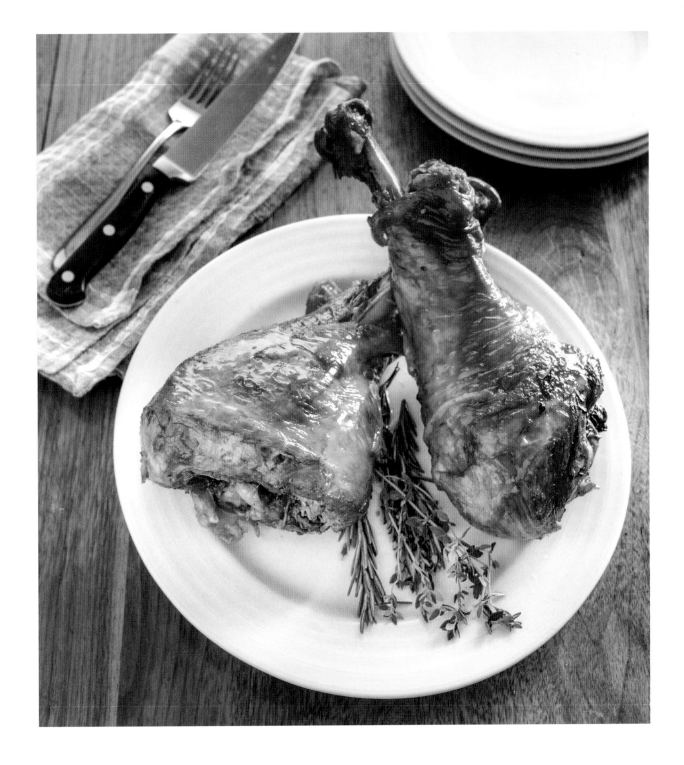

NOTES: ────────

You can buy jarred duck fat (Epic brand is available at Whole Foods, for example), but you may be able to get it cheaper from your butcher. Some butchers sell it frozen for a much lower price than grocery stores, so it's worth asking.

RED WINE–BRAISED DUCK LEGS

SERVES: 4 | **PREP TIME:** 15 minutes | **COOK TIME:** 3 hours

Duck is so festive and delicious, and braising it makes it fall-off-the-bone tender. It's a crowd-pleaser because it's technically poultry, but it's rich and meaty, so steak lovers tend to enjoy it, too. Duck also provides as much iron as red meat. Make this dish for company; most of the work is done in advance.

4 duck leg quarters (about 3 pounds), patted dry

Fine sea salt and freshly ground black pepper

3 medium carrots, chopped (about 1 cup)

3 small ribs celery, chopped (about ¾ cup)

1 medium shallot, sliced (about ¾ cup)

5 cloves garlic, peeled and smashed with the side of a knife

¾ cup dry red wine

3 cups chicken bone broth

4 sprigs fresh thyme

1 dried bay leaf

1. Preheat the oven to 300°F.

2. Prick the duck skin all over with the tip of a paring knife. Season the duck generously all over with salt and pepper. Preheat a Dutch oven over medium-high heat until hot. Put the duck leg quarters in the pot skin side down and cook undisturbed until the skin is crisp and deep golden, 10 to 15 minutes. Be sure to leave space between the quarters; sear them in batches, if needed. Carefully turn the duck over and sear on the other side until browned, 2 to 3 minutes longer. Transfer the duck to a platter. Pour off all but 1 tablespoon of the fat (reserve it for another use).

3. Add the carrots, celery, shallot, and garlic to the pot, season well with salt and pepper, and cook, stirring occasionally, until very tender and beginning to caramelize, 5 to 7 minutes. Pour in the wine and stir to pull any browned bits off the bottom. Boil until the wine has reduced and thickened to a syrupy consistency, about 2 minutes. Add the broth, thyme, and bay leaf. Lower the heat to medium and bring to a simmer. Add the duck legs skin side up, making sure the legs aren't fully submerged; keep the seared part of the skin above the liquid.

4. Cover the pot, transfer to the oven, and braise until the meat is very tender, 2 to 2½ hours. Transfer the duck to a rimmed baking sheet; preheat the broiler. Strain the braising liquid into a measuring cup and let stand until the fat rises. Skim the fat off the top and pour the liquid into a medium saucepan. Place over high heat and boil until the sauce has thickened and reduced by about one-third (to about ⅔ cup), 3 to 4 minutes.

5. Meanwhile, broil the duck legs to crisp the skin, 1 to 2 minutes, watching carefully so it doesn't burn. Serve the duck with the sauce.

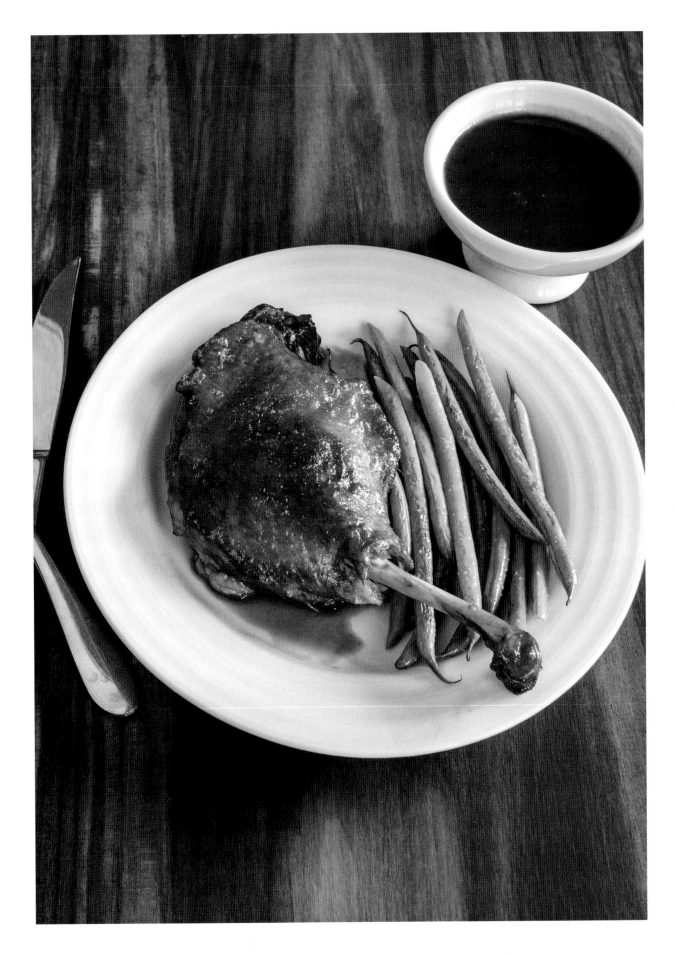

STIR-FRIED CHICKEN AND VEGETABLES

SERVES: 4 | **PREP TIME:** 25 minutes | **COOK TIME:** 12 minutes

The trick with stir-frying is to have all of your ingredients and your sauce ready to go before you start cooking, known as mise en place. This is a high-heat cooking method, so things move quickly; you don't want to be chopping vegetables while your protein is getting overcooked. Swap in different vegetables and protein to suit your tastes and to use up what you have on hand.

¼ cup kosher salt

1½ pounds chicken breast tenders, patted dry and cut into 1-inch pieces

3 tablespoons coconut aminos

1 tablespoon mirin

1 to 2 teaspoons Sriracha sauce (optional)

¼ teaspoon freshly ground black pepper

1 teaspoon arrowroot powder

2 tablespoons avocado oil, divided

1 medium head broccoli, stem peeled and sliced ¼ inch thick on a diagonal, florets cut into bite-sized pieces (about 3 cups)

Fine sea salt

1 medium red bell pepper, seeded and chopped (about ¾ cup)

6 scallions, sliced on a diagonal (about ⅔ cup; reserve dark green parts for garnish if desired)

1 cup snow peas, trimmed and cut in half crosswise on a diagonal (or into thirds if large)

4 cloves garlic, minced (about 4 teaspoons)

1½ tablespoons minced fresh ginger

2 tablespoons toasted sesame oil

Cauliflower Rice (That Doesn't Suck) (page 268) or Zucchini Noodles (That Don't Suck) (page 270), for serving

1. In a large bowl, stir the kosher salt into 2 cups of warm water until the salt dissolves. Stir in 2 cups of cold water. Add the chicken. Let stand at room temperature while you prepare the rest of the ingredients. (Alternatively, you can cover the bowl and refrigerate it for up to 2 hours.)

2. In a small bowl, whisk together the coconut aminos, mirin, Sriracha (if using), and pepper. Combine the arrowroot with 1 teaspoon of water in a small cup, stirring until the arrowroot dissolves. Whisk the arrowroot mixture into the aminos mixture.

3. Remove the chicken from the brine and pat it thoroughly dry (discard the brine). Warm 1 tablespoon of the avocado oil in a large skillet (or a wok, if you have one) over medium-high heat. Add the chicken to the pan and cook, turning once, until golden on both sides, 3 to 5 minutes. Transfer to a bowl.

4. Warm the remaining 1 tablespoon of oil in the same skillet; lower the heat to medium. Add the broccoli, sprinkle with salt, and cook, stirring, until bright green, about 1 minute. Add the bell pepper, white and light green parts of the scallions, and the snow peas. Sprinkle with salt and cook, stirring, until just beginning to get tender, about 1 minute. Add the garlic and ginger; sauté until fragrant, about 1 minute.

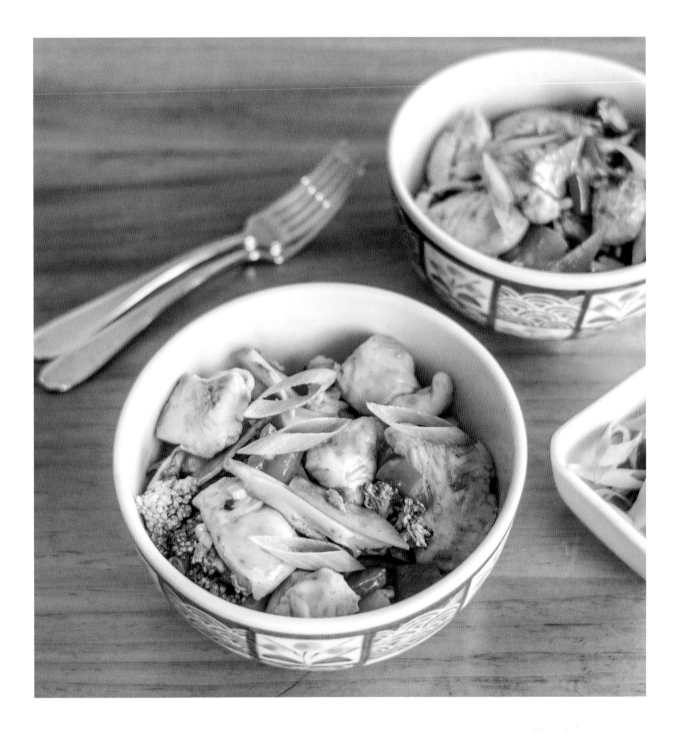

5. Return the chicken and any collected juices to the skillet. Whisk the aminos mixture, then pour it into the pan, stirring to pull up any browned bits from the bottom. Cook, stirring, until the sauce thickens and coats all of the other ingredients, 1 to 2 minutes. Remove the pan from the heat and drizzle with the sesame oil.

6. Divide the cauliflower rice among four shallow bowls. Top with the stir-fry mixture. Sprinkle with the sliced dark green parts of the scallions, if desired, and serve.

AIR FRYER BUFFALO CHICKEN NUGGETS

SERVES: 4 | **PREP TIME:** 20 minutes | **COOK TIME:** 12 minutes per batch

This is a fun recipe to make with another person (it's great to do with kids) because you can set up an assembly line for all of the dipping. If you're going it alone, use one hand for dredging in the dry ingredients and the other for dipping into the wet. Use your left hand to dredge in the cassava, your right to dip in the egg mixture, then your left again to dredge in the panko. This way, you don't get your fingers covered in sticky batter that you have to rinse off every couple of minutes. (It's also great for working your eye-hand coordination.)

1½ pounds boneless, skinless chicken breast tenders, patted dry and cut into 1½-inch pieces

Fine sea salt and freshly ground black pepper

½ cup cassava flour

½ teaspoon garlic powder

1 large egg

¼ cup Frank's RedHot Buffalo Wings Sauce or other Buffalo-style hot sauce

1½ cups pork panko

Bacon ranch dip, homemade (page 344) or store-bought, for serving (optional)

1. Season the chicken lightly with salt and pepper. In a shallow bowl, combine the cassava flour, garlic powder, ½ teaspoon of salt, and ¼ teaspoon of pepper. In another shallow bowl, beat the egg with the hot sauce. Put the panko in a third shallow bowl.

2. Dip each chicken piece in the flour mixture, then the egg mixture, then the panko, shaking off the excess after each. Place the breaded chicken pieces on a rimmed baking sheet or plate.

3. Preheat the oven to 200°F; fit a rimmed baking sheet with a cooling rack and place in the oven. Preheat an air fryer to 350°F for 5 minutes. Mist the air fryer basket with cooking spray. Place as many chicken nuggets as you can in a single layer in the basket. Air-fry until crisp, golden, and cooked through, 10 to 12 minutes, turning over halfway through. Put the cooked nuggets on the rack in the oven to keep warm while you cook the remaining nuggets.

4. Serve hot with bacon ranch dip, if desired.

NOTES:

You can make the nuggets ahead and freeze them uncooked. Place the breaded nuggets on a tray and freeze, then transfer to a freezer bag. They'll keep in the freezer for up to 3 months. You can cook the nuggets from frozen following Step 3, but increase the cooking time to 18 to 20 minutes.

If you like, you can drizzle more hot sauce on the nuggets just before serving, or offer hot sauce on the side.

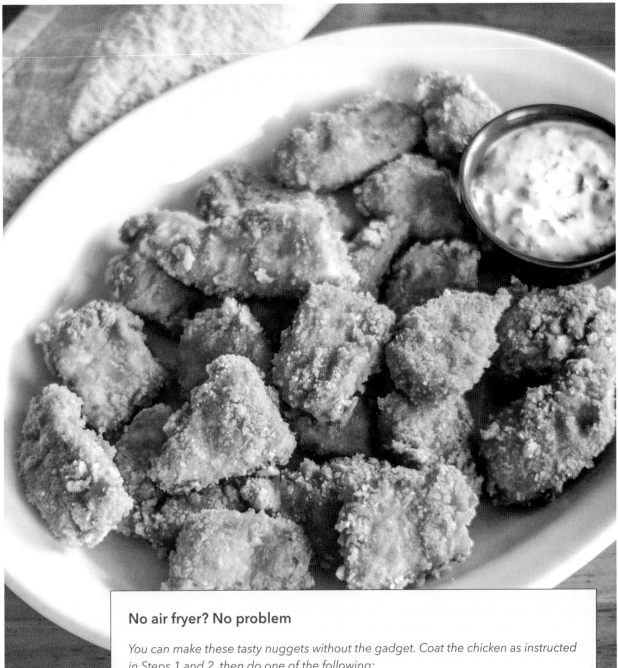

No air fryer? No problem

You can make these tasty nuggets without the gadget. Coat the chicken as instructed in Steps 1 and 2, then do one of the following:

To bake, preheat the oven to 400°F. Fit a rimmed baking sheet with a cooling rack. Coat the rack with cooking spray. Place the nuggets on the rack, mist the tops with cooking spray, and bake until golden and cooked through, about 20 minutes. (No need to turn them.)

To fry, warm about ¼ inch of avocado oil in a medium cast-iron skillet until it reaches 350°F on an instant-read thermometer (or, if you flick a little bit of water in the skillet, it will sizzle when hot enough). Working in batches, fry the nuggets until golden, crisp, and cooked through, about 3 minutes per side. Do not overcrowd the skillet; that will reduce the oil temperature too much and you'll end up with soggy nuggets.

FIVE-SPICE DUCK BREAST WITH ORANGE AND RED WINE JUS

SERVES: 4 | **PREP TIME:** 10 minutes, plus 1 hour to marinate | **COOK TIME:** 20 minutes

The key to a really good duck breast? Crisp skin. And the key to crisp skin is scoring it—that is, cutting into the skin—before cooking. This helps the fat to render and the skin to crisp. The deeper you cut, the more fat will render. How deep you go is your choice (do you want to leave more of the fat on the breast to eat or cook more of it off?), but never cut into the meat, which will expose it to heat and cause it to overcook.

4 (10- to 12-ounce) duck breasts

2 cloves garlic, minced (about 2 teaspoons)

1 tablespoon grated fresh ginger

2 teaspoons five-spice powder

Fine sea salt

1 tablespoon bacon fat or avocado oil

¼ cup dry red wine, such as Rioja

2 tablespoons fresh orange juice

1 teaspoon coconut aminos

Parsnip Mash (page 272), for serving (optional)

1. Pat the duck breasts thoroughly dry. Using a sharp knife, make parallel cuts into the skin on a diagonal. (You can cut again in perpendicular lines to make a crosshatch; this looks nice but isn't technically necessary.) In a large bowl, combine the garlic, ginger, five-spice powder, and ¾ teaspoon of salt. Add the duck breasts and rub the mixture all over them. Cover and refrigerate for at least 1 hour or up to 12 hours.

2. Preheat the oven to 400°F; place a large cast-iron or other heavy bottomed ovenproof skillet in the oven as it preheats. Once the oven reaches temperature, place the skillet on the stove over medium-high heat. Swirl the bacon fat in the skillet. Add the duck breasts, skin side down, season with salt, and sear until the skin is golden brown, 4 to 5 minutes. Turn and sear on the other side, 3 to 4 minutes longer. Turn over again, transfer the skillet to the oven, and cook until the duck reaches the desired doneness; for medium-rare, an instant-read thermometer stuck into the thickest part should read 135°F, 5 to 10 minutes. Transfer to a cutting board, cover loosely with foil, and let rest while you make the sauce.

3. Pour off the fat from the skillet and place the pan over medium-high heat. Add the wine and stir to scrape up any browned bits from the skillet. Cook until the wine has reduced by half, about 1 minute. Stir in the orange juice and aminos; cook until reduced and syrupy, about 1 minute longer. Transfer to a cup; season with salt to taste.

4. Slice the duck on a diagonal and put a breast on each plate. Drizzle with the wine jus and serve with parsnip mash, if desired.

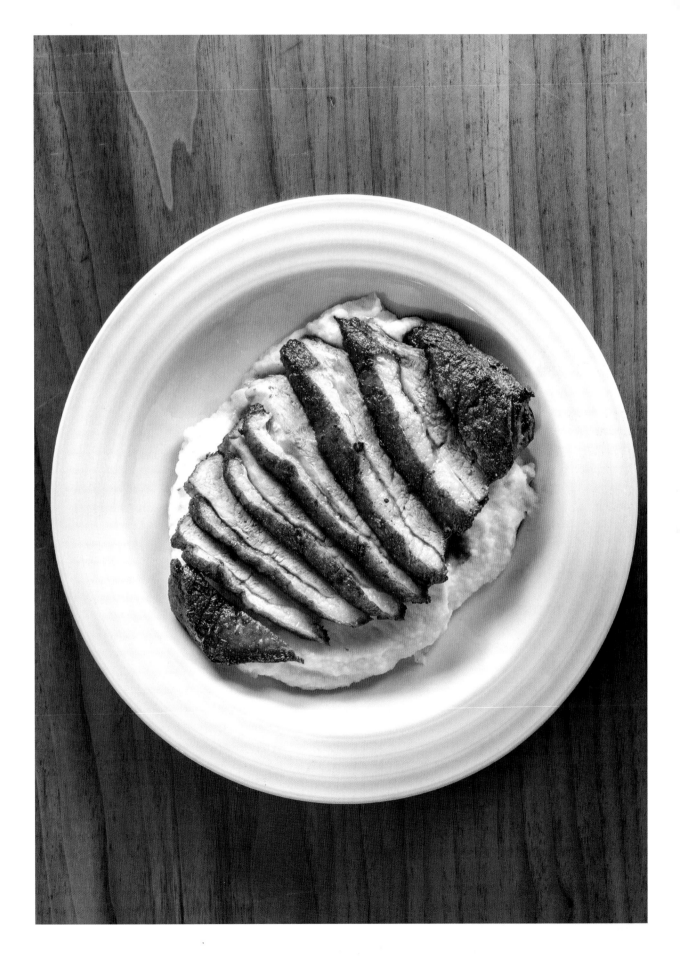

ROAST CHICKEN WITH VEGETABLES

SERVES: 4 | **PREP TIME:** 20 minutes, plus 12 hours to dry-brine chicken | **COOK TIME:** 1 hour 30 minutes

A perfect roast chicken is at once comforting, homey, and a culinary delight. The secret to the most flavorful roast chicken is a dry brine: coating it in salt and letting it sit in the fridge uncovered overnight. It's more than worth the time and the fridge real estate—your chicken will have crisp skin and deeply flavored meat. Don't wipe off the salt; leave it on, brush the bird with olive oil, and then season it again. It seems like too much salt, but it isn't. It's perfect, we promise.

1 (4- to 6-pound) whole chicken, trimmed of excess fat and thoroughly patted dry

Fine sea salt

10 to 12 sprigs mixed fresh woody herbs, such as rosemary, thyme, and/or sage

6 cloves garlic, peeled and smashed with the side of a knife

1 lemon, quartered

Freshly ground black pepper

1 large onion, cut into thick slices

1 large bulb fennel, halved and cut into wedges

1 pound Brussels sprouts, trimmed and halved (or quartered if large)

1 tablespoon extra-virgin olive oil, plus more for brushing the bird

1. Season the chicken thoroughly inside and out with salt. Place on a large plate and refrigerate uncovered for at least 12 hours or up to 1 day.

2. Preheat the oven to 425°F.

3. Fill the chicken cavity with half of the herb sprigs, 3 cloves of garlic, and as much of the lemon as you can fit. Tie the legs together with kitchen twine. Brush the chicken all over with olive oil; season generously with salt and pepper.

4. Put the onion, fennel, Brussels sprouts, and remaining 3 cloves of garlic in a roasting pan. Toss with the olive oil; season with salt and pepper. Tuck the remaining herb sprigs around the vegetables. Place a roasting rack on top of the vegetables. Set the chicken on the rack.

5. Roast the chicken until golden with crisp skin, 1 hour 15 minutes to 1 hour 30 minutes; an instant-read thermometer stuck into the thickest part of the thigh away from the bone should read 165°F. Stir the vegetables once or twice during roasting.

6. Cover the chicken loosely with foil and let rest for 10 to 15 minutes. Remove the herb sprigs from the vegetables. Carve the chicken and serve with the vegetables.

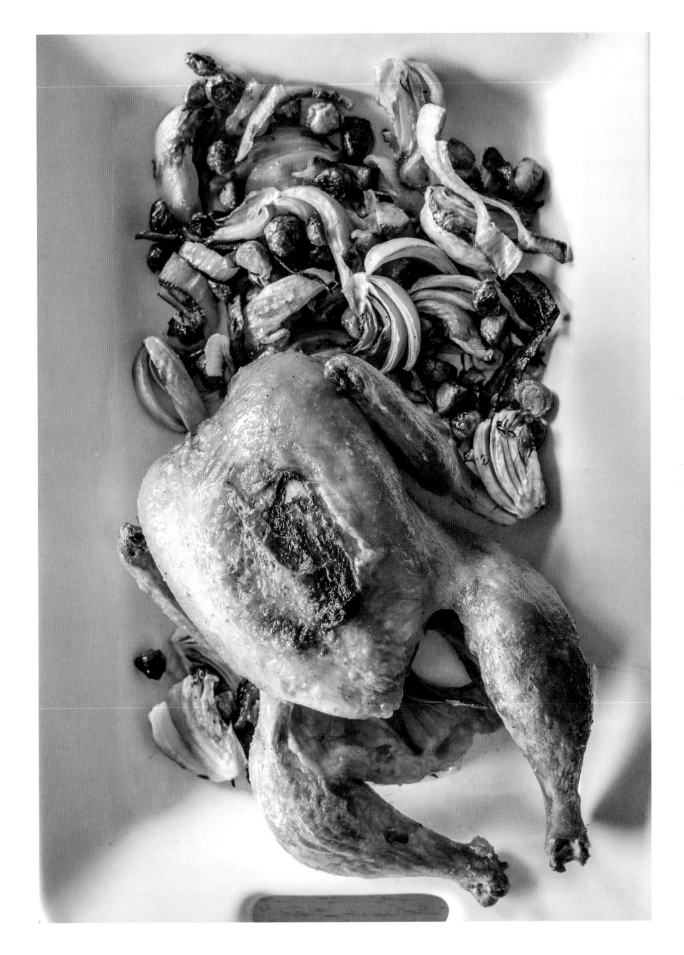

CREAMY CHICKEN, BACON, AND BROCCOLI CASSEROLE

SERVES: 6 | **PREP TIME:** 45 minutes | **COOK TIME:** 50 minutes

We don't want you to follow this recipe. OK, we do…but you don't have to. It takes a lot of prep, so it's a fantastic Sunday cooking project if you're into that. But if you aren't, use your shortcuts. Precooked chicken (or, hey, leftover holiday turkey), precut broccoli florets, presliced mushrooms, preshredded cheese—do what you like to make it quicker. Our favorite shortcut to employ? Frozen riced cauliflower.

4 ounces bacon (about 4 slices)

3 tablespoons avocado oil, divided

1 pound boneless, skinless chicken thighs, trimmed and thoroughly patted dry

1 large head broccoli (about 1 pound), stems peeled and sliced, florets cut into bite-sized pieces (about 4½ cups)

3 cloves garlic (peel left on but thin, papery skin removed)

Fine sea salt and freshly ground black pepper

4 ounces cremini mushrooms, sliced (about 2 cups)

1 medium onion, chopped (about 1⅓ cups)

¾ cup avocado oil mayonnaise

¾ cup sour cream

2 tablespoons fresh lemon juice

1 teaspoon chili powder

½ teaspoon sweet paprika

1 (12-ounce) package frozen riced cauliflower, thawed

1 cup shredded cheddar cheese (about 4 ounces)

Chicken bone broth, if needed

1. Place the bacon in a large unheated skillet; cook over medium-low heat, turning occasionally, until just browned and crisp, about 10 minutes. Transfer the bacon to a cutting board using a slotted spoon, leaving the fat in the skillet.

2. Preheat the oven to 425°F; place 2 rimmed baking sheets in the oven as it preheats.

3. Rub the chicken with 1 tablespoon of the avocado oil and toss the broccoli and garlic cloves with the remaining 2 tablespoons of oil; season both the chicken and broccoli moderately with salt and pepper. Spread the chicken on one hot baking sheet and the broccoli and garlic on the other. Roast until the chicken is cooked through and the broccoli is tender and lightly caramelized in spots, turning the chicken and stirring the broccoli once halfway through, 20 to 25 minutes (remove the broccoli sooner if it begins to brown too much).

4. Meanwhile, add the mushrooms to the skillet with the bacon fat and season lightly with salt. Raise the heat to medium and cook, stirring occasionally, until the mushrooms have released their water, 6 to 7 minutes. Add the onion, sprinkle with salt, and cook, stirring occasionally, until the onion is tender and the mushrooms are turning golden in spots, 6 to 7 minutes longer. Remove the pan from the heat and set aside.

5. In a large bowl, whisk together the mayonnaise, sour cream, lemon juice, chili powder, paprika, ¾ teaspoon of salt, and ¼ teaspoon of pepper. Add the riced cauliflower to the bowl.

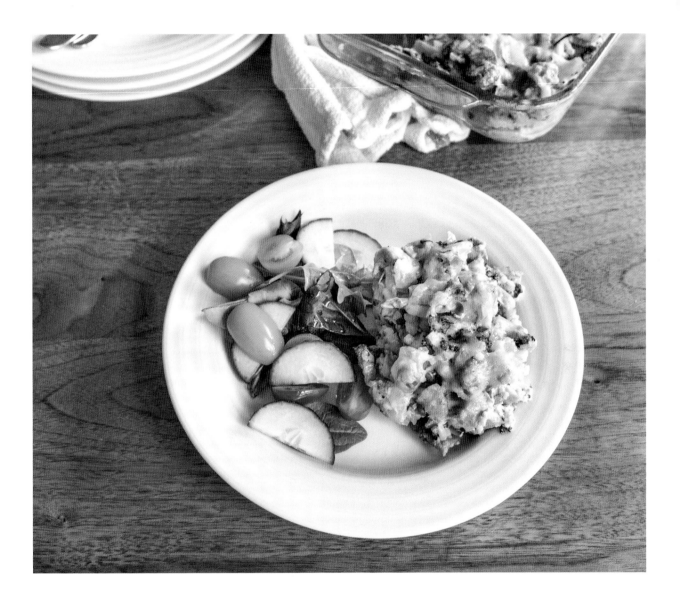

6. When the chicken and broccoli are done, remove the pans from the oven and reduce the oven temperature to 375°F. Transfer the chicken to a cutting board and allow to rest for 5 minutes; let the broccoli cool until it's cool enough to handle, then coarsely chop it and add it to the bowl with the mayonnaise mixture. Squeeze the roasted garlic from the skins, mince the garlic, and add it to the bowl along with the onion and mushrooms. Chop the chicken; add it to the bowl, along with any juices that have accumulated on the cutting board. Add ¾ cup of the cheese. Chop the bacon and add it to the bowl. Fold all of the ingredients together. If the mixture is dry, stir in broth ¼ cup at a time until it is creamy.

7. Grease a 9 by 13-inch baking pan. Spread the chicken mixture evenly in the pan. Sprinkle with the remaining ¼ cup of cheese. Bake until the casserole is heated through, bubbling, and golden in spots, 20 to 25 minutes. Let stand for 5 minutes before serving.

VIETNAMESE CHICKEN MEATBALL LETTUCE WRAPS

SERVES: 4 | **PREP TIME:** 25 minutes | **COOK TIME:** 32 minutes

Let's face it: ground chicken on its own isn't all that exciting. But once you mix it with aromatics like scallions, ginger, and lemongrass, flavor it with fish sauce, and form it into meatballs, it's a whole different ballgame. Don't skip the pickled carrots or the herbs; they lend a pop of color and flavor.

PICKLED CARROTS:

¼ cup unseasoned rice vinegar or apple cider vinegar

1½ teaspoons raw honey

½ teaspoon fine sea salt

2 medium carrots, cut into matchsticks (about 1 cup)

MEATBALLS:

1 tablespoon coconut oil

1 serrano chili, seeded and minced (about 2 tablespoons)

3 scallions, white and light green parts, minced (about ¼ cup)

2 tablespoons minced fresh ginger

3 cloves garlic, minced (about 1 tablespoon)

¼ teaspoon plus a pinch of fine sea salt

1½ pounds ground chicken

1½ tablespoons fish sauce

3 tablespoons cassava flour

1 tablespoon drained and minced jarred sliced lemongrass (optional; see Note, opposite)

FOR SERVING:

1 head Bibb lettuce, leaves separated

1 bunch fresh mint, leaves picked

1 bunch fresh basil (preferably Thai), leaves picked and torn or thinly sliced

Hoisin and/or Sriracha sauce or other condiment of choice (optional)

1. Preheat the oven to 350°F. Line a rimmed baking sheet with parchment paper.

2. Make the pickled carrots: In a small saucepan, combine the vinegar, ¼ cup of water, the honey, and salt. Place over low heat and cook, stirring, until the honey and salt dissolve. Put the carrots in a medium heatproof bowl; pour the vinegar mixture over them. Let stand at room temperature. (You can make the pickles up to a day ahead. Let cool, then cover and refrigerate.)

3. Make the meatballs: Warm the coconut oil in a small skillet over medium heat. Add the chili, scallions, ginger, and garlic, season with a pinch of salt, and cook, stirring occasionally, until tender and fragrant, 1 to 2 minutes. Transfer to a small bowl to cool.

4. In a large bowl, combine the ground chicken, fish sauce, cassava flour, lemongrass (if using), and ¼ teaspoon of salt. Add the cooled ginger-scallion mixture. Using your hands, mix gently but thoroughly until the ingredients are evenly distributed. Use a ¼-cup scoop or measuring cup to divide the mixture into 12 equal portions. Roll each portion into a ball and place on the lined baking sheet. Bake until the meatballs are cooked through and golden on the outside, 25 to 30 minutes, turning them over halfway through. (You can use an instant-read thermometer to check for doneness; the temperature in the center of a meatball should be 165°F.)

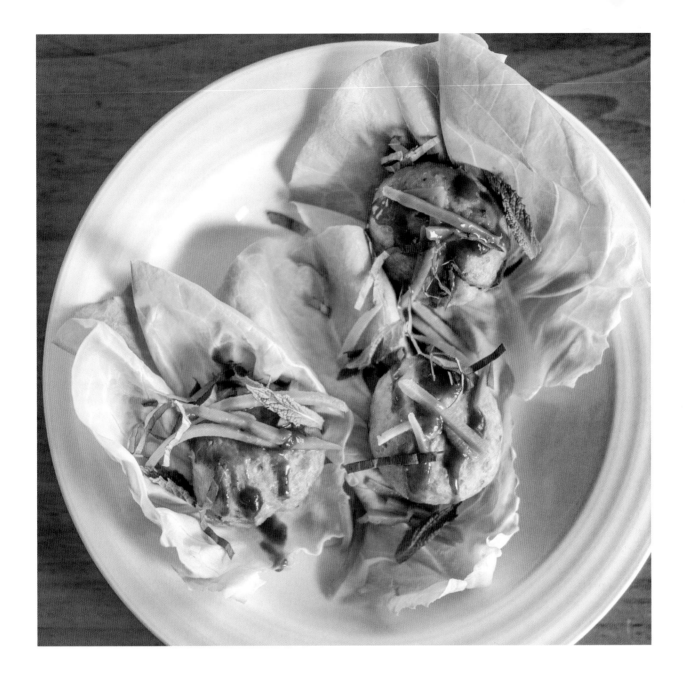

5. Serve the meatballs hot with the lettuce leaves for wrapping, plus the pickled carrots, mint, basil, and condiment(s) of choice, if desired.

NOTE:

You can find jarred sliced lemongrass in Asian markets and online. You may also encounter lemongrass paste or jarred whole stalks. We like the sliced variety because it's simple to use as is or to chop up, but feel free to buy another form if it's easier to find (or leave it out altogether).

SKILLET CHICKEN THIGHS WITH CABBAGE

SERVES: 2 | **PREP TIME:** 5 minutes | **COOK TIME:** 38 minutes

Throw some tasty ingredients in a skillet, let them cook together and marinate in their own delicious juices, and get ready for a fantastic dinner with almost no work. You're welcome.

2 large bone-in, skin-on chicken thighs (about 1¼ pounds)

2 teaspoons fine sea salt, divided

1 teaspoon curry powder

½ teaspoon freshly ground black pepper

¼ teaspoon garlic powder

¼ teaspoon sweet paprika

4 tablespoons avocado oil, divided

½ medium head green cabbage, shredded

3 cloves garlic, minced (about 1 tablespoon)

1. Place a rack in the middle of the oven and preheat the oven to 375°F.

2. Pat the chicken dry and season with 1 teaspoon of the salt, the curry powder, pepper, garlic powder, and paprika.

3. Heat 1 tablespoon of the avocado oil in a large cast-iron or other ovenproof skillet over medium-high heat. Add the chicken skin side down and sear until the skin is deep golden brown, 7 to 8 minutes. Transfer to a plate skin side up.

4. Lower the heat to medium. Add the remaining 3 tablespoons of oil and swirl it in the pan. Add the cabbage, garlic, and remaining
1 teaspoon of salt and cook, tossing occasionally, until the cabbage is just wilted, about 5 minutes.

5. Return the chicken to the skillet skin side up and place the pan in the oven. Bake until the chicken is cooked through and an instant-read thermometer stuck into the thickest part away from the bone reads 165°F, 20 to 25 minutes. Remove from the oven. Taste the cabbage mixture and add additional seasonings, if needed. Serve hot.

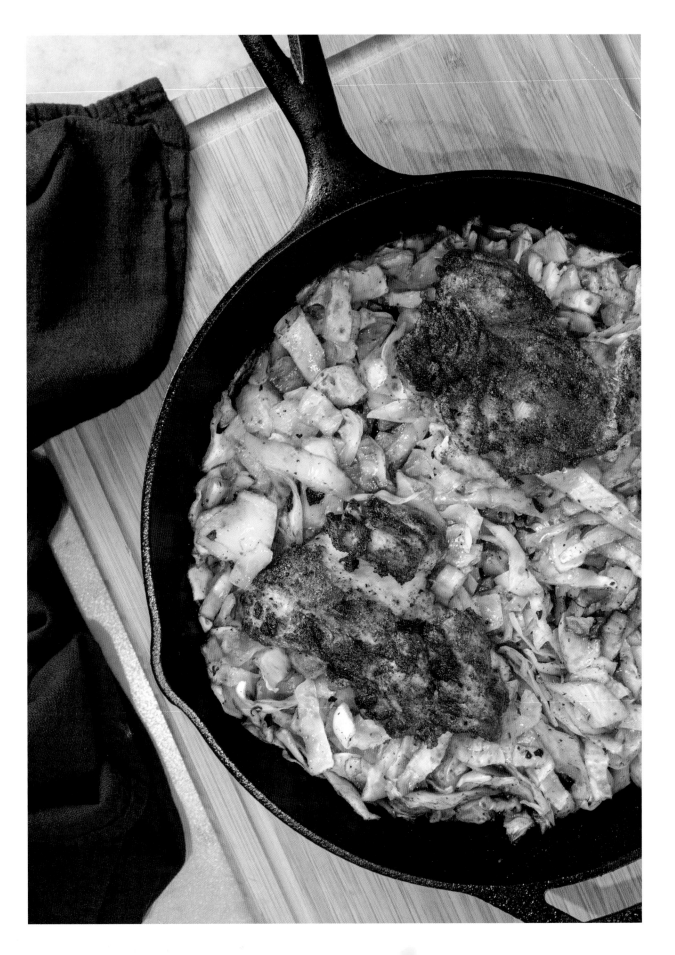

CHICKEN SHAWARMA

SERVES: 4 | **PREP TIME:** 20 minutes, plus at least 1 hour to marinate |
COOK TIME: 25 minutes

Chicken shawarma is a Mediterranean delight. Usually it's cooked on a rotisserie, but we've made it super simple by just roasting it. The spices add layers of luscious flavor and are also great for you. Turmeric has anti-inflammatory benefits, coriander may help with blood sugar regulation, and paprika is loaded with antioxidants. Serve this tasty dish with pita or on top of a salad; it's even better with a drizzle of tahini or a spoonful of tzatziki.

2½ teaspoons turmeric powder

¾ tablespoon ground coriander

¾ tablespoon garlic powder

¾ tablespoon sweet paprika

½ teaspoon cayenne pepper

1½ pounds boneless, skinless chicken thighs

½ teaspoon plus 1 pinch of fine sea salt, divided

1 large white onion, thinly sliced

Juice of 1 lemon, divided

⅓ cup plus 2 tablespoons extra-virgin olive oil, divided, plus more for the pan

1 cucumber

1 tomato

½ cup black olives, pitted

FOR SERVING:

4 gluten-free pitas, warmed and halved, or large lettuce leaves

¼ cup garlic sauce, tahini, or tzatziki, homemade (page 352) or store-bought

Pickled turnips (optional)

1.   In a small bowl, combine the turmeric, coriander, garlic powder, paprika, and cayenne.

2.   Pat the chicken dry and season on both sides with ½ teaspoon of salt, then thinly slice the thighs into bite-sized pieces, about 1 by 2 inches. Put the chicken pieces in a large bowl. Add the spice mix and toss to coat. Add the onion, 1 tablespoon of the lemon juice, and ⅓ cup of the olive oil; toss to combine. Cover and refrigerate for at least 1 hour or up to overnight.

3.   Preheat the oven to 425°F. Take the chicken out of the fridge and let it sit at room temperature while the oven heats up. Lightly oil a rimmed baking sheet.

4.   Spread the chicken mixture in a single layer on the prepared baking sheet and roast until cooked through and golden brown, about 25 minutes. Stir the chicken about halfway through cooking.

5.   While the chicken is roasting, chop the cucumber and tomato into bite-sized pieces and place in a medium bowl. Add the olives, remaining 2 tablespoons of oil, remaining 1 tablespoon of lemon juice, and a pinch of salt; fold together.

6.   Serve the chicken mixture and cucumber salad in pitas or lettuce leaves with garlic sauce, tahini, or tzatziki and pickled turnips, if desired.

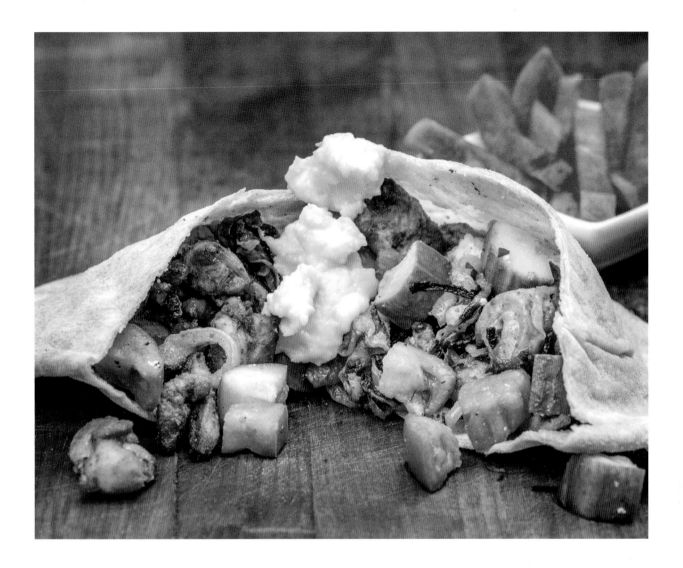

NOTES:

Garlic sauce is a thick, rich sauce made with garlic emulsified in mayonnaise, oil, or butter. It is usually found refrigerated in Middle Eastern grocery stores. You can also try the Garlic and Dill Yogurt Dip on page 354.

Tahini, a Middle Eastern condiment made from ground sesame seeds, can be found in Middle Eastern groceries and increasingly in the condiment aisle at major grocery stores. It varies in consistency; some are quite runny, while others are thick and pastelike. For convenience, we prefer the runny type for drizzling over foods and whisking into dressing. But if the thicker kind is what's available to you, it's easy to thin it by whisking in hot water (or a combo of hot water and lemon juice) a bit at a time until it reaches the consistency you want.

Look for pickled turnips at Middle Eastern grocery stores. They add a bright crunch to any chicken dish.

HOT HONEY CHICKEN WINGS

SERVES: 4 | **PREP TIME:** 10 minutes | **COOK TIME:** 40 minutes

Spicy and sweet wings are the perfect food for a party, of course—but who's to say you can't also have them for dinner when you feel like it? Place the bowl of wings on the table, have plenty of napkins ready, and a regular dinner will feel like a fun event. You can buy premade hot honey (basically a mix of honey and hot sauce), but we like to mix up our own.

2 pounds whole chicken wings

3 cloves garlic, minced (about 1 tablespoon)

1 teaspoon ginger powder

1 teaspoon smoked paprika

1 teaspoon fine sea salt

⅓ cup raw honey

2 tablespoons coconut aminos

2 tablespoons hot sauce

1. Preheat the oven to 425°F. Line a rimmed baking sheet with parchment paper.

2. Pat the chicken wings dry and place in a large bowl. Add the garlic, ginger, smoked paprika, and salt; toss to coat.

3. Lay the wings flat in a single layer on the lined baking sheet. Roast until golden brown and cooked through, about 40 minutes; turn them over halfway through roasting.

4. Meanwhile, make the sauce: In a large bowl, combine the honey, coconut aminos, and hot sauce.

5. After removing the wings from the oven, let them cool for 5 minutes. Transfer them to the bowl with the sauce and toss to coat. Serve immediately.

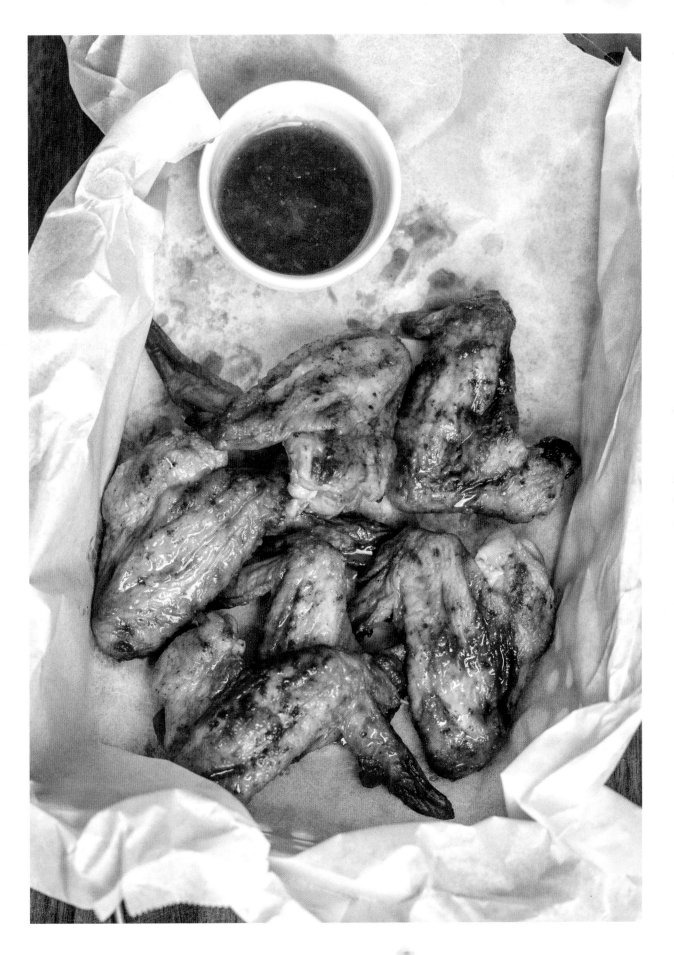

SPICY AIR FRYER CHICKEN THIGHS

SERVES: 4 | **PREP TIME:** 5 minutes, plus at least 1 hour to marinate | **COOK TIME:** 30 minutes

This is one of those "so simple it's barely a recipe" recipes, but we wanted to include it to show you just how easily you can prepare juicy, flavorful, and versatile protein. This chicken tastes excellent thrown on top of a salad, dunked in Garlic and Dill Yogurt Dip (page 354), or as finger food for your kiddos (you can ease up on the spice if needed). It's easy to stress over the details, thinking a meal must have a certain number of components or a snack has to look a certain way, but we're here to tell you that a perfectly cooked, crisp-skinned chicken thigh needs nothing more and is perfect for whenever hunger strikes. We like to use an air fryer for this recipe because not only is it super easy, but it yields incredibly juicy meat and crisp skin. But an air fryer isn't required. Using an alternative two-step method of oven and stovetop, you can still get a very good result (see the method opposite).

4 boneless chicken thighs, preferably skin-on (about 1½ pounds)

1 tablespoon hot sauce

1 teaspoon garlic powder

1 teaspoon smoked paprika

½ teaspoon cayenne pepper

½ teaspoon onion powder

½ teaspoon fine sea salt

1. Pat the chicken thighs dry and put them in a 9 by 13-inch glass baking dish or a large bowl with a lid. Sprinkle with the hot sauce, garlic powder, smoked paprika, cayenne, onion powder, and salt. Stir to coat and place in the fridge to marinate for at least 1 hour or up to overnight.

2. Preheat an air fryer to 380°F for 5 minutes. Once the air fryer is preheated, mist the basket with cooking spray. Place the chicken thighs in a single layer in the basket, skin side down, and cook for 8 to 10 minutes, or until the meat is cooked through. (Work in batches if all of the chicken doesn't fit in a single layer.)

3. Turn the chicken thighs over and cook until the skin is crisp and golden and an instant-read thermometer stuck into the thickest part reads 165°F (you can also cut one open and eyeball it for doneness), 7 to 8 minutes longer.

4. Let the chicken rest for 5 minutes before serving.

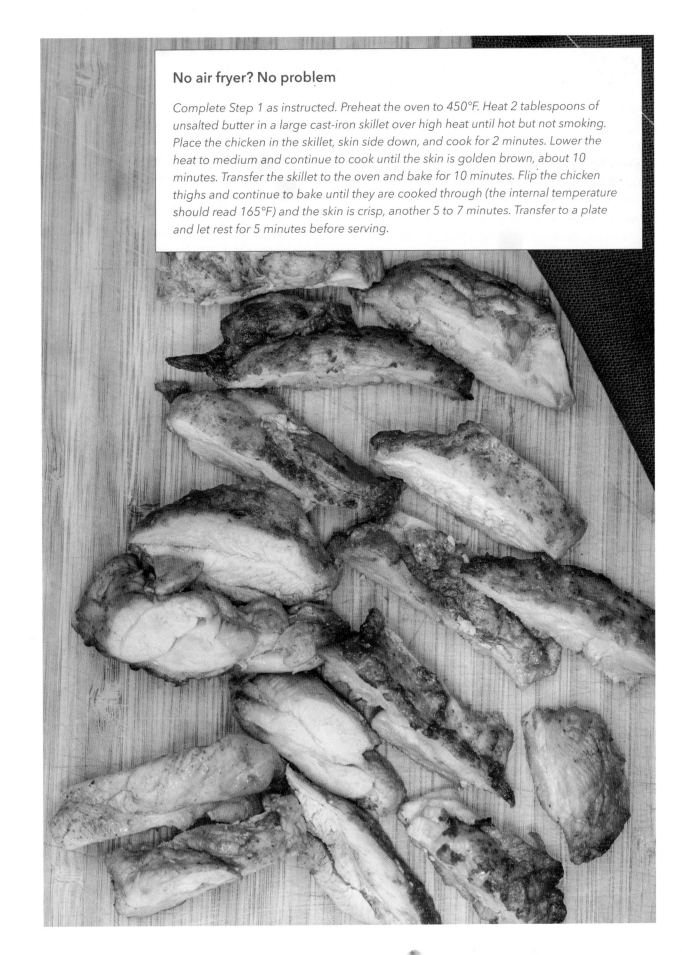

No air fryer? No problem

Complete Step 1 as instructed. Preheat the oven to 450°F. Heat 2 tablespoons of unsalted butter in a large cast-iron skillet over high heat until hot but not smoking. Place the chicken in the skillet, skin side down, and cook for 2 minutes. Lower the heat to medium and continue to cook until the skin is golden brown, about 10 minutes. Transfer the skillet to the oven and bake for 10 minutes. Flip the chicken thighs and continue to bake until they are cooked through (the internal temperature should read 165°F) and the skin is crisp, another 5 to 7 minutes. Transfer to a plate and let rest for 5 minutes before serving.

MEXICAN-STYLE SHREDDED CHICKEN BOWL

SERVES: 2 | **PREP TIME:** 15 minutes | **COOK TIME:** 2 hours

This simple but flavorful dish may remind you of a healthier, less salty version of your favorite Mexican fast-food establishment's burrito bowl. You can add rice or leave it low-carb, as here. Cauliflower rice also would work well (see the recipe on page 268). It wouldn't be wrong to sprinkle it with some shredded cheddar or Jack cheese (or both).

2 boneless, skinless chicken breasts (about 1 pound)

½ cup chicken bone broth

¼ teaspoon chili powder

¼ teaspoon ground cumin

¼ teaspoon onion powder

¼ teaspoon freshly ground black pepper

1 large green bell pepper, seeded

1 medium yellow onion

¼ cup extra-virgin olive oil

½ cup salsa

Fine sea salt

GUACAMOLE:

1 large avocado, peeled and pitted

¼ cup diced tomatoes

⅛ teaspoon garlic powder

⅛ teaspoon onion powder

¼ teaspoon fine sea salt, plus more for finishing

⅛ teaspoon freshly ground black pepper

1 teaspoon fresh lime juice

1. Put the chicken in a 6-quart slow cooker. Pour in the broth and add the chili powder, cumin, onion powder, and pepper. Cover and cook on high until the chicken is cooked through and comes apart easily with a fork, about 2 hours.

2. Meanwhile, roast the vegetables: Preheat the oven to 375°F. Cut the bell pepper and onion into ½-inch-thick slices. Put the pepper and onion slices in a 10 by 15-inch glass baking dish; toss with the olive oil. Spread the vegetables out in a single layer and roast until they are tender and the onion is lightly caramelized in spots, stirring once or twice, about 50 minutes.

3. When the chicken is nearly done, make the guacamole: Put the avocado in a medium bowl; mash with a fork. Stir in the tomatoes, garlic powder, onion powder, salt, pepper, and lime juice. Mash and stir until it's as chunky (or smooth) as you like it.

4. Transfer the chicken to a cutting board and shred with two forks; season to taste with salt. Divide the chicken between two serving bowls. Add the roasted pepper and onion and a dollop of salsa and guacamole to each bowl and serve.

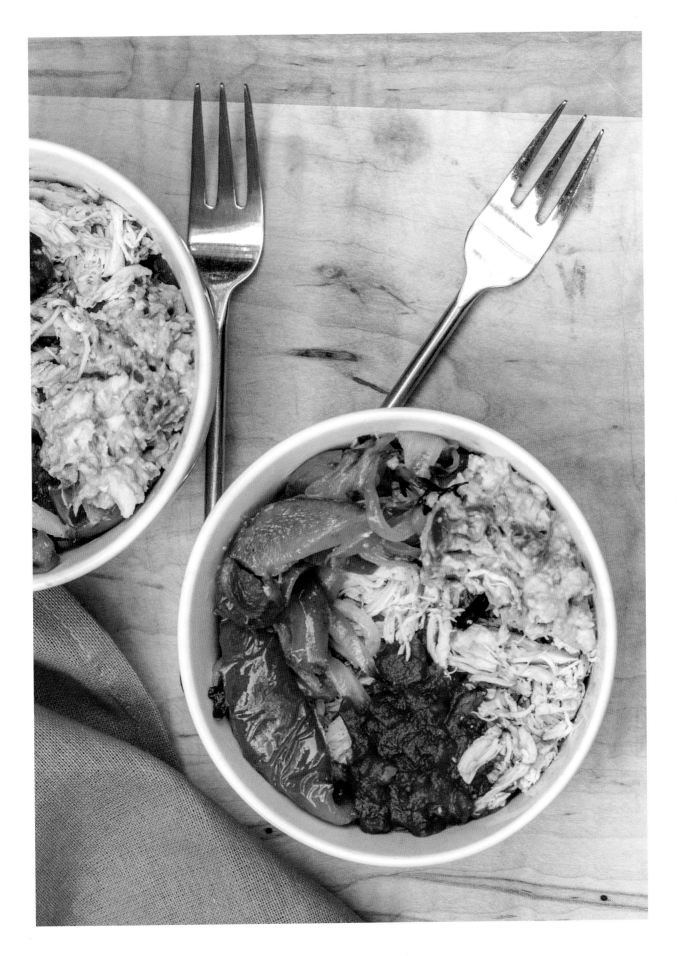

SHREDDED CHICKEN TOSTADAS

SERVES: 4 | **PREP TIME:** 10 minutes | **COOK TIME:** 2 hours

Everyone loves taco (or, in this case, tostada) night, and it's even easier when you've prepared the chicken in advance. Put all of the ingredients on the table and let everyone build their own. We like the open-faced crunch of these store-bought tostadas (you can find them most anywhere you'd buy hard taco shells), but for a lower-carb option, serve the chicken and other toppings in Bibb lettuce leaves or on a bed of shredded romaine lettuce.

2 boneless, skinless chicken breasts (about 1 pound)

½ cup chicken bone broth

¼ cup fresh orange juice (from 1 small orange)

¼ teaspoon freshly ground black pepper

¼ teaspoon ground cumin

¼ teaspoon garlic powder

¼ teaspoon dried oregano leaves

¼ teaspoon smoked paprika

Fine sea salt

8 (6-inch) hard corn tortillas

1 cup shredded cheddar cheese (about 4 ounces)

½ medium red onion, diced

FOR FINISHING:

1 large avocado, pitted and diced

Sliced jalapeño peppers

Hot sauce of choice

Lime wedges

1. Put the chicken in a 6-quart slow cooker. Add the broth, orange juice, pepper, cumin, garlic powder, oregano, and paprika. Cover and cook on high until the chicken is cooked through and comes apart easily with a fork, about 2 hours.

2. Transfer the chicken to a cutting board and shred with two forks; season to taste with salt. Turn the oven on to the broil setting.

3. Assemble the tostadas: Place the tortillas on a rimmed baking sheet. Top each with ½ cup of the shredded chicken, some cheese, and a few pieces of onion and broil for 5 minutes. Remove and finish with diced avocado, sliced jalapenos, hot sauce, and a squeeze of lime juice.

How to make simple shredded chicken

We love taking a basic component like shredded chicken and customizing it to create easy yet flavorful dishes like this one. Here's our basic method: Place boneless chicken breast(s) in a 6-quart slow cooker, then pour in chicken broth and season with dried herbs and/or spices of choice. Cover and cook on high until the chicken is cooked through and comes apart easily with a fork, about 2 hours. For every pound of chicken, you will need ½ cup broth and a total of ¾ to 1¼ teaspoons dried herbs/spices. You can vary the flavor further by adding other liquids, such as citrus juice, along with the broth or using fresh herbs instead of dried.

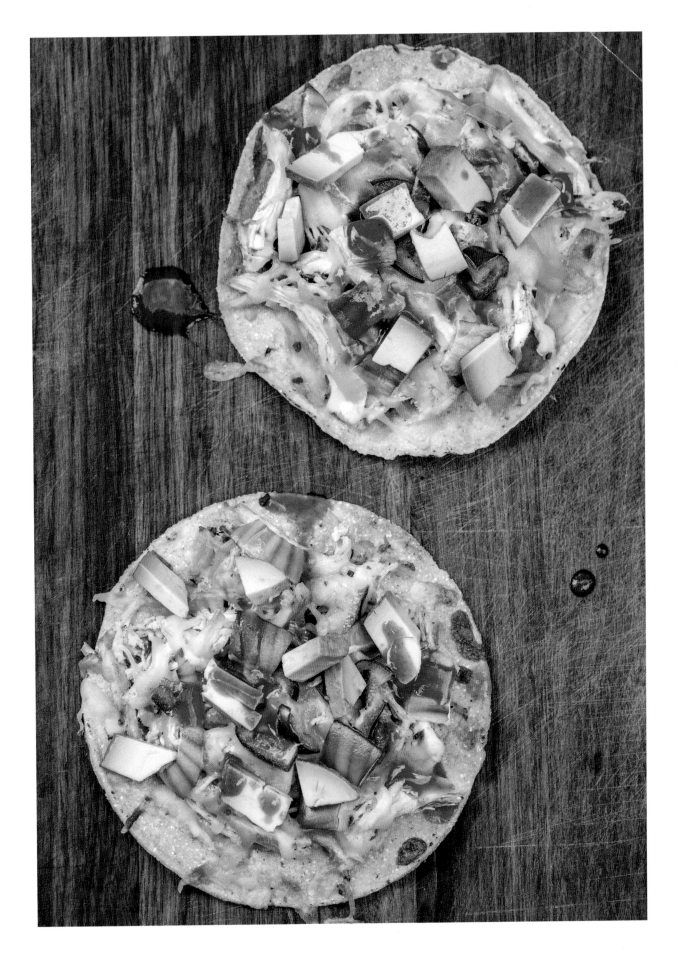

CHICKEN SALAD WITH FENNEL AND ASIAN PEAR

SERVES: 2 | **PREP TIME:** 8 minutes

Some days, nothing tastes better than cold leftover roast chicken (with the skin on, of course). When you just don't have the time or energy for anything other than leftovers, this recipe elevates cold chicken to something even more delicious and picnic-worthy. We love the subtle sweetness and crunch of Asian pear, but feel free to swap in another type of pear or an apple if you like.

3 tablespoons stone-ground mustard

2 tablespoons avocado oil mayonnaise or extra-virgin olive oil

1 teaspoon fresh lemon juice

Fine sea salt and freshly ground black pepper

2 cups shredded roast chicken (white and dark meat, with skin on, about 8 ounces)

1 bulb fennel, finely chopped (about ½ cup)

1 Asian pear, cored and chopped (about 2 cups)

2 ounces raw walnuts, chopped (about ½ cup)

Iceberg lettuce leaves, for serving (optional)

1. In a small bowl, combine the mustard, mayonnaise, and lemon juice. Season with salt and pepper to taste.

2. In a large bowl, combine the chicken, fennel, pear, and walnuts. Add the mustard mixture and stir until well combined. Taste and season with additional salt and pepper, if needed.

3. Serve as is, or spoon into iceberg lettuce wraps.

NOTE:

Leftovers of our roast chicken recipe on page 122 work well here, as does store-bought rotisserie chicken. If your fennel bulb came with the fronds, reserve some to garnish this salad.

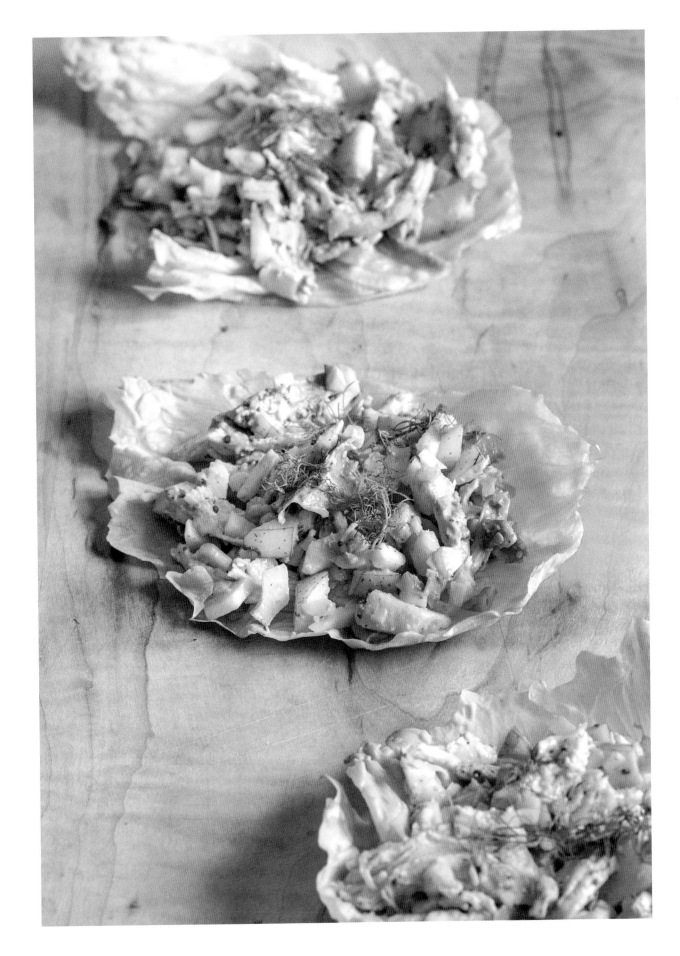

SWEET CHILI AND ORANGE DUCK WINGS

SERVES: 2 | **PREP TIME:** 5 minutes | **COOK TIME:** 35 minutes

Chicken wings are great, but duck wings? Sublime. Crisp skin and rich, gamey meat...they're so good. Toss with a few simple seasonings, roast, and serve—and don't forget to have plenty of napkins handy.

3 tablespoons grated orange zest

¼ cup fresh orange juice (from 1 small orange)

½ cup sweet red chili sauce

2 teaspoons coconut aminos

1 to 3 teaspoons harissa paste, depending on desired spice level (optional)

2 teaspoons sweet paprika

1 pound whole duck wings

2 scallions, green parts only, thinly sliced

¼ cup chopped raw cashews

1.   Preheat the oven to 425°F. Line a rimmed baking sheet with parchment paper.

2.   In a large bowl, whisk together the orange zest, orange juice, sweet chili sauce, coconut aminos, 1 teaspoon of the harissa (if using), and the sweet paprika. Taste and add more harissa if you want more heat. Transfer half of the sauce to a separate large bowl.

3.   Put the wings in one of the bowls of sauce and toss to coat. Spread the wings in a single layer on the lined baking sheet; discard any remaining sauce in the bowl. Roast the wings, turning once, until the meat is cooked through and the sauce starts to caramelize and thicken, about 35 minutes.

4.   Remove the wings from the oven. Add the cooked wings to the remaining bowl of sauce and toss to coat. Pile the wings onto a platter, sprinkle with the scallions and cashews, and serve.

NOTE:

Duck wings may not be quite as easy to source as chicken, but their rich, deep flavor makes them worth the extra effort. They can usually be found in Asian markets and many butcher shops.

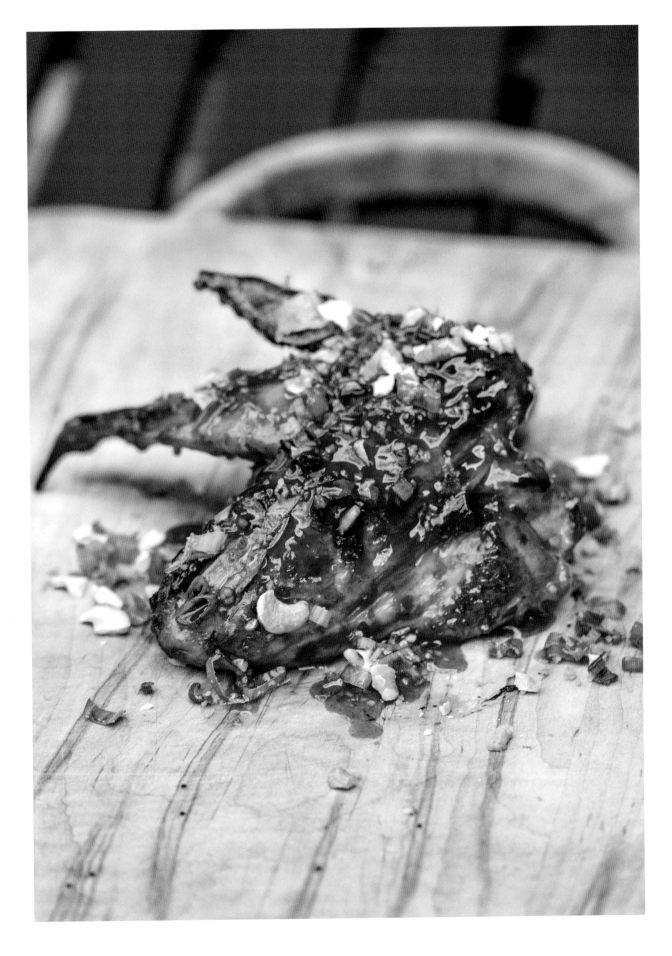

AIR FRYER HERBED BUTTER TURKEY BREAST

SERVES: 4 | **PREP TIME:** 10 minutes | **COOK TIME:** 30 minutes

We recognize that not everyone has the deep-seated love of dark meat that we do (and that's OK; more thighs and drumsticks for us), so we look for ways to make the white meat, which tends to be bland and dry, more delicious. Of course, heavy sauces, breading, or frying would work, but you might not want all that. So we turned to the air fryer and made sure to use plenty of butter and seasoning. The result: juicy and flavorful skin-on turkey breast that you will not want to wait for a holiday to eat. (Pro tip: You don't have to.) We prefer using an air fryer for this recipe because it's so much faster than the conventional oven-roasting method and gives the absolute best results, but if you don't own one, you can simply roast the turkey breast in the oven (see the method opposite).

1 (2-pound) boneless turkey breast, skin on

2 teaspoons fine sea salt

1½ teaspoons freshly ground black pepper

3 tablespoons (1½ ounces) unsalted butter, melted

3 cloves garlic, minced (about 1 tablespoon)

2 teaspoons chopped fresh rosemary

2 teaspoons chopped fresh thyme

1. Pat the turkey breast dry and season both sides with the salt and pepper.

2. Preheat an air fryer to 350°F for 5 minutes. Mist the air fryer basket with cooking spray. Place the turkey breast in the basket, skin side down, and cook at 375°F for 15 minutes.

3. Meanwhile, in a small bowl, combine the melted butter, garlic, rosemary, and thyme.

4. Flip the turkey breast skin side up. Brush the skin with the butter mixture. Continue to air-fry until an instant-read thermometer stuck into the thickest part reads 165°F, about 15 minutes longer.

5. Transfer the turkey to a cutting board, tent with foil, and let rest for at least 5 minutes before slicing and serving. Wrap leftovers tightly and store in the fridge for up to 5 days.

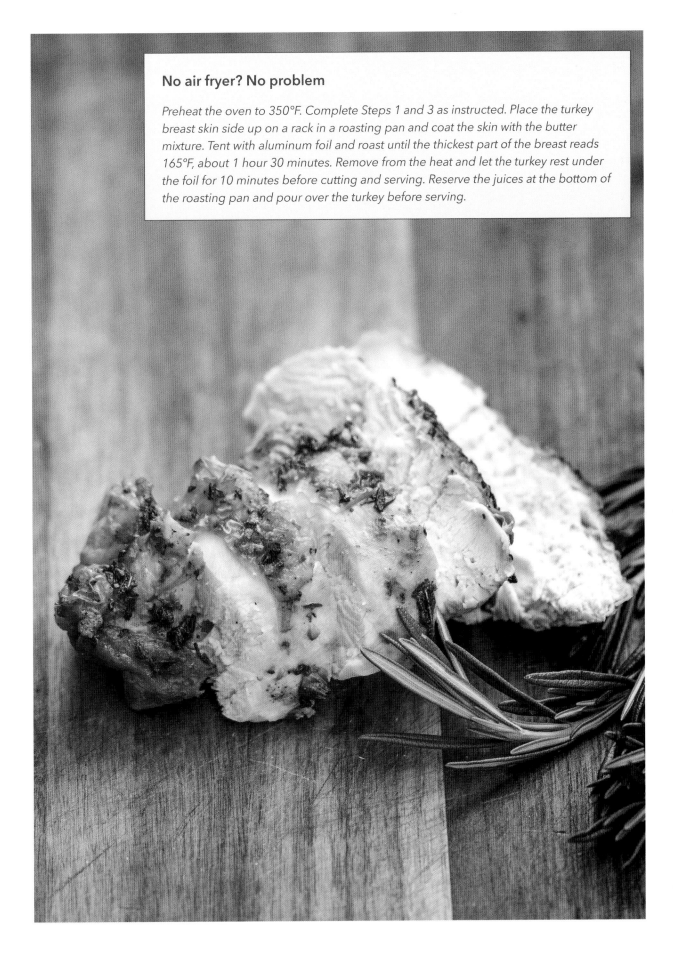

No air fryer? No problem

Preheat the oven to 350°F. Complete Steps 1 and 3 as instructed. Place the turkey breast skin side up on a rack in a roasting pan and coat the skin with the butter mixture. Tent with aluminum foil and roast until the thickest part of the breast reads 165°F, about 1 hour 30 minutes. Remove from the heat and let the turkey rest under the foil for 10 minutes before cutting and serving. Reserve the juices at the bottom of the roasting pan and pour over the turkey before serving.

TURKEY AND CABBAGE BOWL

SERVES: 4 | **PREP TIME:** 5 minutes | **COOK TIME:** 15 minutes

Get a good night's sleep. Drink plenty of water. Call your mom. Sometimes the best advice is...not sexy. The same is true about food—sometimes the recipes we love the most and turn to again and again are just simple and good. That's this recipe: five ingredients, inexpensive, fast, easy, and nourishing.

2 tablespoons avocado oil, divided

½ head large purple cabbage, shredded or chopped (about 4 cups)

Fine sea salt

¼ cup coconut aminos

1 pound ground turkey (85% lean)

1 tablespoon toasted sesame seeds

Freshly ground black pepper

1. Preheat a large skillet (or a wok, if you have one) over medium heat until hot. Pour in 1 tablespoon of the avocado oil; swirl the oil around in the pan. Add the cabbage, season generously with salt, and cook, stirring occasionally, until it begins to soften, about 5 minutes. Stir in the coconut aminos. Cover and continue to cook, stirring occasionally, until the cabbage is very soft, about 10 minutes longer.

2. Meanwhile, warm the remaining tablespoon of oil in a separate large skillet over medium heat. Add the ground turkey. Cook, stirring often, until cooked through and browned in spots, about 8 minutes.

3. Add the turkey to the cabbage and stir to combine. Divide the cabbage and turkey mixture among four bowls, top with the sesame seeds, and season with salt and pepper to taste. Serve hot.

How to toast sesame seeds

You can buy pretoasted sesame seeds at Asian markets, but it's easy to toast them yourself. To toast sesame seeds, spread them in a large cast-iron skillet and place over medium-low heat. Cook, stirring occasionally, until they begin to brown and release their oil, 5 to 7 minutes. Remove them from the skillet immediately to prevent burning.

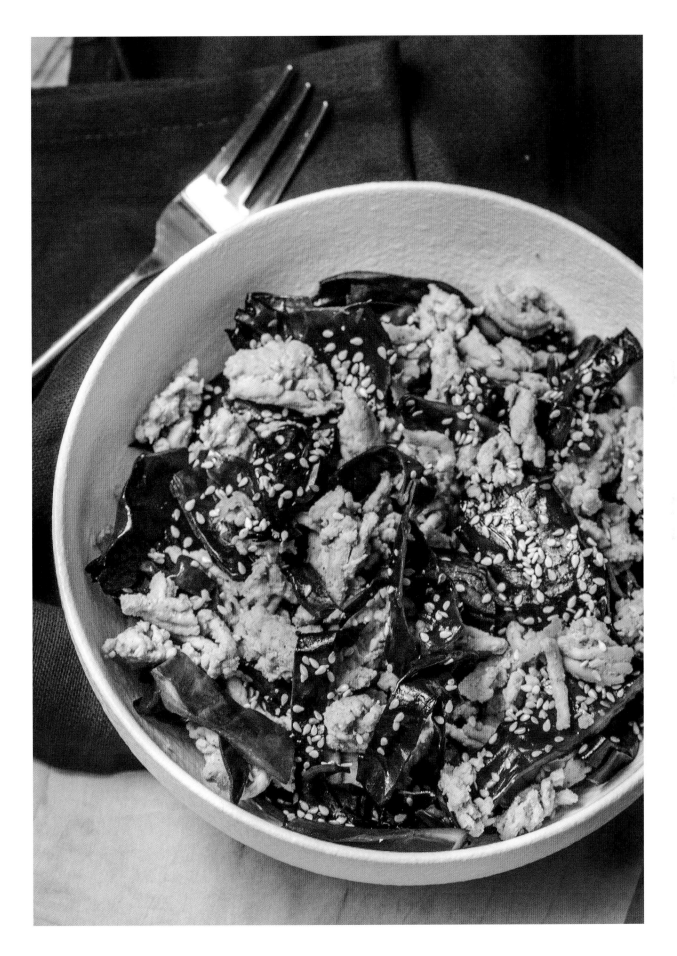

STUFFED PEPPERS

SERVES: 4 | **PREP TIME:** 15 minutes | **COOK TIME:** 50 minutes

We like ground turkey mixed with bacon in these peppers, but you can swap in any ground meat you like. You can prep these in advance, cover and refrigerate, and then bake them at mealtime (add a few extra minutes if you're cooking them right out of the fridge).

8 small bell peppers (any color), tops sliced off, seeds and ribs removed

1 tablespoon (½ ounce) unsalted butter or avocado oil

4 ounces bacon (about 4 slices), chopped

½ red onion, chopped (about 1 cup)

1 (12-ounce) package cremini mushrooms, diced

1 pound ground turkey

1 cup shredded mozzarella cheese (about 4 ounces)

Fine sea salt and freshly ground black pepper, for finishing

1. Preheat the oven to 400°F. Grease a 3-quart baking dish. Place the peppers cut side up in the dish. (Trim the bottoms a little bit if needed so they stand upright.)

2. Warm the butter in a large skillet over medium heat. Add the bacon and cook, stirring, until the fat in the bacon slices becomes translucent, about 5 minutes. Add the onion and mushrooms and cook, stirring, until the onion becomes translucent and the mushrooms soften, about 5 minutes.

3. Add the turkey and cook, stirring and breaking up the meat with a wooden spoon, until no longer pink, 7 minutes. Using a slotted spoon, transfer the turkey mixture to a large bowl. Pour off the excess liquid from the bowl.

4. Divide the turkey mixture evenly among the peppers. Top with the shredded cheese. Cover the baking dish with foil.

5. Bake until the peppers are tender, about 30 minutes. Uncover and bake until the cheese is bubbly, about 5 minutes longer. Finish with salt and pepper and serve.

NOTE: ———————————————————————————

Swap in another cheese if you prefer.

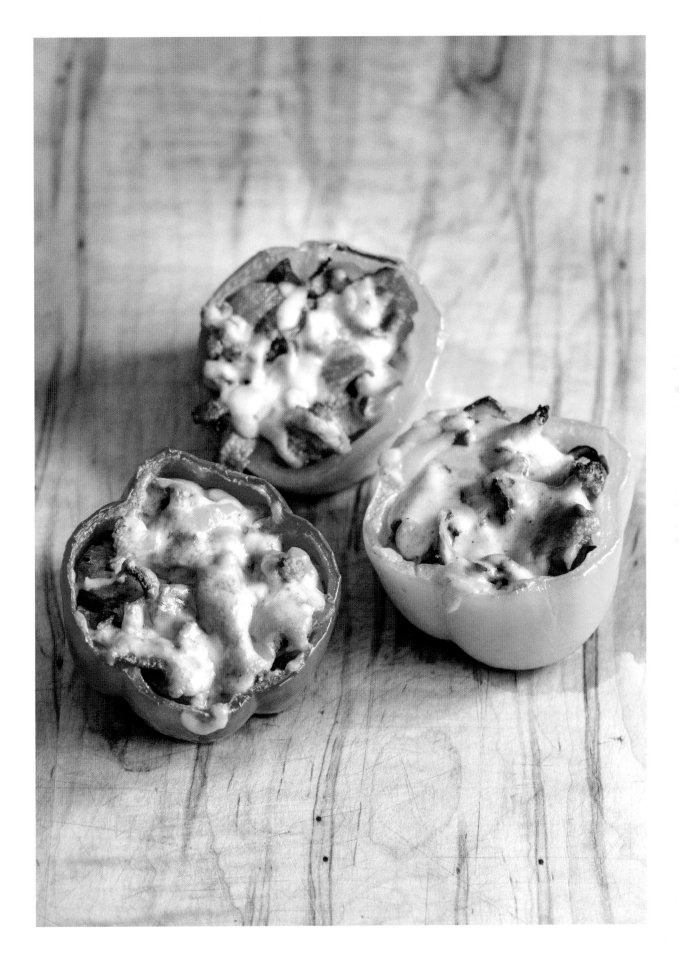

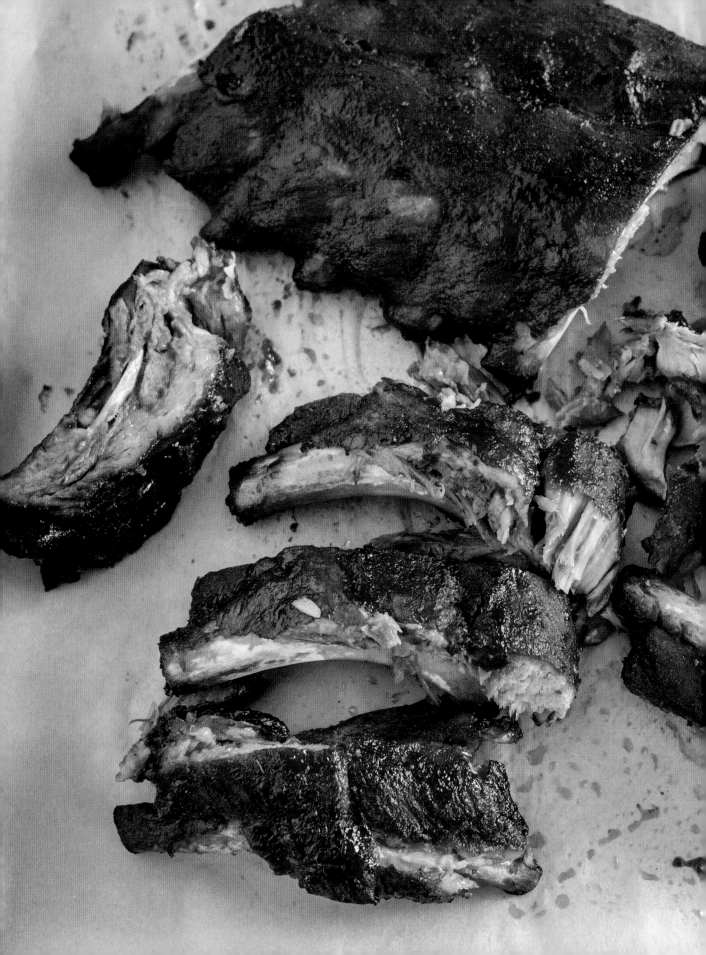

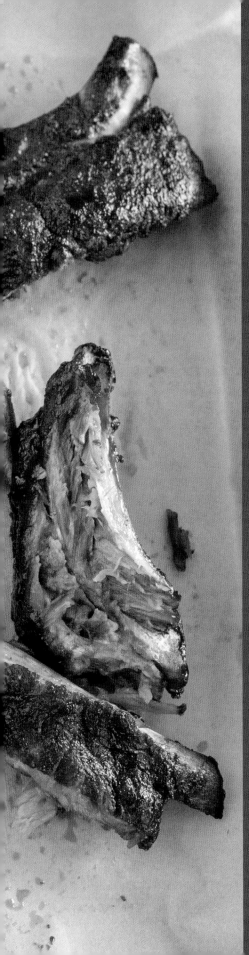

CHAPTER 5:

PORK

MU SHU PORK BOWLS

SERVES: 4 | **PREP TIME:** 20 minutes | **COOK TIME:** 20 minutes

Mu shu pork is a takeout favorite. Meat and vegetables stir-fried with ginger and garlic, drizzled with hoisin? Yes, please. Here we give it a carnivore-ish spin with a higher protein-to-vegetable ratio. This bowl version skips the traditional thin pancakes, though you could wrap it in tortillas or serve it over rice if you like. We made the hoisin optional, but we highly recommend using it. Its tangy sweetness, combined with a hit of heat from the Sriracha, really elevates this dish.

3 tablespoons plus 1 teaspoon coconut aminos

1 tablespoon mirin

1 teaspoon fish sauce

1 teaspoon arrowroot powder

4 tablespoons avocado oil, divided

6 ounces shiitake mushrooms, destemmed and caps thinly sliced

Fine sea salt

1 pound boneless pork loin chops, cut into thin strips

Freshly ground black pepper

3 large eggs, beaten

4 scallions, white and light green parts, sliced on a diagonal (about ¼ cup)

3 cloves garlic, minced (about 1 tablespoon)

1½ tablespoons minced fresh ginger

1 (12-ounce) bag coleslaw mix

1 tablespoon toasted sesame oil

Gluten-free hoisin, for serving (optional)

Sriracha sauce, for serving (optional)

1. In a small bowl, whisk together 3 tablespoons of the coconut aminos, the mirin, and fish sauce. In a small cup, dissolve the arrowroot in 1 teaspoon of water.

2. Warm 1 tablespoon of the avocado oil in a large skillet (or wok, if you have one) over medium-high heat. Add the mushrooms, sprinkle with salt, and cook, stirring occasionally, until tender and golden in spots, 6 to 7 minutes. Transfer to a bowl. Add another tablespoon of the oil to the pan and swirl to coat. Add the pork, season lightly with salt and pepper, and cook, stirring, until just cooked through with no spots of pink left, 1 to 2 minutes. Transfer to the bowl with the mushrooms and cover to keep warm. Pour off any liquid in the pan.

3. Lower the heat to medium. Add another tablespoon of the oil to the pan and swirl to coat. Whisk the remaining teaspoon of coconut aminos into the eggs. Add to the skillet, sprinkle with salt, and cook, stirring, until just cooked through, about 2 minutes. Break up into small pieces and transfer to a separate small bowl.

4. Raise the heat to medium-high. Add the remaining tablespoon of oil to the pan and swirl to coat. Add the scallions, garlic, and ginger; sauté until fragrant, about 1 minute. Add the coleslaw mix, season lightly with salt, and stir-fry until the cabbage begins to wilt, 2 to 3 minutes.

5. Return the mushrooms, pork, and any accumulated liquid to the pan. Pour in the aminos mixture and stir to pull up any browned bits from the bottom of the skillet. Return the cooked eggs to the pan, then drizzle in the arrowroot slurry. Cook, stirring, until the sauce thickens and coats all of the ingredients, about 1 minute. Remove the pan from the heat; drizzle with the sesame oil. Divide among four bowls, drizzle with hoisin and Sriracha, if using, and serve.

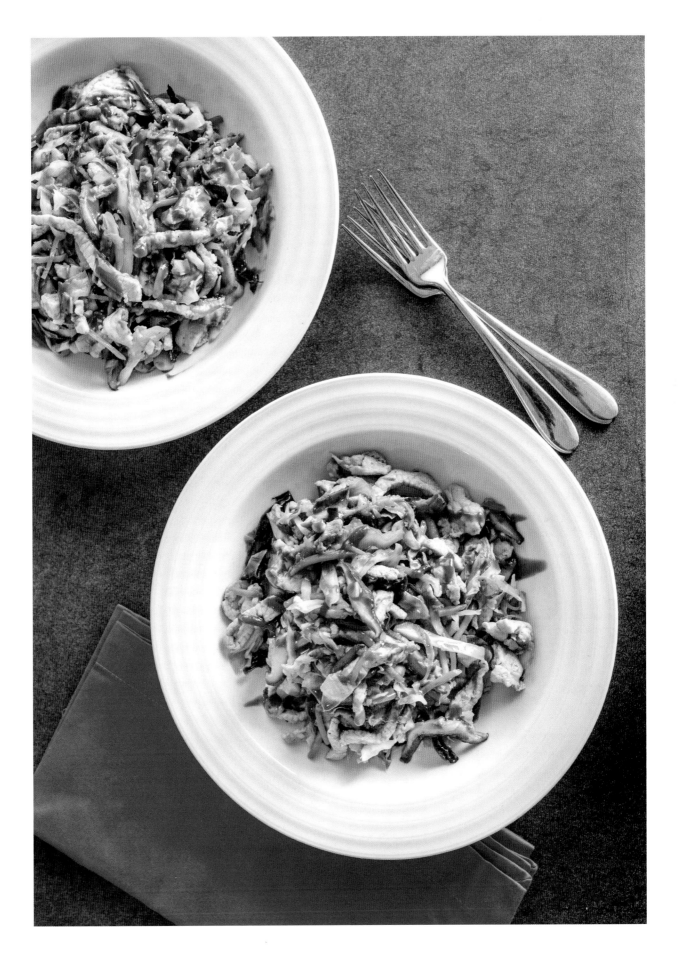

PORK MEDALLIONS WITH MUSTARD PAN SAUCE

SERVES: 4 | **PREP TIME:** 15 minutes | **COOK TIME:** 20 minutes

A pan sauce is a deceptively simple way to make even a quick weeknight meal feel special. Use a liquid like broth and/or wine to pull up the browned bits in the skillet left over from searing your protein—in this case, pork loin (those bits are called the "fond"), and you're most of the way there. The fond is loaded with flavor, so it doesn't take much more to make a really beautiful sauce happen.

½ cup chicken bone broth

1 tablespoon Dijon mustard

1½ teaspoons maple syrup

½ teaspoon arrowroot powder

1 (1½-pound) pork tenderloin, cut into ½-inch-thick slices (about 16)

2 tablespoons avocado oil, plus more if needed

Fine sea salt and freshly ground black pepper

1 medium shallot, chopped (about ½ cup)

1 teaspoon minced fresh rosemary

1 tablespoon chopped fresh flat-leaf parsley, for garnish (optional)

1. In a bowl, whisk together the broth, mustard, and maple syrup. In a small cup, dissolve the arrowroot in ½ teaspoon of water.

2. Pat the pork slices thoroughly dry and place on a cutting board. Put the side of a chef's knife on top of a pork slice. Use the heel of your hand to push down on the side of the blade, pressing the pork to a ¼-inch thickness. Repeat with the remaining pork slices.

3. Warm the avocado oil in a large skillet over high heat. Season the pork all over moderately with salt and pepper. Place the pork slices in the skillet and cook until seared on both sides, turning once, 2 to 3 minutes total. Transfer the pork to a plate; tent with foil to keep warm. (Work in batches if needed to avoid crowding; add more oil to the skillet between batches.)

4. Lower the heat to medium. If there is less than 1 tablespoon of fat in the skillet, add more oil to equal about 1 tablespoon. Add the shallot to the pan, sprinkle lightly with salt, and cook, stirring, until tender and turning golden, 2 to 3 minutes. Whisk the broth mixture and pour it into the skillet, stirring to pull any browned bits from the bottom. Lower the heat to medium-low, add the rosemary, and simmer until the mixture has reduced by about one-third, 3 to 4 minutes.

5. Stir the arrowroot mixture, then pour it into the skillet and stir to combine. Add the pork slices along with any juices that have collected on the plate. Cook until the pork is warmed through and the sauce has thickened, 2 to 3 minutes longer, turning the pork once or twice to coat it with sauce. Serve hot, topped with spoonfuls of the sauce and a sprinkling of parsley, if desired.

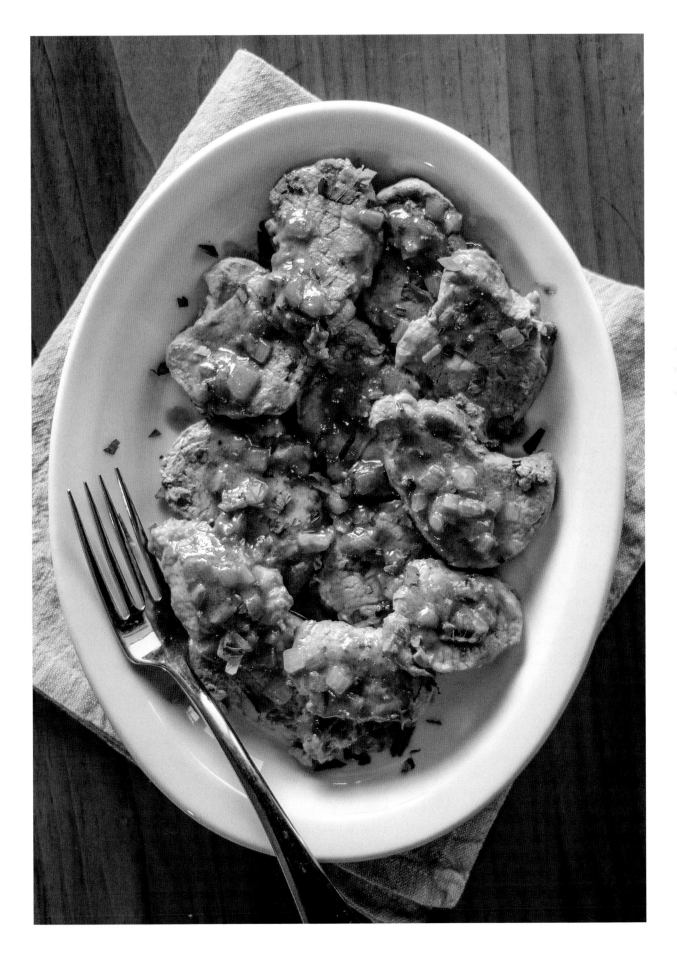

LOADED SWEET POTATOES

SERVES: 4 | **PREP TIME:** 5 minutes | **COOK TIME:** 1 hour

We love stuffing good things with other good things—hence these sweet potato jackets filled with cooked ground pork and topped with two cheeses. Ultimate comfort food. Sprinkle on the pork panko if you'd like some crunch. If you have ground chicken, turkey, or beef on hand, feel free to swap in any of those for the pork.

4 medium sweet potatoes, scrubbed and patted dry

2 tablespoons avocado oil, divided

Fine sea salt

1 pound ground pork

Freshly ground black pepper

1 cup shredded cheddar cheese (about 4 ounces)

1 cup shredded mozzarella cheese (about 4 ounces)

¼ cup thinly sliced scallions

¼ cup pork panko (optional)

1. Preheat the oven to 400°F. Line a rimmed baking sheet with parchment paper.

2. Prick the sweet potatoes all over with a fork. Rub the potatoes with 1 tablespoon of the avocado oil and sprinkle with salt. Place on the lined baking sheet and bake until easily pierced with a knife, about 1 hour.

3. Meanwhile, warm the remaining 1 tablespoon of oil in a large cast-iron skillet over medium heat. Add the pork and cook, stirring and breaking up the meat, until cooked through and no longer pink, about 10 minutes. Season with salt to taste.

4. Remove the sweet potatoes from the oven and let cool for about 10 minutes, or until cool enough to handle but still warm. Using a sharp knife, make a slit lengthwise across the top of each potato and fluff the flesh with a fork. (You can remove and save some of the baked sweet potato flesh to allow more room for filling if you like.) Season with salt and pepper to taste.

5. Divide the cooked pork among the sweet potatoes. Sprinkle with the cheeses, scallions, and panko, if using. Serve immediately.

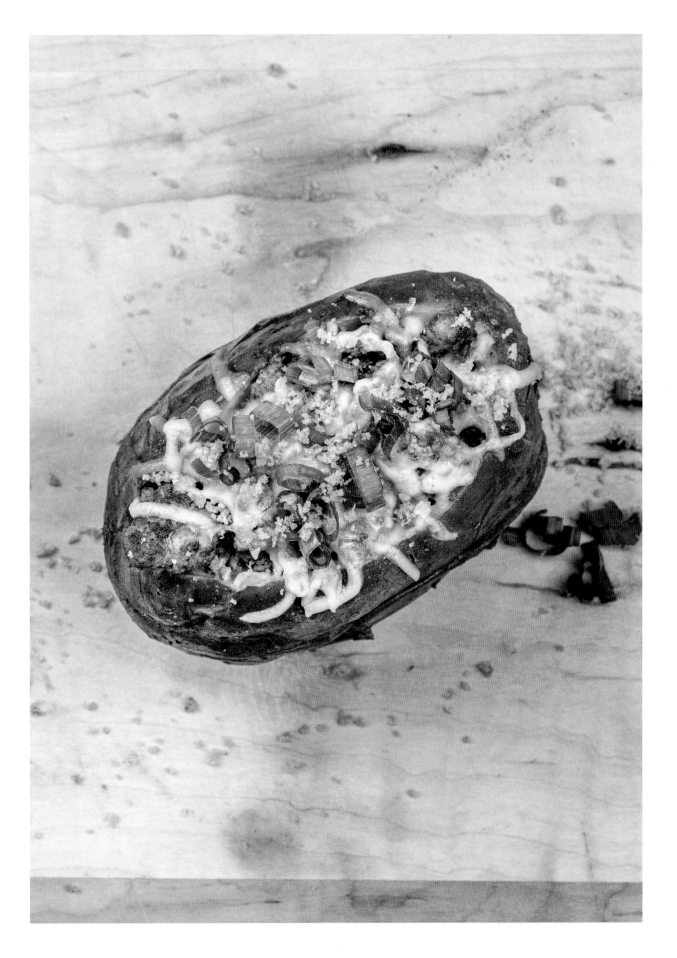

SLOW-BAKED RIBS

SERVES: 4 | **PREP TIME:** 15 minutes | **COOK TIME:** 3½ hours

We. Love. Ribs. On a work trip to Austin a few years back, we were eating at a famous barbecue place, and Beth ordered ribs. The rack was huge and seemed like too much—but of course, we polished it off along with a plate of brisket (#teamwork). As well as being delicious and satisfyingly primal (you have no choice but to pick them up and eat with your hands), ribs are budget-friendly and easy to cook. Rub on a few spices, let the rack hang out in the oven on a low temperature for a few hours, brush the ribs with your favorite barbecue sauce, and get ready to feast.

3 tablespoons coconut sugar

1 tablespoon sweet paprika

1½ teaspoons smoked paprika

2 teaspoons garlic powder

2 teaspoons fine sea salt

½ teaspoon freshly ground black pepper

½ teaspoon ground celery seed (see Note)

2¼ to 2½ pounds baby back pork ribs (see "How to prep ribs," opposite)

½ cup barbecue sauce

1. Preheat the oven to 275°F. Line a rimmed baking sheet with parchment paper.

2. In a small bowl, combine the sugar, sweet and smoked paprikas, garlic powder, salt, pepper, and ground celery seed. Pat the ribs dry. Place the ribs on the lined baking sheet and rub the spice mixture all over them. Cover the pan with foil and bake until the ribs are cooked through and falling off the bones, 2½ to 3 hours.

3. Remove the foil. Brush the ribs with the barbecue sauce. Return the baking sheet to the oven and bake until the sauce is hot and sticky on the ribs, 20 to 30 minutes longer. Serve hot (with plenty of napkins).

NOTE:

You can usually find ground celery seed in the spice section of your supermarket. If your local store doesn't have it, pick it up online from a spice purveyor such as Penzeys.

How to prep ribs

Pork ribs have a thin membrane, called the silverskin, attached to their underside that should be removed before cooking. Some meat purveyors remove this membrane when processing ribs. Check to see if the ribs you purchased have a thin membrane; if so, slip a paring knife under it, slice it, then use your fingers to pull it off. Cut away any bits of membrane that are left after you pull it off. (If you're lazy like us, you can ask your butcher to do this task for you.)

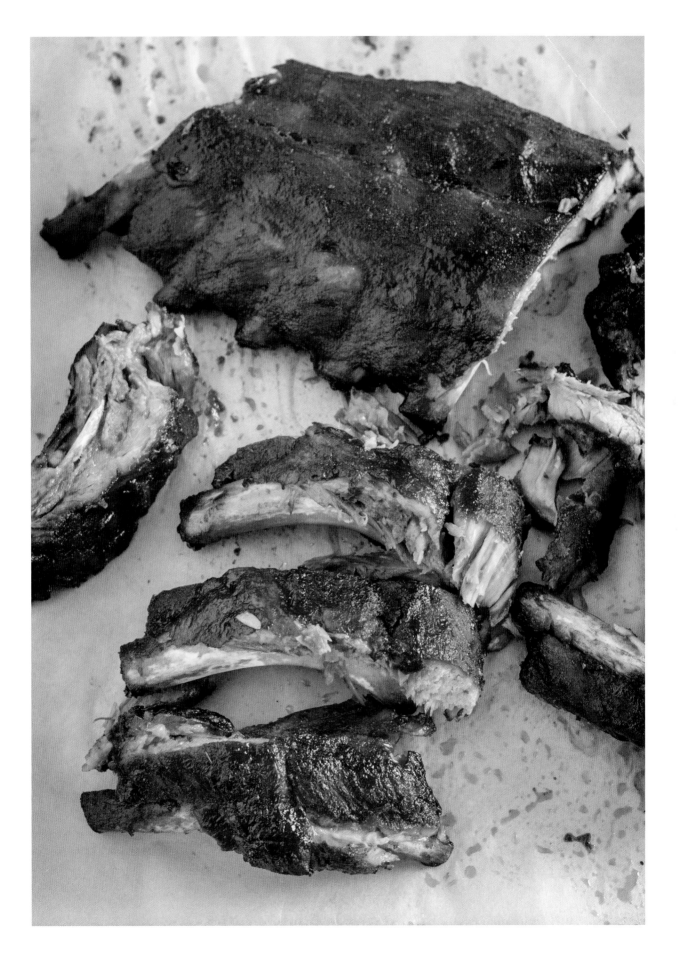

PULLED PORK

MAKES: About 6 cups (6 to 8 servings) | **PREP TIME:** 15 minutes |
COOK TIME: 2¾ to 3¼ hours

Controversial opinion: a Dutch oven is far better for making pulled pork than a slow cooker. We love the texture so much more this way; you just don't get those crispy bits with a slow cooker. There isn't much hands-on cooking with a Dutch oven, either. Try it this way—we swear, it's so good, you'll never go back.

3 tablespoons coconut sugar

2 teaspoons sweet paprika

1 teaspoon smoked paprika

2 teaspoons garlic powder

1½ teaspoons dried oregano leaves

1 teaspoon chili powder

1 teaspoon fine sea salt

½ teaspoon freshly ground black pepper

4 pounds boneless pork shoulder, trimmed of excess fat and cut into 2- to 3-inch pieces

2 tablespoons bacon fat or avocado oil, plus more if needed

½ cup chicken bone broth

Barbecue sauce, for serving (optional)

1. Preheat the oven to 300°F.

2. In a large bowl, combine the sugar, sweet and smoked paprikas, garlic powder, oregano, chili powder, salt, and pepper. Pat the pork pieces thoroughly dry, then toss in the spice mixture until well coated.

3. Heat the bacon fat in a Dutch oven over medium-high heat. Working in batches, add the pork pieces to the pot and cook, turning with tongs, until golden on all sides, 5 to 7 minutes. (Do not overcrowd the pot. Add more fat between batches as needed.)

4. Once all of the pork is seared, return all of the pork to the pot (along with any juices that have collected), pour in the broth, cover, and place in the oven. Bake until the meat is cooked through and shreds easily, nearly all of the liquid has cooked off, and the fat has rendered, 2½ to 3 hours. The meat should be well moistened with some crispy bits.

5. Let cool slightly, then shred the meat. Taste and season with additional salt and pepper, if needed. Eat right away, or let cool, cover, and refrigerate to serve later (it will keep for up to 4 days). Serve with barbecue sauce, if desired.

NOTE:

If, after 3 hours of cooking, there's still too much liquid in the pot, remove the lid and bake the pork for an additional 15 to 20 minutes.

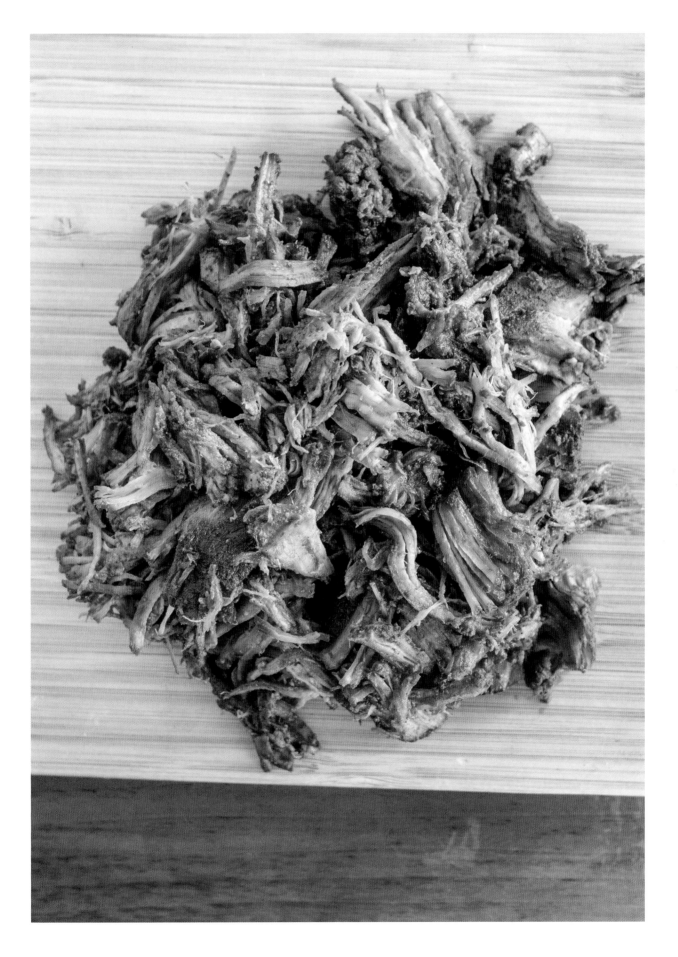

SAUSAGE AND APPLE-STUFFED PORK LOIN ROAST

SERVES: 6 to 8 | **PREP TIME:** 30 minutes | **COOK TIME:** 1½ hours

If you looked at the photo of this roast and thought, "There's no way I could do that," well, you absolutely can. It's simple to execute, and the result is beautiful and delicious, perfect for a holiday meal or dinner party. Make the stuffing a day ahead, cover, and refrigerate. You can even roll the roast up to a few hours in advance and sear and roast it when you're ready. A green vegetable such as Brussels sprouts is a nice foil for the rich, meaty pork.

2 tablespoons avocado oil, divided, plus more if needed

8 ounces sweet Italian sausage, casings removed

2 medium shallots, diced (about ¾ cup)

2 small ribs celery, diced (about ½ cup)

Fine sea salt and freshly ground black pepper

1 small tart green apple, cored and diced (about 1 cup)

2 cloves garlic, minced (about 2 teaspoons)

¼ cup blanched almond flour

1 tablespoon minced fresh sage

1 tablespoon (½ ounce) unsalted butter, at room temperature

1 (3-pound) boneless pork loin roast, butterflied (see Notes)

½ cup chicken bone broth

1. Preheat the oven to 375°F.

2. Warm 1 tablespoon of the avocado oil in a large skillet over medium heat. Add the sausage and cook, breaking up the meat and stirring, until cooked through and browned in spots, 7 to 9 minutes. Use a slotted spoon to transfer the sausage to a medium bowl. If there is less than 1 tablespoon of fat left in the skillet, add oil to equal about 1 tablespoon.

3. Add the shallots and celery to the skillet, sprinkle with salt and pepper, and cook, stirring occasionally, until tender, 3 to 4 minutes. Add the apple and garlic, season lightly with salt, and cook, stirring occasionally, until the apple is tender but not mushy, about 2 minutes longer. Transfer to the bowl with the sausage. Wipe out the skillet.

4. Add the almond flour, sage, and butter to the bowl. Stir until the ingredients are well combined and the butter has melted.

5. Lay the roast on the counter with the narrow side facing you and pat it dry. If the roast is thicker than ¼ inch, place it between two sheets of parchment paper and use a rolling pin or wine bottle to pound it to an even ¼-inch thickness. Season generously with salt and pepper. Spread the sausage mixture over the pork, leaving a 1-inch border on all sides. Roll the meat up tightly. Tie pieces of kitchen twine around the roast at 1-inch intervals to secure it. Trim off any excess twine.

6. Warm the remaining 1 tablespoon of oil in the skillet over high heat. Add the roast and sear, turning with tongs, until golden on all sides, 8 to 10 minutes. Transfer the roast to a rack set inside a

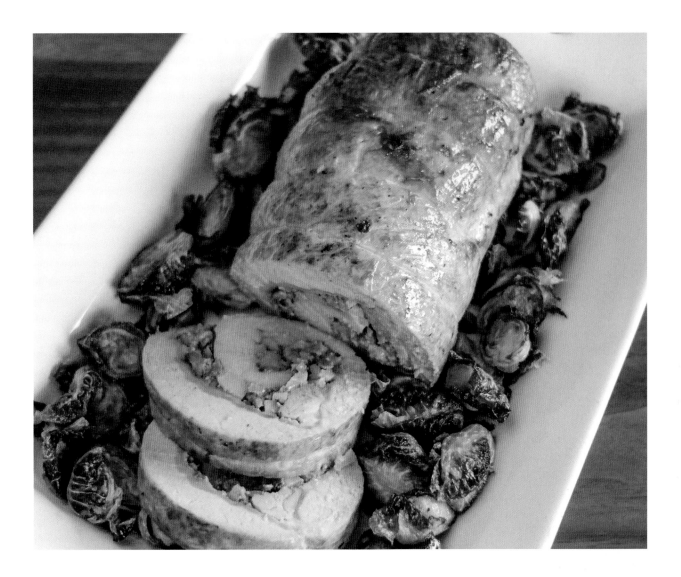

roasting pan, pour the broth into the bottom of the pan, place in the oven, and roast, uncovered, until an instant-read thermometer inserted in the center reaches 145°F, 55 to 65 minutes. Transfer the roast to a cutting board, tent loosely with foil, and let rest for 10 minutes. Snip off the twine, slice the roast, and serve.

NOTES:

To remove sausage from its casing, simply hold one end and squeeze the meat out. If the end is sealed and the meat doesn't come out easily, snip off the end with kitchen shears.

Ask the butcher to butterfly the pork for you. Yes, you can do it yourself, but why? The butcher will do it better and faster.

If there's liquid left over in the roasting pan, strain it and serve it at the table for spooning over the roast.

AIR FRYER PORK KATSU

SERVES: 4 | **PREP TIME:** 25 minutes, plus at least 30 minutes to brine |
COOK TIME: 12 minutes

Deep-fried breaded pork chops—what could be better? How about breading them in pork rinds and air-frying: this way, you get crisp, ultra-porky chops with far fewer carbs and less oil/mess. Brining the chops infuses them with flavor, definitely worth the step. And the sweet and tangy sauce, which comes together quickly, is an absolute must.

KATSU:

¼ cup kosher salt

¼ cup hot water

4 (4- to 5-ounce) boneless pork chops, pounded to ¼ inch thickness

Freshly ground black pepper

¼ cup cassava flour

1 large egg

1 tablespoon coconut aminos

1¼ cups pork panko

TONKATSU SAUCE:

¼ cup unsweetened ketchup

1½ tablespoons Worcestershire sauce

1 tablespoon coconut aminos

1 teaspoon Dijon mustard

¼ teaspoon garlic powder

¼ teaspoon ginger powder

¼ teaspoon freshly ground black pepper

½ to ¾ teaspoon raw honey

1. Make the katsu: In a large heatproof bowl, stir the kosher salt into the hot water until dissolved. Stir in 3 cups of cold water. Add the chops, cover, and refrigerate for at least 30 minutes or up to 2 hours.

2. Make the sauce: In a small bowl, whisk together the ketchup, Worcestershire sauce, coconut aminos, mustard, garlic powder, ginger powder, pepper, and ½ teaspoon of honey. Taste and add another ¼ teaspoon of honey, if needed. You can make the sauce up to 1 day ahead; cover and refrigerate until ready to use.

3. Drain the chops; discard the brine. Pat the chops thoroughly dry, then season lightly with pepper. Put the cassava flour in a shallow bowl. In another shallow bowl, beat the egg with the coconut aminos. Put the panko in a third shallow bowl. Preheat an air fryer to 360°F for 5 minutes.

4. Working one at a time, dip the chops into the flour, shaking off the excess. Then dip in the egg mixture, shaking off the excess. Dip in the panko, pressing to adhere. Place the breaded chops on a platter.

5. Mist the air fryer basket with cooking spray. Place the chops in the basket and air-fry for 8 minutes, turning once halfway through. Raise the temperature to 400°F and air-fry until the chops are golden and crisp, 3 to 4 minutes longer, turning once. Open the fryer but let the chops rest there undisturbed for 1 to 2 minutes, then transfer to a cutting board. Slice the chops and serve with the sauce.

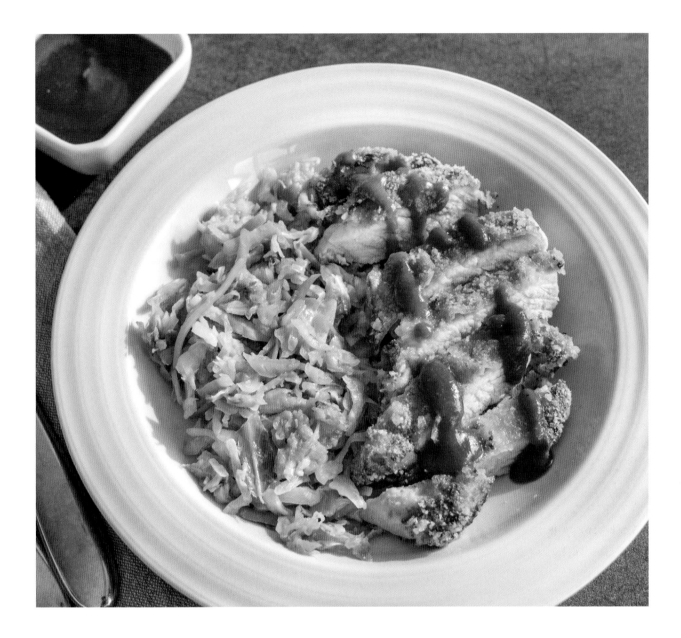

NOTES:

To pound the chops, place them between sheets of parchment paper and hit them with a rolling pin or full wine bottle. Strike firmly but not too hard; too much force will cause the chops to tear.

If you can't fit all of the chops in your air fryer in a single layer, work in batches. Place the first completed batch on a cooling rack set inside a rimmed baking sheet and keep warm in a 200°F oven while you fry the second batch.

For a quick side dish, stir-fry coleslaw mix in a skillet with avocado oil. Add a bit of minced ginger and garlic if you like. Mix in a little of the tonkatsu sauce on the plate.

PORK BREAKFAST SAUSAGE PATTIES

SERVES: 4 | **PREP TIME:** 5 minutes | **COOK TIME:** 15 minutes

We're calling this breakfast sausage since it contains maple syrup and will taste wonderful alongside any of our egg dishes (like the Easy Ham and Egg Mug Omelet pictured; see the recipe on page 214). But the beauty of animal protein (and making your own food rules, really) is that you can eat any type of food at any time. So go ahead and have these breakfast patties at dinner, maybe alongside our Parsnip Mash (page 272) or with a paffle or two (page 294).

1 pound ground pork

2 tablespoons maple syrup

1½ teaspoons fine sea salt

1 teaspoon freshly ground black pepper

1 teaspoon garlic powder

½ teaspoon dried rubbed sage

¼ teaspoon ground cinnamon

2 tablespoons ghee, for the pan

1.   Put the ground pork, maple syrup, salt, pepper, garlic powder, sage, and cinnamon in a large bowl and use your hands to combine the ingredients.

2.   Divide the meat mixture into 8 even portions. Roll each into a ball, then flatten with your palms into 1-inch-thick patties.

3.   Melt the ghee in a large skillet over medium-high heat. Add the patties (work in batches if needed to avoid crowding) and cook until one side is browned, 3 to 4 minutes. Carefully flip the patties and cook until browned on the other side and cooked through, 2 to 3 minutes longer.

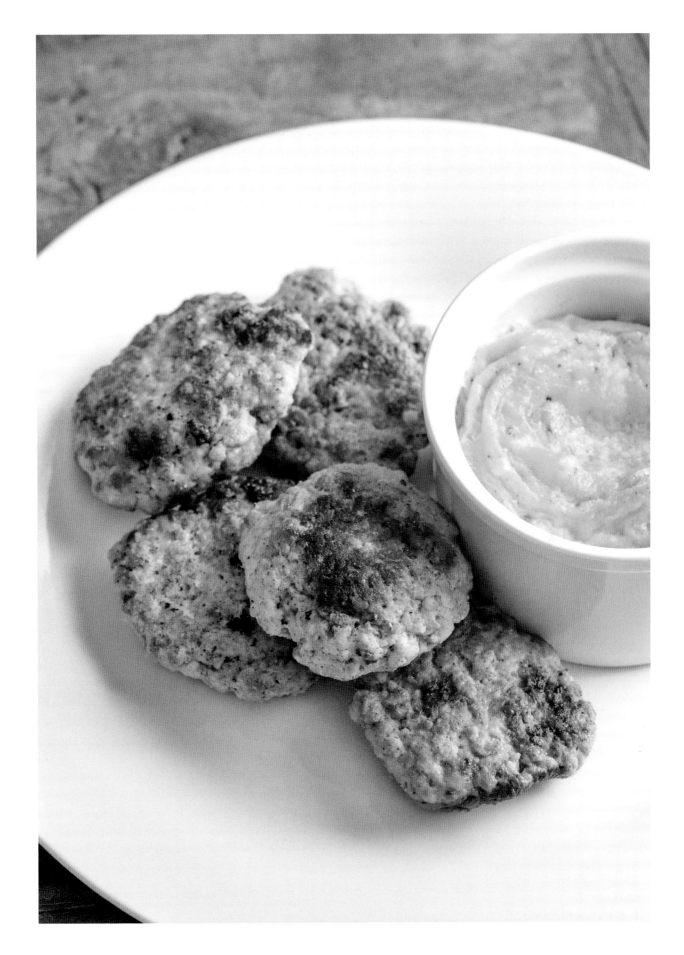

VIETNAMESE-STYLE ROAST PORK LETTUCE WRAPS

SERVES: 12 | **PREP TIME:** 10 minutes, plus at least 1 hour to marinate | **COOK TIME:** 5 hours 20 minutes

This recipe is a perfect example of how lower-carb, protein-forward meals can still be colorful and full of texture (and vegetables). This is a fun family-style meal—the kids can help with the setup and put together their own lettuce wraps.

SAUCE:

¼ cup coconut aminos

2 tablespoons fresh lime juice

2 tablespoons coconut sugar

2 tablespoons apple cider vinegar

2 tablespoons chili garlic sauce

1 tablespoon fish sauce

1 tablespoon raw honey

WRAPS:

2½ pounds boneless pork shoulder, trimmed of excess fat

1 cup chicken or pork bone broth

2 cups shredded carrots

1 cup roasted peanuts, chopped (salted or unsalted, your preference)

½ cup chopped fresh mint

1 head Bibb or butter lettuce, separated into leaves

1 large or 2 small limes, cut into wedges, for serving (optional)

1. In a small bowl, combine the ingredients for the sauce.

2. Put the pork shoulder in a 3-quart baking dish and pat thoroughly dry. Pour half of the sauce over the pork and rub it into the surface with your hands. Cover and refrigerate for at least 1 hour or up to overnight. Reserve the other half of the sauce.

3. Preheat the oven to 450°F. Remove the pork from the fridge and set on the counter to temper for about 30 minutes.

4. Put the pork shoulder fat side down in a roasting pan at least 2 inches deep; pour the broth into the pan around the pork. Roast uncovered for 20 minutes, then lower the temperature to 250°F and continue to cook until the outside is browned and caramelized and a fork goes through the middle of the pork smoothly, about 5 hours. Remove the pan from the oven and let the pork rest, tented with foil, for 30 minutes.

5. Chop the pork into 1-inch pieces; transfer to a large bowl. Serve the pork with the carrots, peanuts, mint, and reserved sauce, along with the lettuce leaves for wrapping. Serve with lime wedges, if desired. The pork will keep in an airtight container in the fridge for up to 1 week; store other ingredients separately.

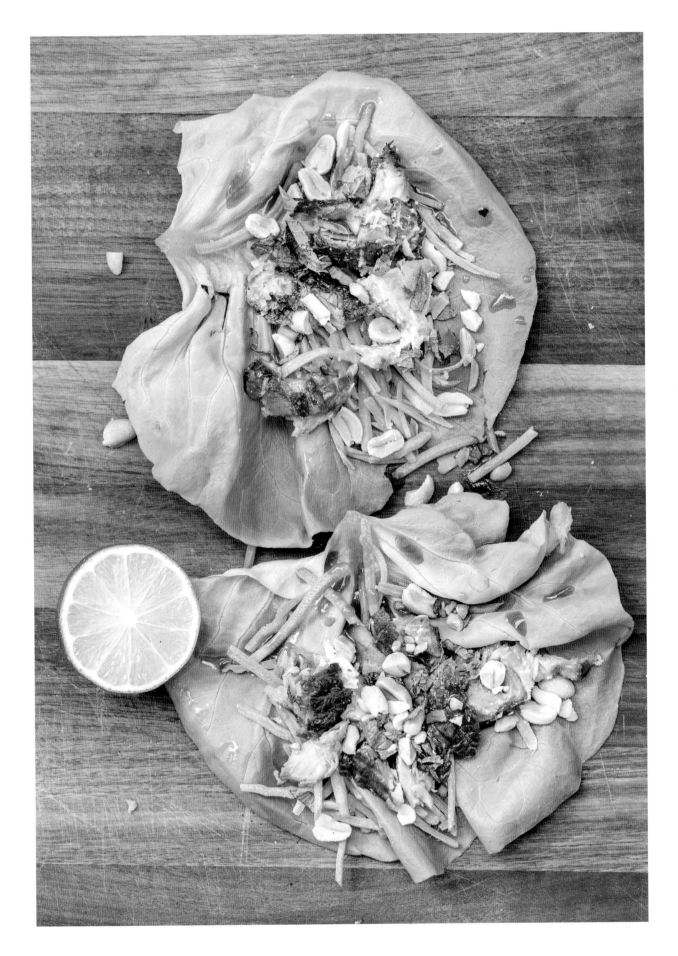

SAUSAGE AND PEPPERS

SERVES: 4 | **PREP TIME:** 10 minutes | **COOK TIME:** 25 minutes

This is a classic combination for a reason—sweet bell peppers and sautéed onion are a perfect foil for rich pork sausage. At the annual Feast of San Gennaro in New York's Little Italy, this is usually served on hero bread, but we love the sausage and peppers' flavor so much that we prefer not to dilute it with bread. Sweet Italian sausage (it isn't actually "sweet," just not spicy) is traditional, but go for hot sausage if you like heat, or try a different flavor depending on your taste.

2 teaspoons avocado oil

1 pound sweet Italian pork sausage links

1 white onion, sliced

3 cloves garlic, sliced

3 bell peppers (any color), seeded and sliced

¾ teaspoon fine sea salt

½ teaspoon freshly ground black pepper

¼ teaspoon red pepper flakes

½ cup chicken bone broth

1. Heat the avocado oil in a large cast-iron skillet over medium-high heat. Add the sausage and cook, turning the links occasionally, until they brown on the outsides, about 4 minutes (they will not be fully cooked). Transfer the sausage to a cutting board, slice, and set aside.

2. Add the onion and garlic to the skillet. Cook, stirring occasionally, until softened, about 3 minutes. Add the bell peppers, salt, black pepper, and red pepper flakes. Cook, stirring often, until the onions are translucent and the peppers are soft, about 5 minutes.

3. Pour the broth into the skillet and scrape the bottom to release all of the browned bits. Return the sausage to the skillet, lower the heat to medium, and cover. Simmer until all of the veggies are fully soft and cooked through, about 10 minutes. Uncover the skillet, increase the heat to medium-high, and cook until the liquid has evaporated and the sausage is cooked through, about 3 minutes longer.

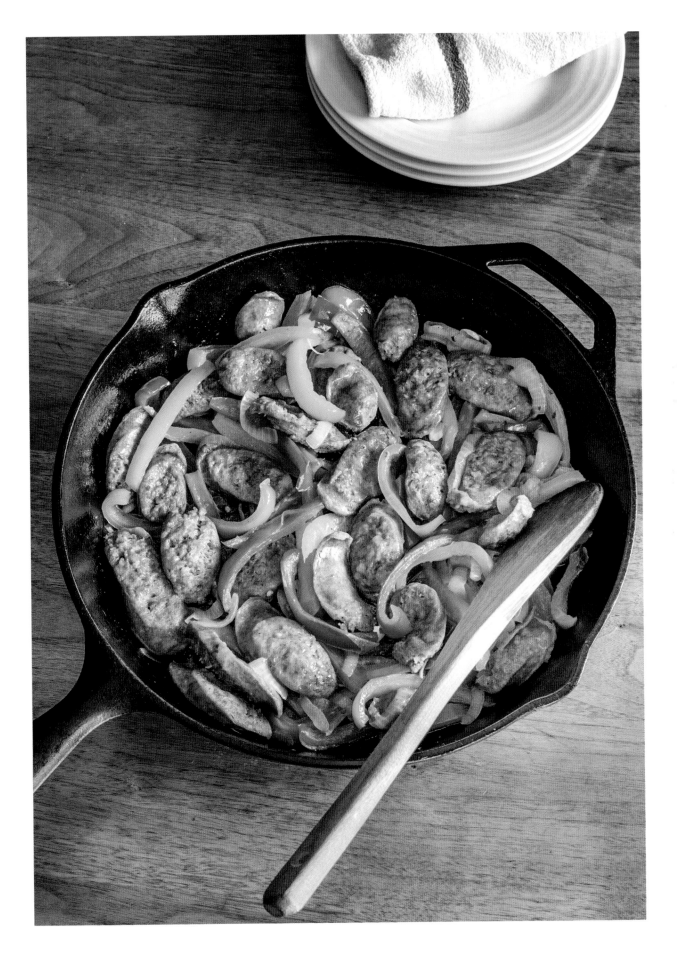

BREADLESS CROQUE MONSIEUR

SERVES: 4 | **PREP TIME:** 5 minutes | **COOK TIME:** 14 minutes

This is our take on the rich decadence of the classic croque monsieur sandwich, without the bread but with the addition of mushrooms for extra texture and umami flavor. We promise, this version is just as satisfying: it has all of the hammy, cheesy goodness you're craving.

2 tablespoons (1 ounce) unsalted butter

8 ounces button mushrooms, chopped (about 2 cups)

1 small shallot, chopped (about ¼ cup)

2 cloves garlic, minced (about 2 teaspoons)

Pinch of fine sea salt

⅛ teaspoon freshly ground black pepper

1 (1-pound) fully cooked boneless ham steak, cut into 4 slices

1 cup shredded Gruyère cheese (about 4 ounces)

1 tablespoon minced fresh flat-leaf parsley (optional)

1. In a large nonstick skillet, melt the butter over medium-high heat. Add the mushrooms and shallot; cook, stirring, until tender, 4 to 6 minutes. Add the garlic, salt, and pepper; cook, stirring, until the garlic is fragrant, 1 minute longer. Transfer the mixture to a bowl; cover to keep warm. Wipe the skillet clean.

2. Place the skillet over medium heat. Put the ham slices in the pan and cook until they begin to brown around the edges, about 3 minutes. Flip the ham; sprinkle with the cheese and cover. Cook until the cheese is melted and the ham is heated through, 2 to 4 minutes.

3. Place the pieces on four plates, top with the mushroom mixture, sprinkle with the parsley, if using, and serve.

NOTE:

These are best eaten right away. Let's face it, reheated melted cheese just isn't the same.

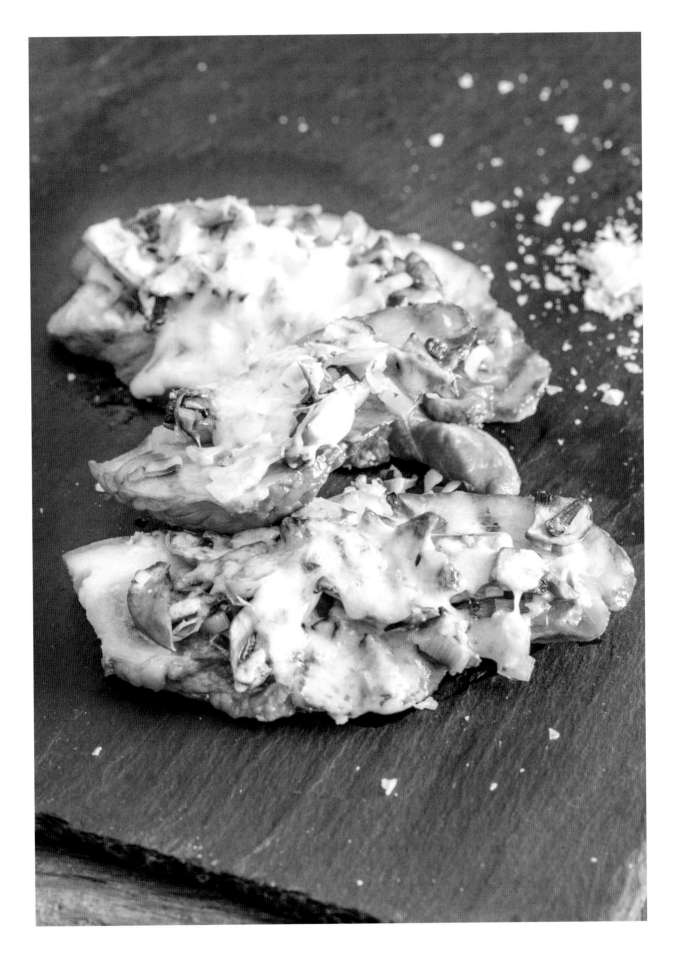

GRILLED PORK CHOPS
WITH SPICY FRUIT SALSA

SERVES: 4 | **PREP TIME:** 5 minutes, plus 1 hour to marinate | **COOK TIME:** 15 minutes

This is a perfect summer meal—fire up the grill and enjoy the balance of sweet, meaty pork with a bright, spicy fruit salsa. These chops also taste great alongside our Garlicky Spaghetti Squash (page 278).

4 bone-in pork chops, about 2 inches thick (about 2 pounds)

¼ cup extra-virgin olive oil

1 tablespoon coconut sugar

2 teaspoons Dijon mustard

1 tablespoon coconut aminos

1 teaspoon fresh lemon juice

½ teaspoon fine sea salt

½ teaspoon freshly ground black pepper

2 cups Spicy Fruit Salsa (page 360)

1. Put the pork chops in a glass bowl or gallon-sized resealable bag. In a medium bowl, whisk together the olive oil, sugar, mustard, coconut aminos, lemon juice, salt, and pepper. Pour the marinade over the meat; rub the marinade into both sides of the meat to ensure even coating. Cover and refrigerate for at least 1 hour or up to overnight. Remove the chops from the fridge about 15 minutes before cooking to temper.

2. Preheat an outdoor grill or indoor grill pan to medium heat. Remove the chops from the marinade; discard the marinade. Set the chops on the grill or in the grill pan. Cook, turning once, until you see grill marks and an instant-read thermometer inserted into the thickest part of a chop away from the bone registers 145°F, 6 to 8 minutes per side.

3. Transfer the chops to a cutting board, tent with foil, and let rest for 5 minutes. Plate the chops and serve with the salsa.

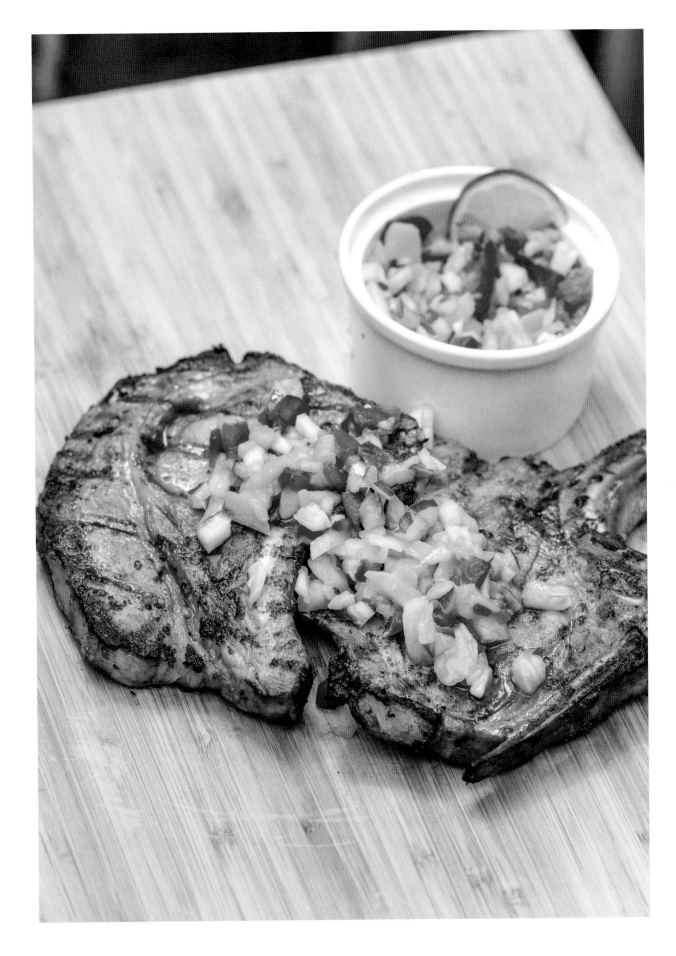

ITALIAN SUB SALAD

SERVES: 2 | **PREP TIME:** 5 minutes, plus 8 hours to marinate

Despite mostly giving up sandwiches, we love a hearty, zesty Italian sub–the layers of flavorful meats and cheeses cut through with some vinegary dressing, peppers, onions, and olives make a perfect picnic-ready meal. The carnivore-ish solution: a high-protein, low-carb deconstructed sub–aka, a salad. Feel free to sub in (pun intended) other meats like capicola, cheeses like mozzarella, hot peppers, giardiniera, and other vegetables you like.

2 ounces thick-sliced ham

2 ounces salami

2 ounces mortadella

3 ounces provolone cheese, sliced

½ red onion, sliced thinly

3 to 4 vine tomatoes, quartered

¼ cup marinated banana peppers

¼ cup black olives, such as kalamata, pitted and minced

2 tablespoons extra-virgin olive oil

2 tablespoons balsamic vinegar

¼ teaspoon freshly ground black pepper

Chop the meats and cheese into 1-inch-square pieces and finely slice the banana peppers. Toss in a large bowl with the onion, tomatoes, and olives. Drizzle with the olive oil and balsamic vinegar, sprinkle with the pepper, and toss until thoroughly mixed. Cover and refrigerate until you're ready to eat.

NOTE:

If you have Italian dressing on hand, you can skip the oil, vinegar, and black pepper and use 3 to 4 tablespoons of the prepared dressing instead.

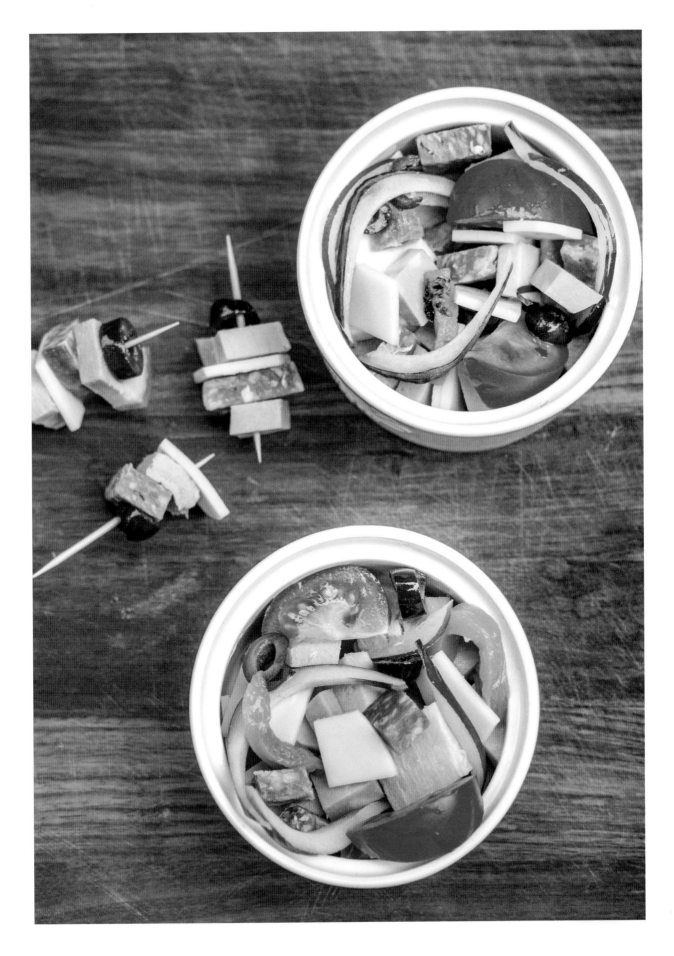

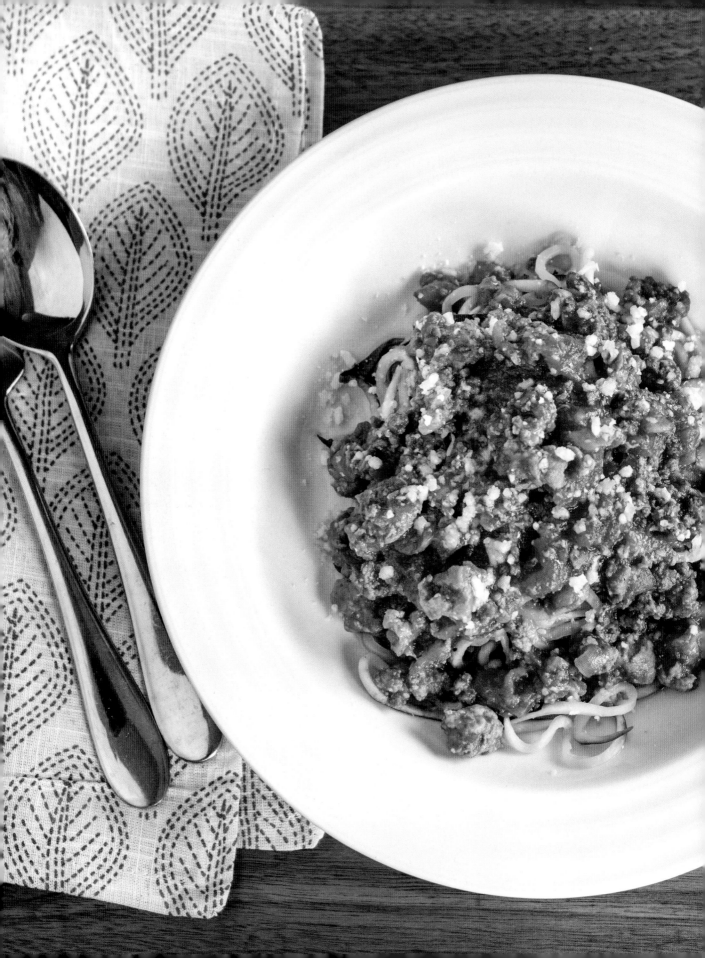

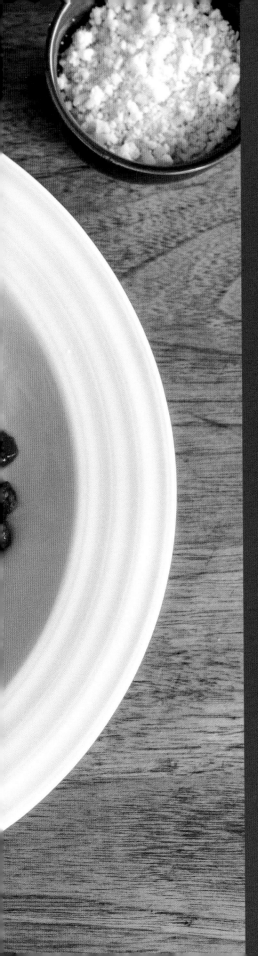

CHAPTER 6:
GAME

COFFEE-RUBBED VENISON DENVER LEG

SERVES: 4 | **PREP TIME:** 10 minutes, plus 3 hours to season meat |
COOK TIME: 10 minutes

The Denver leg of venison is the deer's hind leg, deboned and cut into various pieces. Venison in general is lean, and this part of the animal, which moves a lot, has very little fat. As such, you don't want to cook it past medium-rare or it can get tough. That's why this recipe is so fast and unfussy: the meat is flavorful on its own, so all it needs is a nice spice rub, a quick sear, and a few minutes in the oven to finish.

1½ pounds venison Denver leg

2 tablespoons finely ground coffee

1½ tablespoons coconut sugar

1½ teaspoons smoked paprika

1 teaspoon fine sea salt

1 teaspoon garlic powder

½ teaspoon chili powder

¼ teaspoon freshly ground black pepper

¼ teaspoon ginger powder

1 tablespoon avocado oil

1. Place a cooling rack inside a rimmed baking sheet. Pat the venison thoroughly dry.

2. In a small bowl, combine the coffee, sugar, paprika, salt, garlic powder, chili powder, pepper, and ginger. Rub the mixture all over the venison. Place it on the cooling rack and put the baking sheet in the fridge for at least 3 hours or up to 6 hours. Remove the venison from the fridge and let stand for 30 minutes before cooking.

3. Preheat the oven to 400°F; put a large cast-iron skillet in the oven as it preheats. When the oven reaches temperature, carefully remove the skillet and place it over high heat. Swirl the oil in the pan. Add the venison and cook until seared on one side, about 2 minutes. Flip and sear on the other side, 1 to 2 minutes longer. Flip again and transfer the skillet to the oven. Cook until an instant-read thermometer stuck into the thickest part of the leg reads 120 to 125°F for medium-rare, 4 to 6 minutes.

4. Transfer the venison to a cutting board, tent with foil, and let rest for 5 to 10 minutes. Slice against the grain and serve.

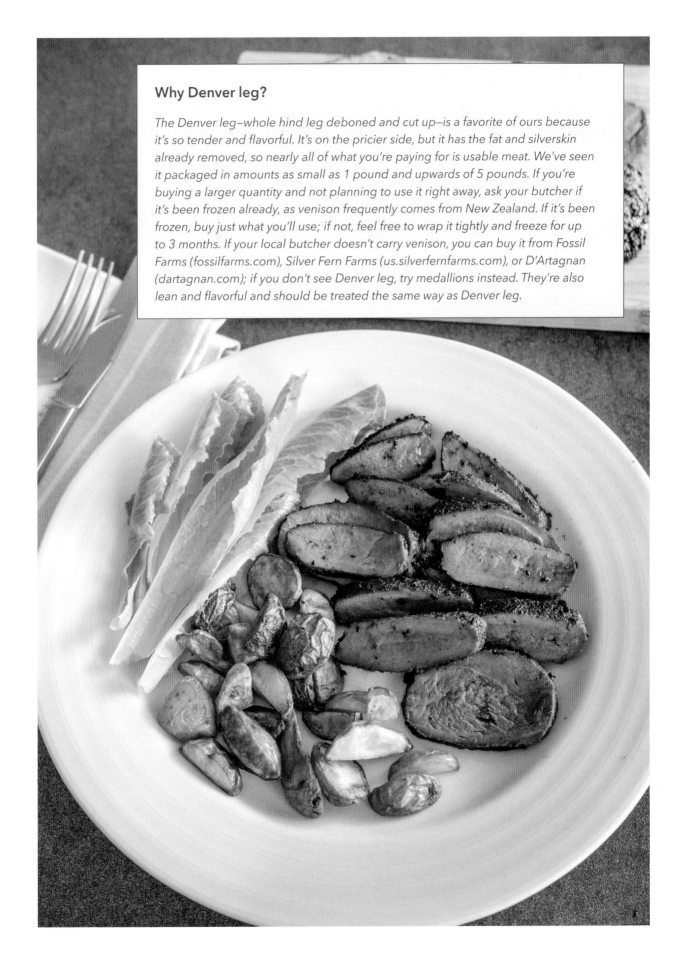

Why Denver leg?

The Denver leg—whole hind leg deboned and cut up—is a favorite of ours because it's so tender and flavorful. It's on the pricier side, but it has the fat and silverskin already removed, so nearly all of what you're paying for is usable meat. We've seen it packaged in amounts as small as 1 pound and upwards of 5 pounds. If you're buying a larger quantity and not planning to use it right away, ask your butcher if it's been frozen already, as venison frequently comes from New Zealand. If it's been frozen, buy just what you'll use; if not, feel free to wrap it tightly and freeze for up to 3 months. If your local butcher doesn't carry venison, you can buy it from Fossil Farms (fossilfarms.com), Silver Fern Farms (us.silverfernfarms.com), or D'Artagnan (dartagnan.com); if you don't see Denver leg, try medallions instead. They're also lean and flavorful and should be treated the same way as Denver leg.

BISON SLOPPY JOE

SERVES: 4 | **PREP TIME:** 10 minutes | **COOK TIME:** 40 minutes

The good old-fashioned sloppy joe gets a modern spin with bison and clean ingredients like unsweetened ketchup and coconut aminos, but it's just as sweet/savory as you remember it. And since we think the meat is the best part, we forgo the hamburger buns (though we do have some serving suggestions; see below). Leftovers are even better. Pro tip: Try it with a runny fried egg on top.

2 tablespoons bacon fat or avocado oil

1 large onion, finely diced (about 1¾ cups)

1 large red bell pepper, seeded and finely diced (about 1 cup)

Fine sea salt

3 cloves garlic, minced (about 1 tablespoon)

1½ pounds ground bison

Freshly ground black pepper

¾ cup unsweetened ketchup

⅓ cup coconut aminos

3 tablespoons tomato paste

1 teaspoon raw honey

½ teaspoon fish sauce or Worcestershire sauce

1. Heat the bacon fat in a large skillet over medium heat. Add the onion and bell pepper, season lightly with salt, and cook, stirring occasionally, until tender, 5 to 7 minutes. Add the garlic and sauté until fragrant, about 1 minute.

2. Add the ground bison and season moderately with salt and pepper; cook, stirring and breaking up the meat with a wooden spoon, until the meat is cooked through and beginning to brown in spots and most of the liquid has cooked off, 8 to 10 minutes.

3. Stir in the ketchup, coconut aminos, tomato paste, honey, and fish sauce. Reduce the heat to low and simmer until the sauce has thickened and the flavors have melded, 15 to 20 minutes.

NOTE:

Even though we don't go for hamburger buns, it's nice to have something to spoon the meat mixture over. (Of course, if you want to eat it on its own or just with an egg on top, carnivore-style, go for it.) Good serving options include Cauliflower Rice (That Doesn't Suck) (page 268), Zucchini Noodles (That Don't Suck) (page 270), Keto Egg Breads (page 300), and Tostones (page 282).

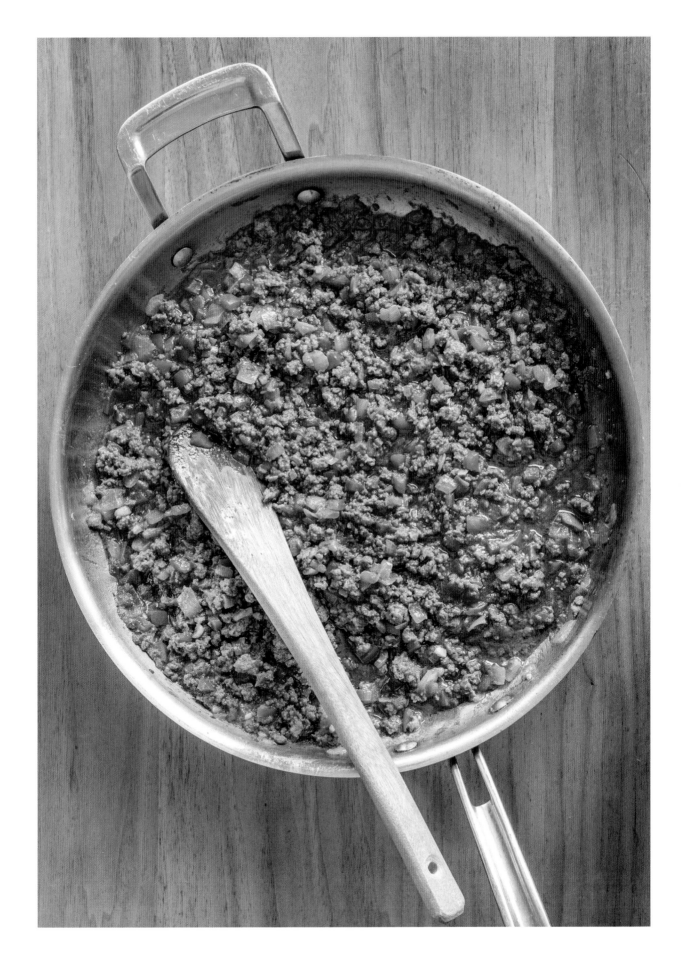

OPEN-FACED BISON PATTY MELTS

SERVES: 4 | PREP TIME: 15 minutes | COOK TIME: 30 minutes

Bison makes delicious burgers, but you have to watch it carefully. Because the meat tends to be lean, it can get really dry if it's overcooked. Timing is everything here, so have the onions and mushrooms done first so you can focus on the burgers. It will seem like a ton of onions and mushrooms at the start, but don't worry, they will cook down a lot. Traditionally, a patty melt has two slices of bread and is grilled, but we prefer to showcase the burger with less bread, and we toast the bread to save a step. Swap in Gruyère for the Swiss cheese if you want to make it a little fancier.

2 tablespoons (1 ounce) unsalted butter, divided

2 tablespoons avocado oil, divided

1 large onion, thinly sliced (about 3 cups)

Fine sea salt

8 ounces cremini mushrooms, thinly sliced (about 4 cups)

2 teaspoons minced fresh sage

1½ pounds ground bison

Freshly ground black pepper

4 slices Swiss cheese

2 grain-free English muffins (such as Mikey's), split, or 4 cauliflower rounds (such as Outer Aisle), toasted

Ketchup, mayo, mustard, or other condiments (optional)

Pickles (optional)

1.   Warm a large cast-iron or other heavy-bottomed skillet over medium-low heat. Melt ½ tablespoon of the butter with ½ tablespoon of the oil. Add the onion, sprinkle with salt, and cook, stirring occasionally, until tender and caramelized, about 20 minutes. (Adjust the temperature as needed if the onion starts to cook too quickly. If it's cooking unevenly, add a few tablespoons of water and stir well until the water evaporates.) Transfer the onion to a small bowl and keep warm; set the skillet aside for the patties.

2.   Meanwhile, warm a medium skillet over medium heat. Melt another ½ tablespoon of the butter with another ½ tablespoon of the oil. Add the mushrooms, sprinkle with salt, and cook, stirring occasionally, until they release their water and turn golden, 10 to 15 minutes. Transfer to a small bowl; keep warm.

3.   Using your fingers, mix the sage into the ground bison. Divide the meat into 4 equal portions and form into ½-inch-thick patties. Season the patties generously with salt and pepper.

4.   In the same large skillet, melt the remaining 1 tablespoon of butter with the remaining 1 tablespoon of oil over medium-high heat. Add the patties and cook, flipping once, until the burgers reach the desired doneness, 3 to 5 minutes per side for medium-rare (an instant-read thermometer inserted into the center should read 140°F). Top with the cheese for the last minute of cooking to melt it.

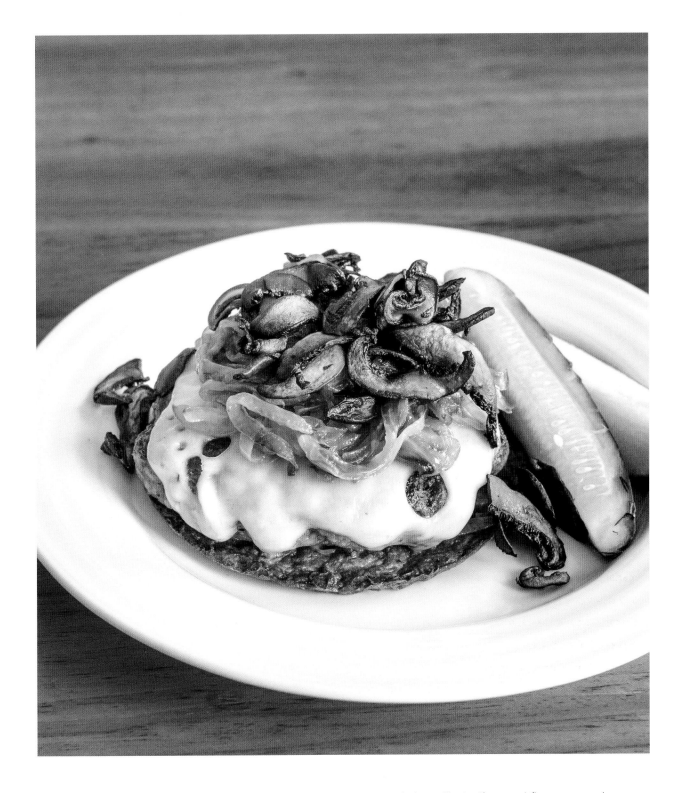

5. To serve, place an English muffin half or cauliflower round on each of four plates. Top each with a burger patty. Divide the onion and mushrooms among the burgers. Serve hot with your favorite condiments and/or pickles, if desired.

BRAISED RABBIT WITH MUSHROOMS AND MUSTARD

SERVES: 4 to 6 | **PREP TIME:** 20 minutes, plus 1 hour to dry-brine rabbit |
COOK TIME: 1 hour 35 minutes

This recipe comes courtesy of Heather Marold Thomason, butcher
extraordinaire and founder of Primal Supply Meats in Philadelphia.
Beth first met Heather (virtually) while interviewing her for an article for
Well+Good and fell in love with Heather's intelligence, thoughtfulness,
and passion for well-raised meat. It comes through in this truly delicious
dish. Take the time to dry-brine the rabbit, which makes it extra juicy
and flavorful; if you're going to the trouble to cook a rabbit, you may
as well get the most out of it. Serve it with Parsnip Mash (page 272),
Cauliflower Rice (page 268), mashed potatoes, or cooked polenta.

1 whole rabbit (3 to 4 pounds),
cut into 6 pieces

Fine sea salt

4 ounces bacon (about 4 slices),
diced

1 tablespoon avocado oil, if
needed

8 ounces shiitake mushrooms,
tough stems removed, caps
sliced (about 4 cups)

1 large onion, diced (about
1¾ cups)

2 tablespoons Dijon mustard

Freshly ground black pepper

1 cup dry white wine

2 cups chicken bone broth

1 teaspoon sherry vinegar

4 sprigs fresh thyme

4 sprigs fresh tarragon

2 tablespoons minced fresh
chives, for garnish (optional)

1.   Pat the rabbit pieces dry and season generously all over with
salt. Place on a plate, cover, and refrigerate for at least 1 hour or up
to overnight.

2.   Preheat the oven to 375°F. Warm a Dutch oven over medium-
low heat. Add the bacon and cook, stirring occasionally, until
it's golden and most of the fat has rendered, 10 to 12 minutes.
Remove the bacon with a slotted spoon and set aside.

3.   Increase the heat under the pot to medium-high. Add the
rabbit and cook, turning, until browned on both sides, 6 to 8
minutes total. (Do not overcrowd the pot; work in batches if
needed.) Remove the browned rabbit pieces to a platter.

4.   If there isn't any fat left in the pot, swirl in a tablespoon of
avocado oil. Add the mushrooms, sprinkle with salt, and cook,
stirring occasionally, until starting to become tender, about
4 minutes. Add the onion, sprinkle with salt, and cook, stirring
often, until the onion and mushrooms are golden and tender, 5 to
6 minutes longer. Stir in the mustard and season with pepper.

5.   Add the wine and stir to deglaze the pot. Stir in the broth,
then bring to a simmer. Remove the pot from the heat and stir in
the vinegar and reserved bacon. Nestle the pieces of rabbit into
the liquid; they should be snug and not quite submerged (pour in
any juices that have collected on the platter). Tuck the herb sprigs
around the rabbit. Cover the pot, transfer to the oven, and bake
until the rabbit is cooked through and fork-tender, about 1 hour.

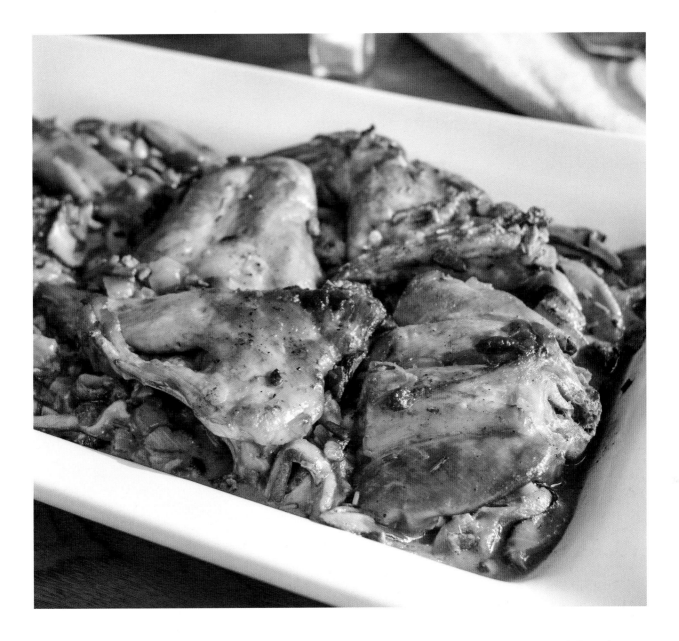

6.   Transfer the rabbit pieces to an ovenproof serving dish and place in the oven while you finish the sauce. Remove the herb sprigs from the braising liquid. Place the Dutch oven over high heat and boil the braising liquid, stirring often, until it reaches a sauce consistency, 6 to 8 minutes. Taste and season with salt and pepper, if needed. Divide the rabbit pieces among four shallow bowls. Top with the mushrooms and sauce, sprinkle with the chives, if using, and serve.

NOTE: ——————————————————————

If you're cutting up the rabbit yourself, the six pieces should be the four legs and the saddle halved.

SAUSAGE AND OSTRICH BOLOGNESE

MAKES: 6 cups (6 to 8 servings) | PREP TIME: 15 minutes | COOK TIME: 1 hour 50 minutes

This rich sauce is a break from tradition in that we used ostrich meat instead of ground beef. Though ostrich is a bird, the meat is red and looks and feels very similar to ground beef; it's also high in vitamins B_6 and B_{12} as well as minerals like iron and zinc. One big difference is that ostrich is much lower in fat, but you won't miss the fat in this sauce, which gets plenty of richness from the olive oil, pork sausage, and a touch of heavy cream. Make this luscious sauce on a Sunday when you have time to let it simmer; you'll be rewarded with amazing aromas. Zucchini noodles (page 270) are a perfect pairing.

2 tablespoons extra-virgin olive oil

1 medium onion, chopped (about 1½ cups)

1 medium carrot, diced (about ½ cup)

1 large rib celery, diced (about ½ cup)

Fine sea salt

8 ounces sweet Italian sausage, casings removed

12 ounces ground ostrich

Freshly ground black pepper

3 cloves garlic, minced (about 1 tablespoon)

2 tablespoons tomato paste

½ teaspoon red pepper flakes

½ cup dry red wine

1 (28-ounce) can crushed tomatoes

2 tablespoons heavy cream, room temperature

2 dried bay leaves

Cooked noodles of choice, for serving

Freshly grated Parmesan cheese, for serving (optional)

1. Warm the olive oil in a large saucepan over medium heat. Add the onion, carrot, and celery, sprinkle with salt, and cook, stirring occasionally, until tender, 5 to 7 minutes. Raise the heat to medium-high, add the sausage, and cook, breaking up the meat, until partway done and the fat begins to render, 4 to 5 minutes. Add the ostrich, season moderately with salt and pepper and cook, stirring and breaking up the meat, until the ostrich and sausage are cooked through and broken up into very small pieces, 4 to 5 minutes longer.

2. Stir in the garlic; cook, stirring, until fragrant, about 1 minute. Stir in the tomato paste and red pepper flakes; cook, stirring, for 1 minute, until heated and well combined. Add the wine and cook, stirring, until nearly cooked off, about 1 minute. Add the crushed tomatoes, stir well, and bring just to a boil. Reduce the heat to low, stir in the cream, tuck in the bay leaves, and let the sauce simmer, uncovered, stirring occasionally, until it thickens, about 1 hour 30 minutes. Remove and discard the bay leaves. Taste and season with salt and pepper.

3. Spoon over noodles and top with grated Parmesan, if desired.

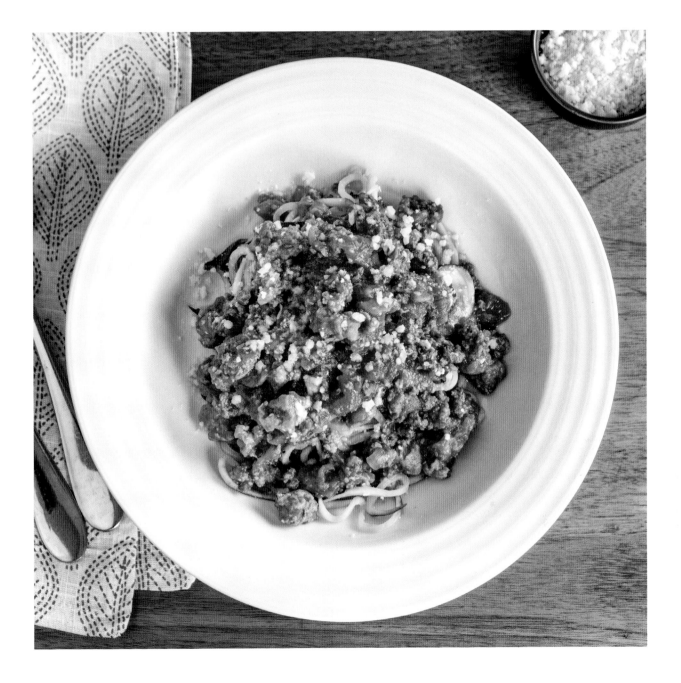

NOTES:

If you're looking to get as much variety into your diet as possible (as we are) but you don't feel like taking a ton of time to learn how to make a kind of meat that's new to you, ostrich is a good option, and ground is the simplest form.

This sauce is delicious the day it's made, but it's even better if it has time to develop. Let it cool, cover, and refrigerate for at least 4 hours or up to overnight. Rewarm gently on the stove.

ELK STEAK SALAD

SERVES: 2 | **PREP TIME:** 15 minutes | **COOK TIME:** 3 minutes

We think everyone should be eating more elk steak. It's similar to beef but more flavorful, though it isn't quite what you'd call gamey. There's something elegant about this game meat, which is why we added it to a sophisticated yet simple salad—although it tastes just as great on its own, sprinkled liberally with salt.

12 ounces top round elk steak

1½ teaspoons fine sea salt

1½ teaspoons freshly ground black pepper

3 tablespoons (1½ ounces) unsalted butter

4 cups mixed salad greens, such as arugula and spinach

1 cup fresh blueberries

2 ounces shelled sunflower seeds, raw or roasted

2 ounces feta cheese, crumbled

1 tablespoon extra-virgin olive oil

1 tablespoon balsamic vinegar

1. Season the elk steak all over with the salt and pepper. Let stand on the counter for about 10 minutes to temper.

2. Melt the butter in a large cast-iron skillet on high heat. Add the steak and sear on each side for 60 to 90 seconds; the inside should still be pink. Transfer the steak to a cutting board, tent with foil, and let rest for 5 to 7 minutes.

3. Meanwhile, make the salad: Put the greens, blueberries, sunflower seeds, and feta in a large bowl. Drizzle with the olive oil and vinegar, season with salt and pepper, if desired, and toss. Divide the salad between two bowls.

4. Slice the steak against the grain into 1-inch-thick strips and divide between the two bowls. Serve right away.

NOTE:

Elk is a delicious and only slightly more adventurous protein for beef lovers. The best way to find elk is to seek out a specialty butcher, order online, or make friends with a hunter. A dark, lean meat, elk is high in protein and low in fat, with a rich taste similar to beef but a little stronger, without any gaminess. Because of its natural rich flavor, it doesn't require much other than a little salt and pepper; in this recipe, a simple salad adds some lightness and texture.

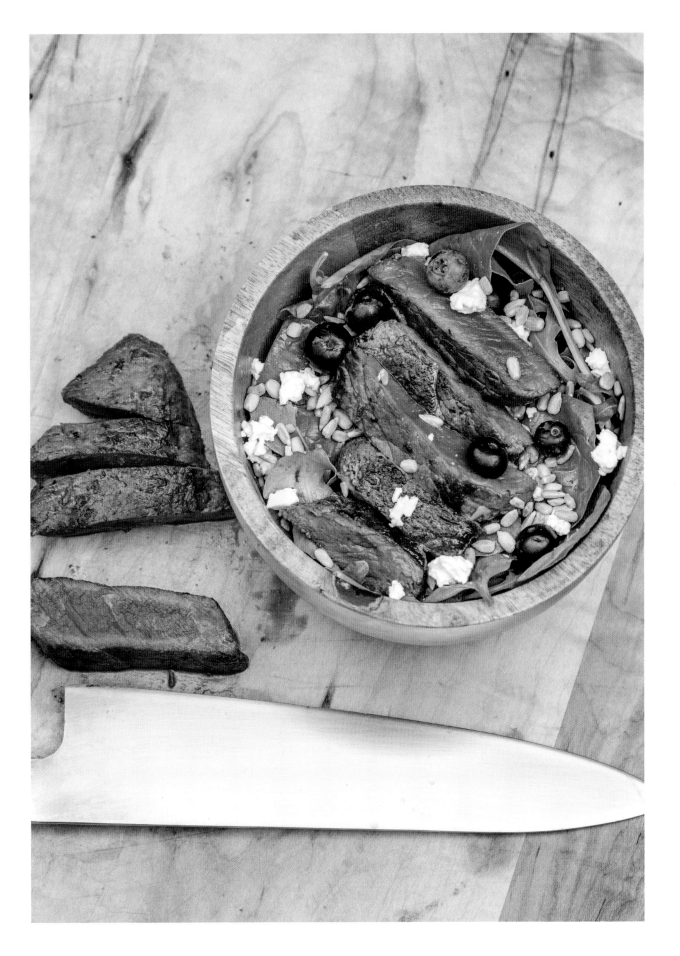

WILD BOAR MEATBALLS

SERVES: 4 | **PREP TIME:** 7 minutes | **COOK TIME:** 20 minutes

If more people knew how delicious wild boar is, it would be on every restaurant menu. Ashleigh first discovered it at a local farmers market and, after making friends with the owners of the boar farm, proceeded to try every cut and preparation she could. With a flavor landing deliciously between pork and beef, wild boar has a minerally richness like red meat with a touch of nutty sweetness like pork. Add the umami cheesiness of Parmesan cheese, and these meatballs have an unforgettable flavor combination. Enjoy them with our Parsnip Mash (page 272) or Cauliflower Rice (page 268).

½ cup pork panko

1 cup heavy cream

1 pound ground wild boar

⅓ cup minced onions

2 cloves garlic, minced (about 2 teaspoons)

¼ cup freshly grated Parmesan cheese (about ¾ ounce), plus more for serving

1 large egg, beaten

1 teaspoon stone-ground mustard

1 teaspoon fine sea salt

½ teaspoon freshly ground black pepper

1. Preheat the oven to 400°F. Line a rimmed baking sheet with parchment paper.

2. In a medium bowl, combine the panko and cream. Stir and set aside to soak for about 5 minutes.

3. Put the ground meat, onions, garlic, Parmesan, egg, mustard, salt, and pepper in a large bowl and use your hands to combine the ingredients. Add the soaked panko (along with the soaking liquid, if there's any left) and mix gently. Moisten your hands and form the mixture into 1-inch balls. Place on the lined baking sheet.

4. Bake the meatballs until browned on the outside and cooked through, turning them over once, 15 to 20 minutes. Serve hot with grated Parmesan.

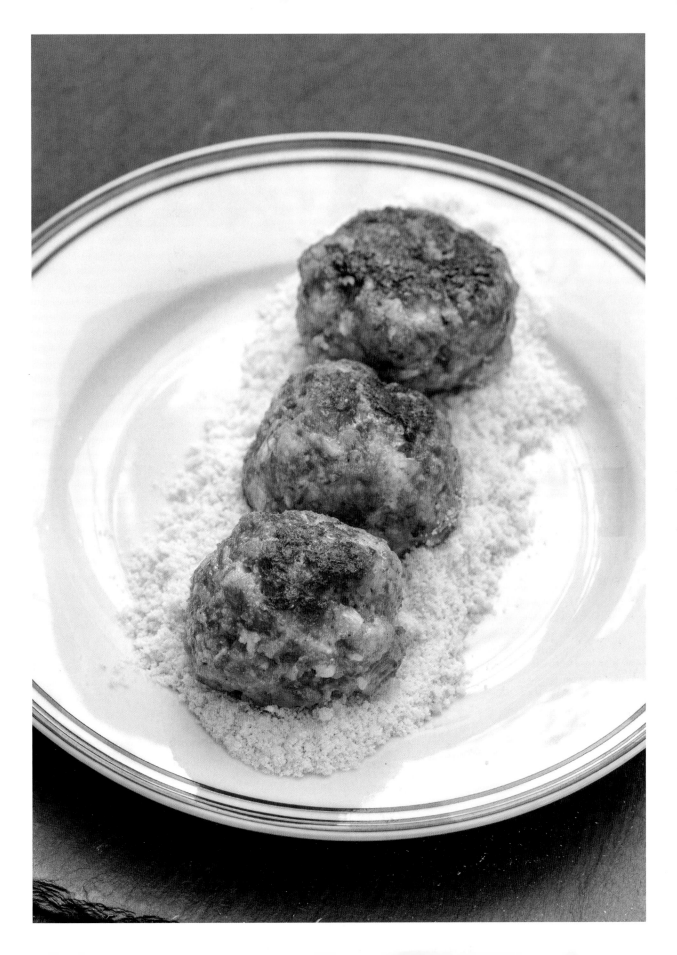

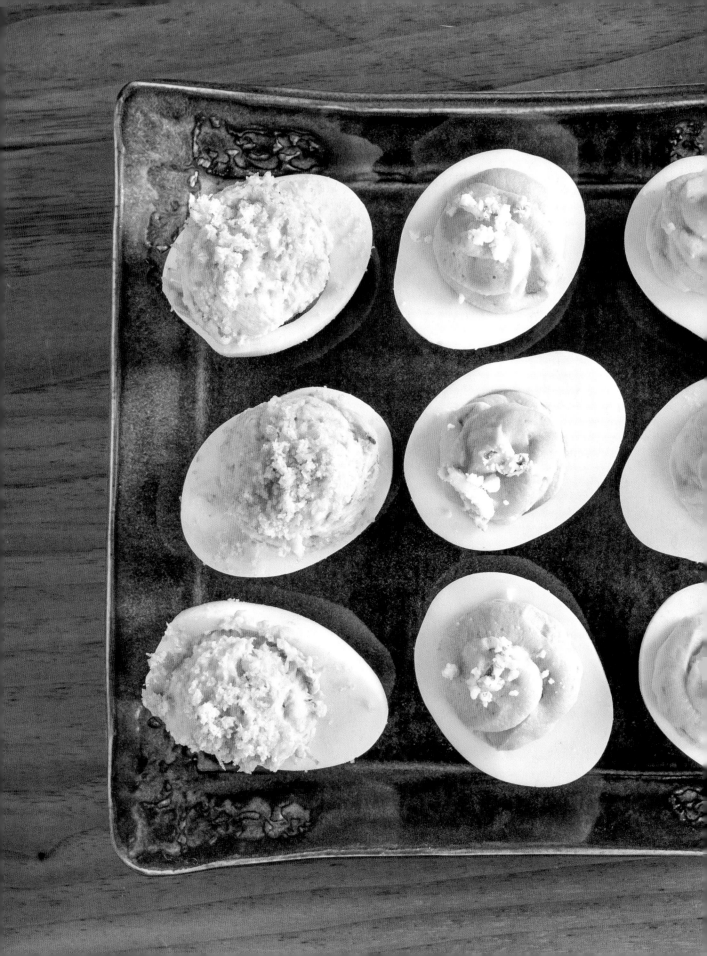

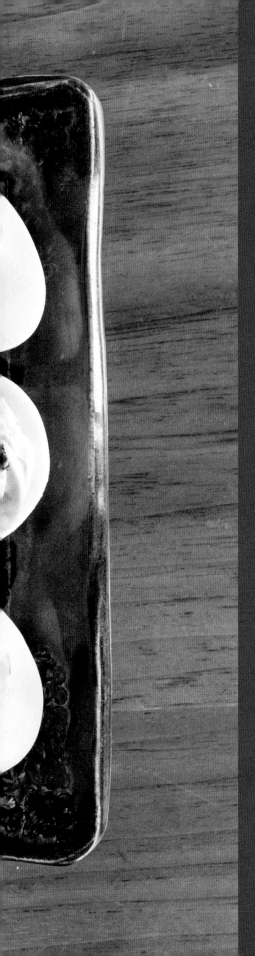

CHAPTER 7:

EGGS

CHEDDAR-CHIVE SOUFFLÉS

SERVES: 4 | **PREP TIME:** 15 minutes | **COOK TIME:** 30 minutes

Soufflés have a rep for being super fussy and difficult, but once you make one, you'll think, "Really? That's it?" The most important thing to remember is that temperature consistency is key, so don't open the oven door until the soufflé is done (if you need to peek, use the oven light). These individual soufflés are fantastic for brunch but also would work for dinner.

3 tablespoons (1½ ounces) unsalted butter, divided

4 tablespoons freshly grated Parmesan cheese (about ¾ ounce)

2 tablespoons cassava flour

Fine sea salt

⅔ cup half-and-half, at room temperature

¾ cup shredded sharp cheddar cheese (about 3 ounces)

½ teaspoon mustard powder

Pinch of cayenne pepper

2 tablespoons minced fresh chives

Freshly ground black pepper

4 large eggs

¼ teaspoon cream of tartar

1. Place a rack in the lowest position of the oven and preheat the oven to 375°F.

2. Melt 1 tablespoon of the butter and brush it all over the insides of four 8-ounce ramekins. Divide the Parmesan evenly among the ramekins and swirl it around until the cheese coats the bottoms and sides. Use a paper towel to wipe off the rims. Refrigerate the ramekins.

3. In a medium saucepan, melt the remaining 2 tablespoons of butter over medium heat. Add the cassava flour, season with a pinch of salt, and whisk until a paste forms. Cook, whisking constantly, until the paste turns light golden, about 30 seconds. Slowly drizzle in the half-and-half, whisking constantly and vigorously, until the mixture is smooth. Reduce the heat to low and cook, stirring and scraping the bottom, sides, and corners of the pan, until the sauce has thickened, about 1 minute (don't let it boil). Remove the pan from the heat and whisk in the cheddar, mustard powder, cayenne, and chives. Whisk until the cheese melts (if it doesn't, place over the lowest heat and whisk until smooth). Taste and season generously with salt and pepper. Transfer to a large bowl.

4. Separate the eggs, placing the yolks in a medium bowl and the whites in a clean, dry large mixing bowl. Whisking vigorously, drizzle a few tablespoons of the cheese sauce into the yolks. Drizzle the yolk mixture back into the sauce, whisking continuously.

5. Using a clean, dry whisk or electric mixer on high speed, beat the whites until they turn foamy. Add the cream of tartar and continue to beat until firm peaks form, 2 to 3 minutes longer.

6. Using a silicone spatula, fold one-fourth of the whites into the yolk mixture. Fold in the remaining whites just until incorporated.

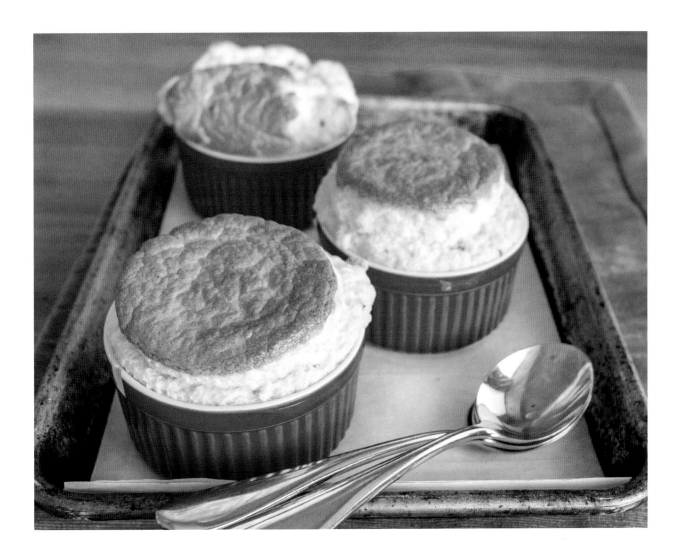

7. Place the ramekins on a rimmed baking sheet. Divide the mixture among the ramekins, filling them about three-quarters full. Bake until the soufflés are puffed and golden, 20 to 23 minutes. Serve immediately.

NOTES:

Make this recipe your own by changing up the cheese and/ or herbs. Gruyère with thyme or sage, Jack with chili powder, Muenster with Dijon mustard and sautéed shallots—the possibilities are endless.

If you're making these for company, prep them in advance. Do everything except beat the egg whites; keep the bowl with the yolk mixture and the bowl with the whites covered and refrigerated. When you're ready to serve, whip the whites and fold in, picking up at Step 5. The soufflés may need a few extra minutes of baking time.

DEVILED EGGS THREE WAYS

It's classic party food—but why wait for a party? Deviled eggs are perfect to whip up on a weekend and keep in the fridge for quick snacks or to go with a meal for an extra shot of protein. There are endless ways to flavor them; here are three of our favorites.

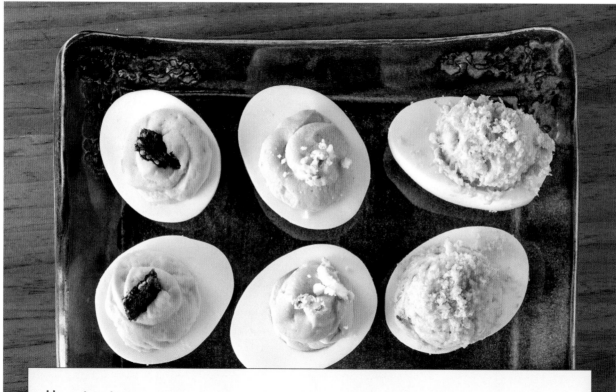

How to steam eggs

We can't believe it took as long as it did for us to try steaming eggs. It takes the same amount of time as traditional hard-cooking, but the eggs are so much easier to peel. No more pulling off whole chunks of the white, no more scraggly-looking deviled eggs, no more keeping eggs in the fridge until they are no longer "too fresh to hard-cook." The steam permeates the shells and gently loosens the whites, so the peels slip right off. Here's how to do it: Put about an inch of water in a saucepan and add a steamer basket. Cover and bring the water to a boil. Lower the heat to medium-low and add the eggs to the basket in a single layer (use tongs so you don't burn your hand). Cover and steam to your desired doneness (9 to 11 minutes will yield yolks that are cooked but still creamy inside, perfect for deviled eggs; go a minute or two longer for more firmly cooked yolks, a few less for softer cooked). Transfer to a bowl of ice water to halt cooking.

Buffalo Deviled Eggs

MAKES: 12 deviled egg halves | **PREP TIME:** 15 minutes

6 hard-cooked large eggs, peeled and halved lengthwise

2 tablespoons avocado oil mayonnaise

1½ tablespoons Frank's RedHot Wings Sauce or other Buffalo-style hot sauce

2 tablespoons crumbled blue cheese, divided

1 medium rib celery, minced (about ¼ cup)

Fine sea salt and freshly ground black pepper

Bacon ranch dip, homemade (page 344) or store-bought, for serving (optional)

1.   Spoon the egg yolks into a medium bowl. Add the mayonnaise, hot sauce, and 1 tablespoon of the blue cheese; mash with a fork until well blended. (Alternatively, you can blend the ingredients in a small food processor.) Fold in the celery. Taste and season with salt and pepper.

2.   Spoon the filling into the egg whites, or place it in a resealable plastic bag, snip off a corner, and pipe the filling into the whites. Crumble the remaining tablespoon of blue cheese on top. Drizzle with bacon ranch dip, if desired, and serve.

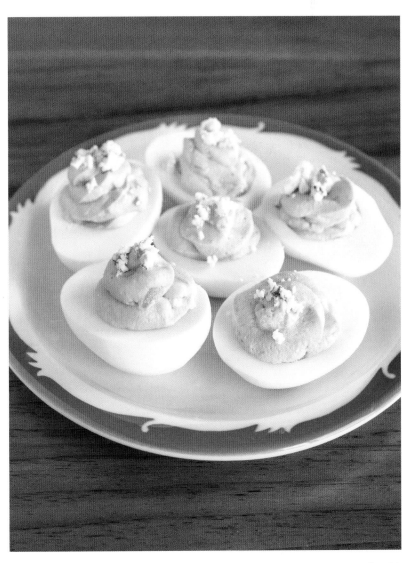

Crab Cake Deviled Eggs

MAKES: 12 deviled egg halves | **PREP TIME:** 20 minutes

2 tablespoons pork panko

1 tablespoon avocado oil

1 tablespoon minced shallots

6 hard-cooked large eggs, peeled and halved lengthwise

2 tablespoons avocado oil mayonnaise

½ teaspoon Dijon mustard

½ teaspoon apple cider vinegar

⅛ teaspoon coconut aminos

Pinch of cayenne pepper (optional)

2 ounces crabmeat, picked over for shells

Fine sea salt and freshly ground black pepper

1. Put the panko in a small unheated skillet. Place over medium-low heat and cook, shaking the pan often, until the panko is lightly toasted, slightly golden, and fragrant, 3 to 4 minutes. Transfer to a cup to cool.

2. Add the avocado oil and shallots to the same skillet. Cook, stirring, until the shallots are tender and fragrant, 1 to 2 minutes. Transfer to a separate cup to cool.

3. Spoon the egg yolks into a medium bowl. Add the mayonnaise, mustard, vinegar, coconut aminos, and cayenne, if using. Mash with a fork until well blended. Stir in the shallots. Fold in the crabmeat. Taste and season with salt and pepper.

4. Spoon the filling into the egg whites. Sprinkle with the toasted panko and serve.

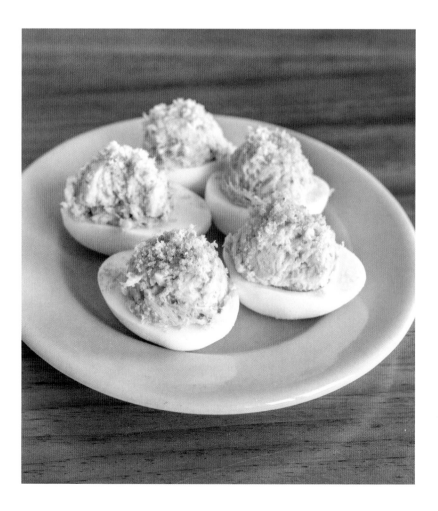

Ginger-Wasabi Deviled Eggs

MAKES: 12 deviled egg halves | **PREP TIME:** 20 minutes

2 tablespoons avocado oil

2 scallions, white and light green parts, minced (about 3 tablespoons)

1 tablespoon minced fresh ginger

1 tablespoon avocado oil mayonnaise

1 teaspoon unseasoned rice vinegar

1 teaspoon coconut aminos

1 teaspoon mirin, plus more if needed

½ teaspoon wasabi paste

Fine sea salt

6 hard-cooked large eggs, peeled, halved lengthwise

12 small pieces torn baked nori (such as SeaSnax), for garnish (optional)

NOTE:

If you don't want to bother with the nori, you can slice the dark green parts of the scallions and garnish the eggs with those instead.

1. Combine the avocado oil, scallions, and ginger in a small unheated skillet. Cook over low heat until the mixture begins to sizzle. Allow to sizzle for 1 minute, then transfer to a medium bowl to cool.

2. Add the mayonnaise, vinegar, coconut aminos, mirin, and wasabi to the bowl with the scallion mixture. Spoon the egg yolks into the bowl. Mash with a fork until well blended. (Alternatively, you can blend the ingredients in a small food processor.) If the mixture needs a little more sweetness, mash in up to 1 teaspoon more mirin. Taste and season with salt.

3. Spoon the filling into the egg whites, or place it in a resealable plastic bag, snip off a corner, and pipe the filling into the whites. Garnish with the nori pieces, if using, and serve.

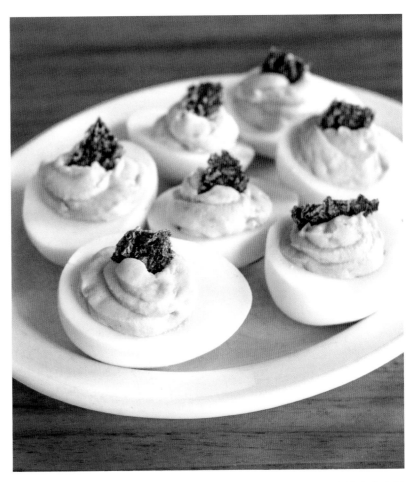

SPICY KIMCHI PICKLED EGGS

MAKES: 6 eggs | **PREP TIME:** 10 minutes, plus 3 days to pickle

Kimchi, a spicy Korean condiment, is a gift: it's tangy and super delicious, and it's fermented, so it's good for gut health. We love it, and we love eggs, so it's no wonder that putting them together is awesome. These eggs make great snacks, or you can turn them into next-level egg salad or add them to Grilled Chicken Heart Cobb Salad (page 262).

1 (16-ounce) jar kimchi, drained, liquid reserved

6 hard-cooked large eggs, peeled

1. Put a layer of kimchi in a 1-quart jar. Place 2 eggs on top. Continue layering the kimchi and eggs until all of the eggs are used up, gently pressing down as you go (be careful here; you don't want to crush the eggs). Top with a final layer of kimchi.

2. Add the reserved kimchi liquid to the jar until the eggs and kimchi are mostly covered. Cover the jar and lightly shake.

3. Refrigerate for 3 days, shaking gently a few times while pickling. Pickled eggs will keep, covered and refrigerated, for up to a month. The longer they sit in the brine, the more pronounced the flavor will get.

NOTES:

If the pieces of cabbage in your kimchi are large, chop them before layering in the eggs. This will help you cover the surface of the eggs more completely.

You can do this with the brine from pickled beets instead of kimchi. The eggs won't be spicy, but they're still really tasty. Bonus: Using beet brine will give the eggs a pretty purple ring around the outsides of the whites.

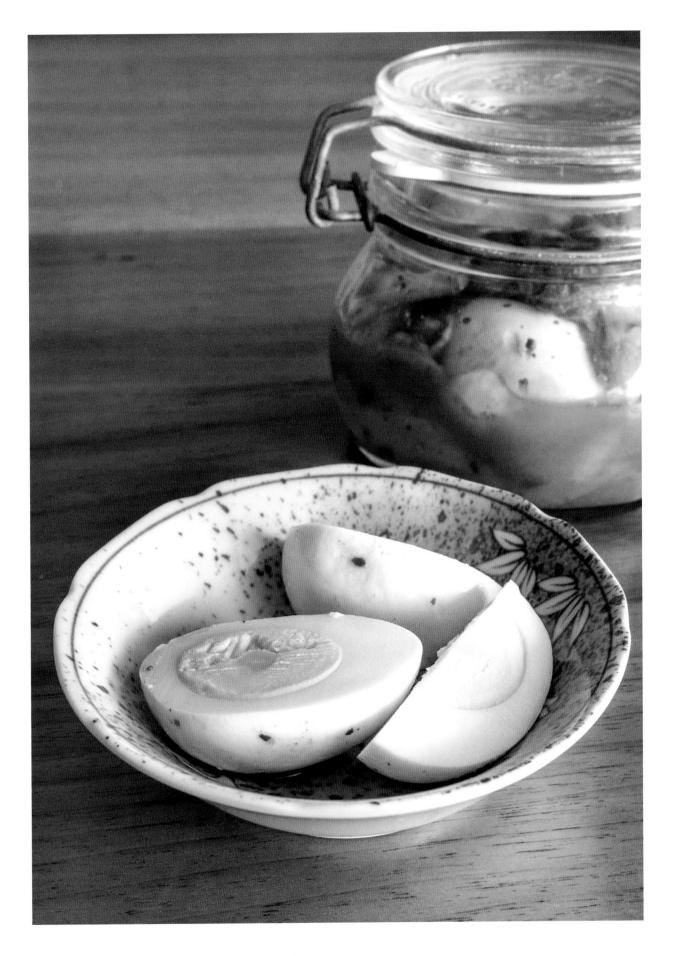

EGG DROP SOUP

MAKES: 5 cups (4 to 6 servings) | **PREP TIME:** 10 minutes | **COOK TIME:** 10 minutes

Beth grew up eating a lot of Chinese food, and egg drop soup was (and still is) a favorite. It manages to be rich, hearty, and slightly complex but also comforting at the same time. Stirring the broth into a whirlpool as you drizzle in the beaten eggs will give you those delicious egg ribbons that make the soup so good.

2 teaspoons arrowroot powder

1 tablespoon avocado oil

2 cloves garlic, minced (about 2 teaspoons)

1 tablespoon grated fresh ginger

3 scallions, sliced on a diagonal (about ⅓ cup; reserve sliced dark green parts for garnish)

4 cups chicken bone broth

2 teaspoons coconut aminos

3 large eggs, beaten

½ teaspoon toasted sesame oil

Fine sea salt and freshly ground black pepper

1. In a small cup, stir the arrowroot with 2 teaspoons of water until smooth.

2. Warm the avocado oil in a medium saucepan over medium heat. Add the garlic, ginger, and white and light green parts of the scallions. Cook, stirring occasionally, until tender and fragrant, about 2 minutes. Pour in the broth and whisk in the arrowroot mixture until it has dissolved. Stir in the coconut aminos.

3. Raise the heat to medium-high and bring the soup just to a boil, 2 to 3 minutes. Turn off the heat. While whisking with one hand to form a whirlpool, use the other hand to slowly drizzle in the beaten eggs, forming ribbons of eggs. Stir in the sesame oil, then taste and season with salt and pepper. Place the pan over medium-low heat and stir to rewarm the soup if needed, about 2 minutes.

4. Ladle the soup into bowls, top with sliced dark green parts of the scallions, and serve.

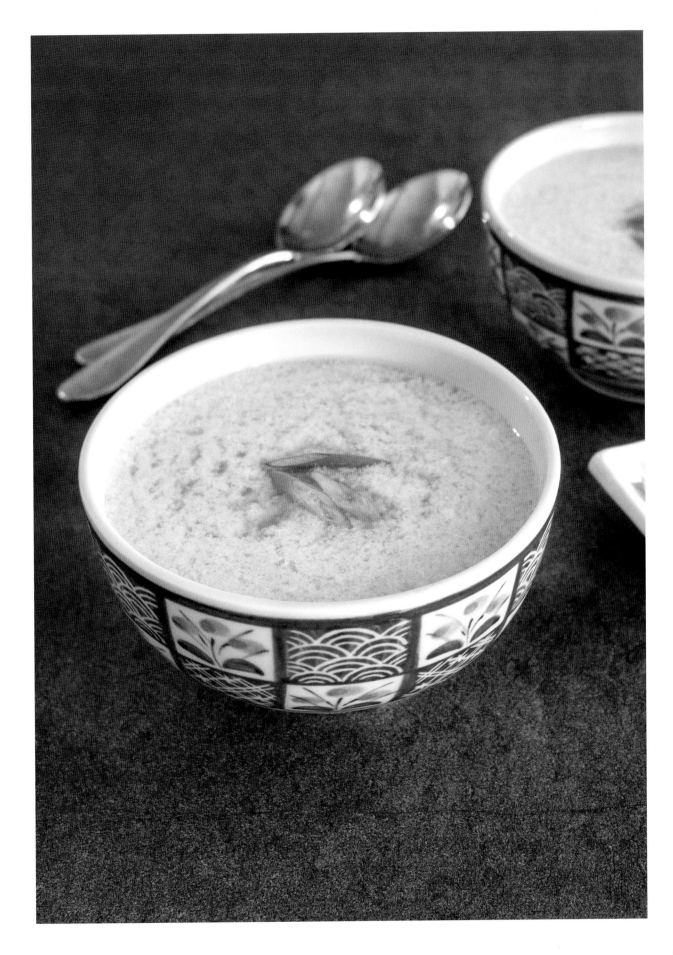

DENVER SCRAMBLE

SERVES: 2 | **PREP TIME:** 10 minutes | **COOK TIME:** 15 minutes

Omelets are lovely, but if you're serving more than one person at a time, omelets can be a hassle. We took the ingredients of a classic Denver omelet and made a scramble instead, so everyone gets to eat at the same time. Canadian bacon, also known as back bacon, is more like ham than what we think of as bacon. It lends a slight sweetness and a gentler flavor than ham. Feel free to swap in ham if you like it better. You can easily double this recipe; it will take a few extra minutes to cook, so plan accordingly.

1 tablespoon ghee or bacon fat

1 small or ½ large onion, chopped (about 1 cup)

1 medium green bell pepper, seeded and chopped (about ¾ cup)

Fine sea salt

3 ounces Canadian bacon, diced

6 large eggs, beaten

Freshly ground black pepper

½ cup shredded sharp cheddar cheese (about 2 ounces)

1. Melt the ghee in a large nonstick skillet over medium heat. Add the onion and bell pepper, season lightly with salt, and cook, stirring often, until tender, about 5 minutes. Add the Canadian bacon and sauté until beginning to brown in spots, about 3 minutes.

2. Reduce the heat to medium-low. Add the eggs, season with salt and pepper, and sprinkle with the cheese. Cook, stirring, until the eggs are cooked to your desired level of doneness; 4 to 5 minutes will give you a scramble that's soft but not wet. Serve hot.

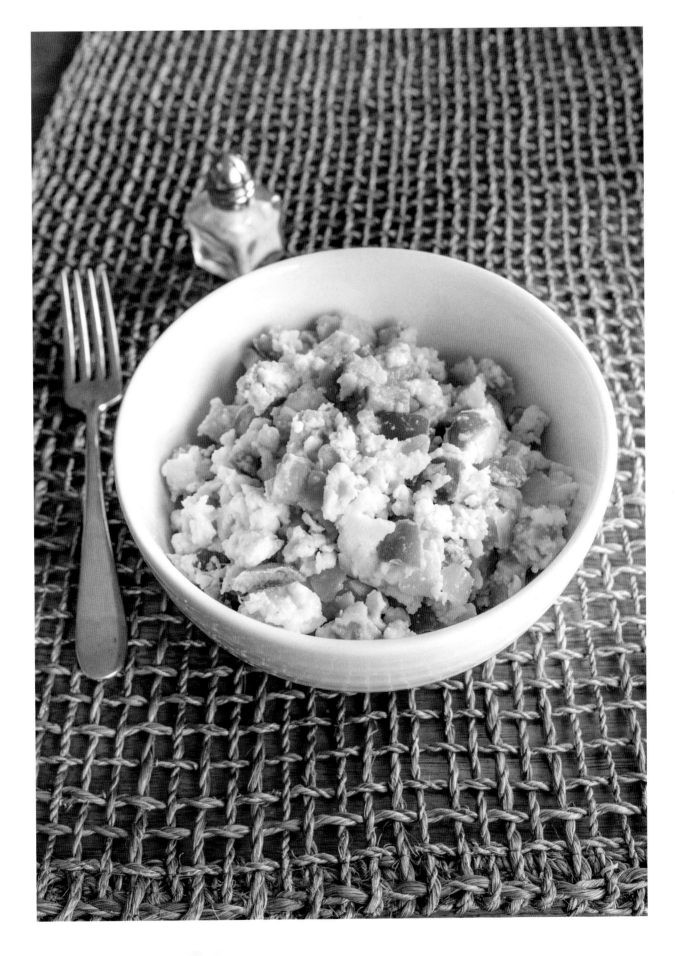

QUICHE LORRAINE

SERVES: 6 | **PREP TIME:** 30 minutes | **COOK TIME:** 1 hour 20 minutes

This classic French dish was already most of the way there, featuring eggs, bacon, cheese, and cream. A crust made from pork panko is the finishing touch it needed to be fully carnivore-ish. This quiche is perfect for special brunch guests, or for a lazy Sunday just for yourself and to enjoy for lunch for a few days.

CRUST:

2 cups pork panko

¾ cup (78 grams) blanched almond flour

¼ cup (36 grams) arrowroot powder

¼ cup (26 grams) flax meal

¼ teaspoon fine sea salt

2 large eggs

FILLING:

4 ounces bacon (about 4 slices)

2 medium shallots, chopped (about 1 cup)

¼ teaspoon plus 1 pinch fine sea salt, divided

3 large eggs

1 cup heavy cream

1 teaspoon fresh thyme leaves

Pinch of ground nutmeg

¼ teaspoon freshly ground black pepper

⅔ cup shredded Gruyère cheese (about 2.6 ounces)

1. Preheat the oven to 375°F.

2. Make the crust: Put the panko in a food processor; process until finely ground. Add the almond flour, arrowroot, flax meal, and salt and pulse to combine. Add the eggs; pulse to mix well. Transfer to a large bowl, then use your hands to finish mixing until the dough just holds together. Press the dough into a 9-inch glass pie plate. Line the crust with parchment paper and fill with pie weights or dried beans. Bake for 10 minutes. Carefully remove the parchment and weights; return the crust to the oven and bake until the edges are turning golden, about 5 minutes longer. Remove the crust from the oven and set aside to cool.

3. Lower the oven temperature to 350°F; place a rimmed baking sheet in the oven.

4. Make the filling: Put the bacon in a large unheated skillet over medium-low heat. Cook, turning once or twice, until browned and crisp, about 10 minutes. Transfer to a cutting board to cool. Pour off all but 1 tablespoon of the fat (reserve for another use, if desired). Add the shallots, season with a pinch of salt, and cook, stirring often, until tender and lightly caramelized, 4 to 5 minutes. Transfer to a small bowl and let cool. Finely chop the bacon.

5. In a medium bowl, whisk together the eggs, cream, thyme, nutmeg, pepper, and remaining ¼ teaspoon of salt. Spread the cheese evenly over the cooled crust. Pour in the custard, then sprinkle with the bacon and shallots. Place the quiche on the hot baking sheet in the oven and bake until the edges are golden and the center jiggles just slightly, 40 to 50 minutes (an instant-read thermometer stuck into the center should read 160°F). Remove to a cooling rack and let cool for at least 1 hour before serving. Keep leftovers covered and refrigerated for up to 3 days.

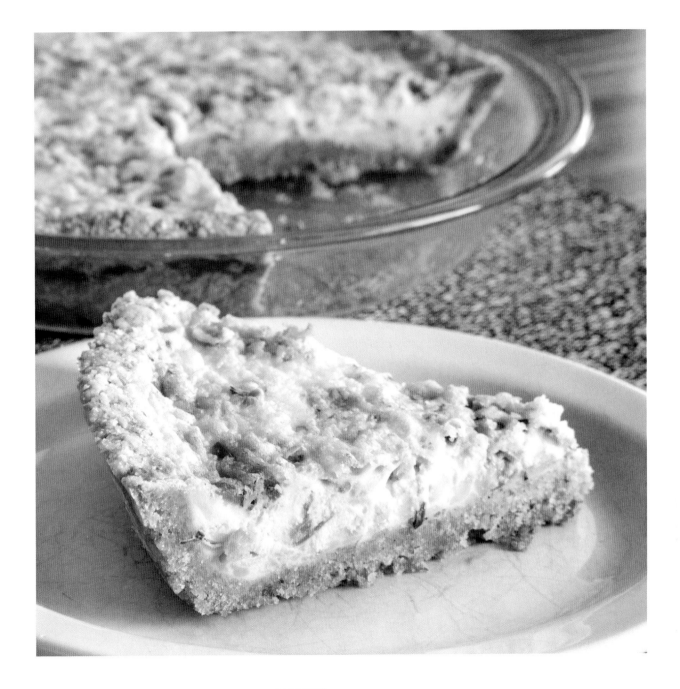

NOTES:

Don't worry if you see fat bubbling out of the crust when it's blind-baking or when you pull the quiche out of the oven. Just leave it alone; it will melt back into the crust as it cools.

To reheat leftover quiche, preheat the oven (or a toaster oven) to 350°F. Take the quiche out of the fridge and let it stand on the counter while the oven preheats. Bake in the pie pan (or, if only warming some of it, place the slices in a baking dish) until warmed through, 15 to 20 minutes. Cover the crust with foil if it starts to brown too much.

CINNAMON BUN CHAFFLES

SERVES: 2 | **PREP TIME:** 15 minutes | **COOK TIME:** 8 minutes

Similar to the paffle on page 294, this low-carb take on a waffle is cheese-based but has a sweet flavor profile. It's like magic: the vanilla protein powder and spices give it a treatlike taste and surprisingly waffle-y texture without all of the carbs and sugar in a typical waffle. These are easy to make and go over great with kids.

1 cup shredded mozzarella cheese (about 4 ounces)

3 tablespoons unsweetened, unsalted sunflower seed butter or nut butter of choice (runnier is better)

2 large eggs

3 tablespoons vanilla-flavored whey protein powder

2 teaspoons ground cinnamon, plus more for sprinkling (optional)

¼ teaspoon vanilla extract

⅛ teaspoon baking powder

⅛ teaspoon stevia extract (optional)

Pinch of fine sea salt

Unsalted butter or Cinnamon and Vanilla–Infused Ghee (page 358) and/or maple syrup, for serving (optional)

1. Preheat a waffle iron to high. In a large bowl, combine the mozzarella, sunflower seed butter, eggs, protein powder, cinnamon, vanilla, baking powder, stevia (if using), and salt.

2. Coat the waffle iron with cooking spray. Spoon half of the batter into the waffle iron, leaving a small gap at the edge to allow the batter to spread. Close the waffle iron and cook until the chaffle is golden brown, about 4 minutes (or as the manufacturer instructs).

3. Open the lid and allow the chaffle to cool for about 30 seconds before carefully removing it at the edges with a silicone spatula and transferring it to a plate. Repeat with more cooking spray and the remaining batter. While warm, sprinkle the chaffles with cinnamon and top with butter, infused ghee, and/or maple syrup, if desired, and serve.

NOTE: ————————————

To ensure your chaffles don't stick, a nonstick waffle iron is ideal; if you're using a waffle iron without a nonstick surface, use a brush to grease it with oil or melted ghee or butter. If using a nonstick waffle iron, remember to use a silicone spatula to avoid scratching it.

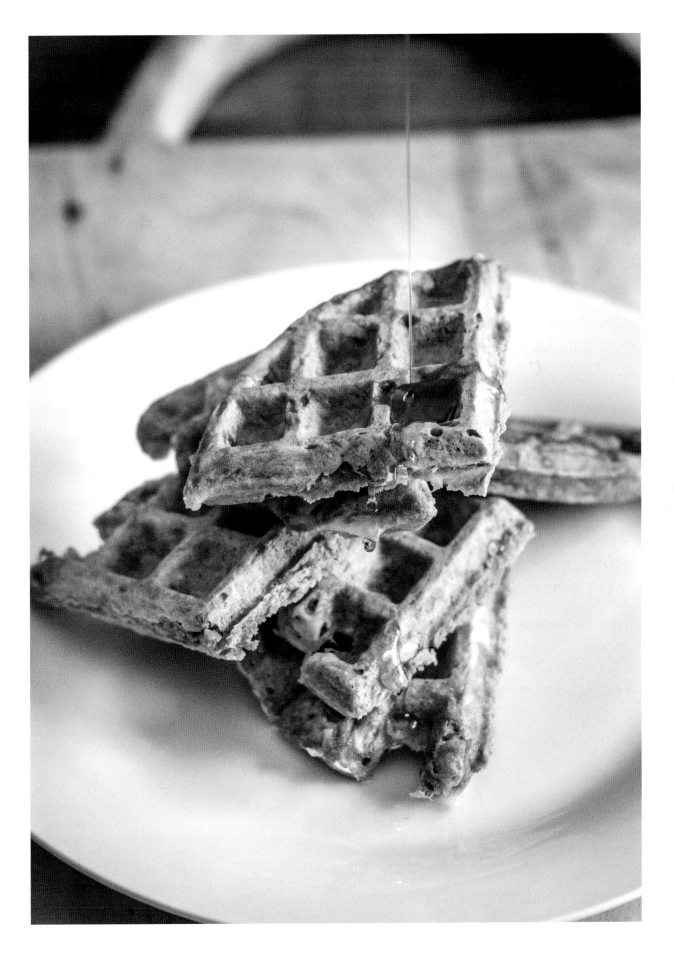

CARAMELIZED ONION AND **LEEK FRITTATA** WITH PROSCIUTTO

SERVES: 4 | **PREP TIME:** 15 minutes | **COOK TIME:** 1 hour 15 minutes

Onions and leeks are in the same botanical family (alliums, thanks for asking), and although they're both antiviral and antibacterial, they taste different. Leeks are milder and more delicate than onions. So combining them in this recipe adds complexity; plus, caramelizing the onion makes it sweet, so it meshes beautifully with the salty prosciutto. If you have leftovers, they're great hot or cold.

3 tablespoons (1½ ounces) unsalted butter, divided

1 small yellow onion, chopped (about 1 cup)

Fine sea salt

2 small leeks, white and light green parts only, trimmed, thoroughly cleaned, and chopped (about ½ cup)

1 bunch hearty greens, such as chard, kale, beet greens, or dandelion greens, torn (about 6 cups)

⅓ cup heavy cream

8 large eggs, beaten

6 thin slices prosciutto, torn

Flaky sea salt and freshly ground black pepper, for finishing

1. Preheat the oven to 375°F.

2. In an 8-inch ovenproof skillet, melt the butter over medium-low heat. Add the onion and a pinch of salt and cook, stirring occasionally, until the onion turns deep brown and caramelizes, about 45 minutes. Add the leeks and greens to the skillet and cook, stirring occasionally, until they have softened, 4 to 5 minutes.

3. Whisk the cream into the beaten eggs, then pour the mixture into the skillet. Scatter the prosciutto pieces on top and cook for about 5 minutes, then transfer to the oven and bake until the eggs are set and a toothpick inserted in the middle of the frittata comes out clean, about 8 minutes longer.

4. Let the frittata cool for 5 minutes. Finish with flaky salt and pepper, slice into wedges, and serve.

NOTE:

To reheat leftover frittata, place it in a baking dish, cover, and warm in a preheated 300°F oven or toaster oven for 10 to 15 minutes. Alternatively, you can steam it for 5 to 10 minutes, which keeps it from drying out.

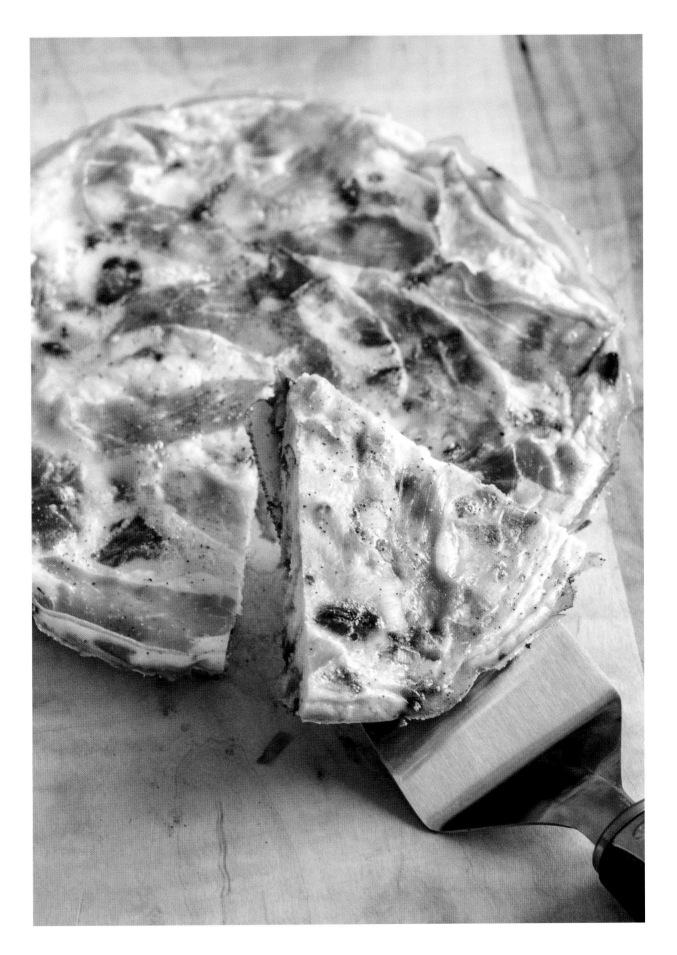

EASY HAM AND EGG MUG OMELETS

SERVES: 2 | **PREP TIME:** 3 minutes | **COOK TIME:** 2 minutes

This recipe proves that you can make a high-protein breakfast (or anytime snack) super quickly, without many steps or a lot of dirty dishes. Switch up the cheese and other additions per your preferences.

4 large eggs

2 ounces honey baked or smoked ham, finely chopped

¼ cup shredded cheddar cheese (about 1 ounce)

Fine sea salt and freshly ground black pepper

1. Mist two 6-ounce microwave-safe mugs or ramekins with cooking spray. In a bowl, whisk the eggs until well blended. Stir in the ham and cheese; season lightly with salt and pepper.

2. Pour the mixture evenly into the mugs and microwave until the eggs are just set in the center, 1½ to 2 minutes. (If they look a little soft in the middle, it's OK; they'll continue to set. You don't want to overcook them and end up with rubbery eggs.)

3. Let stand for a minute, then remove the omelets from the mugs, if desired. Season with additional salt and pepper, if needed, and serve hot.

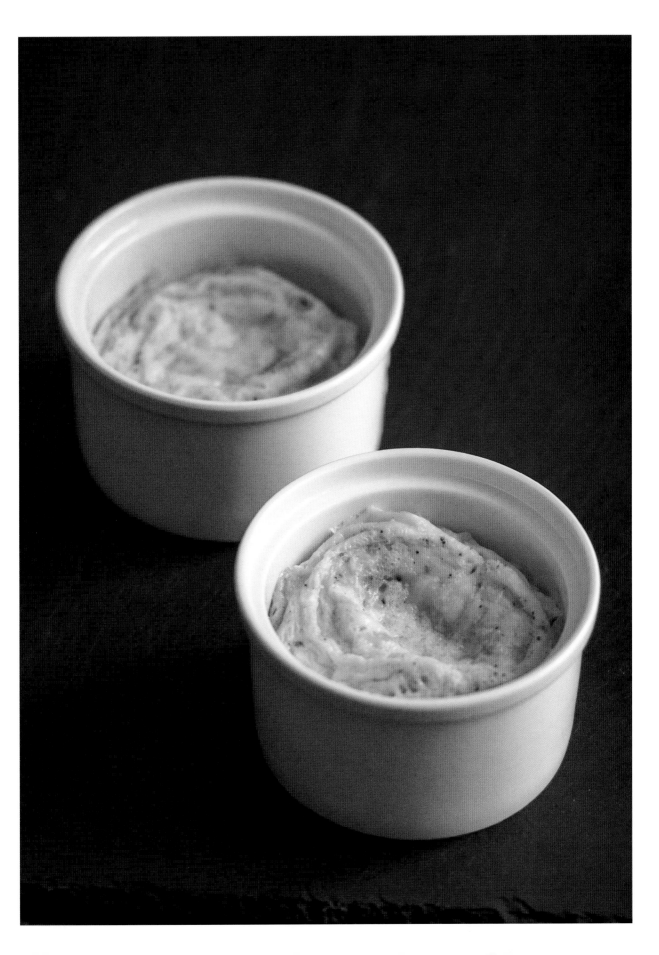

CAULIFLOWER-CHEESE BREAKFAST WRAPS

SERVES: 2 | **PREP TIME:** 10 minutes | **COOK TIME:** 35 minutes

Sometimes, when you make healthier versions of foods you love, you prepare to settle for less than the real thing—maybe the texture is slightly off or the flavor isn't quite there. We're happy to say that with these homemade wraps, you won't feel like you're settling, because they are truly delicious as well as healthy. They hold up well when filled with your favorite breakfast foods and have a pleasantly savory, chewy bite. They can be made a day or so ahead of time, stored in an airtight container in the fridge, and reheated in the oven or in a skillet for a few minutes. We oven-bake the bacon for this recipe because it's a more hands-off method (since the recipe has so many other moving parts), but frying it in a skillet works just as well.

WRAPS:

1 medium head cauliflower, separated into florets, or 1 (12-ounce) package frozen riced cauliflower, thawed

2 large eggs

½ cup shredded mozzarella cheese (about 2 ounces)

½ teaspoon cornstarch

½ teaspoon fine sea salt

FILLING:

4 ounces bacon (about 4 slices)

2 teaspoons unsalted butter, divided

½ white or sweet onion, finely chopped (about ½ cup)

Fine sea salt

4 large eggs, beaten

Freshly ground black pepper

2 cups spinach, large stems removed

Hot sauce, for serving (optional)

1. Make the wraps: Preheat the oven to 375°F and line a rimmed baking sheet with parchment paper.

2. If using frozen riced cauliflower, skip ahead to Step 3. Pulse the cauliflower florets in a food processor until they are the consistency of rice. Transfer the riced cauliflower to a large microwave-safe bowl, cover, and microwave on high for 8 to 10 minutes, or until cooked. (Alternatively, steam the rice using your favorite method.) Let stand until the cauliflower is cool enough to handle.

3. Transfer the cauliflower rice to a cheesecloth or clean kitchen towel, roll up, and squeeze tightly to get rid of as much extra liquid as possible. It should be dense and clumpy.

4. Return the cauliflower to the food processor. Add the eggs, mozzarella, cornstarch, and salt. Process until smooth, about 1 minute.

5. Divide the cauliflower mixture into two equal portions and place on the lined baking sheet. Use a silicone spatula or the back of a spoon to spread into thin circles, about ½ inch thick and 7 inches across. Bake until the edges are dry and the bottoms are golden, about 10 minutes. Carefully flip over, then bake until fully set and cooked through but not crisp, 5 minutes longer. Remove

(continues on page 219)

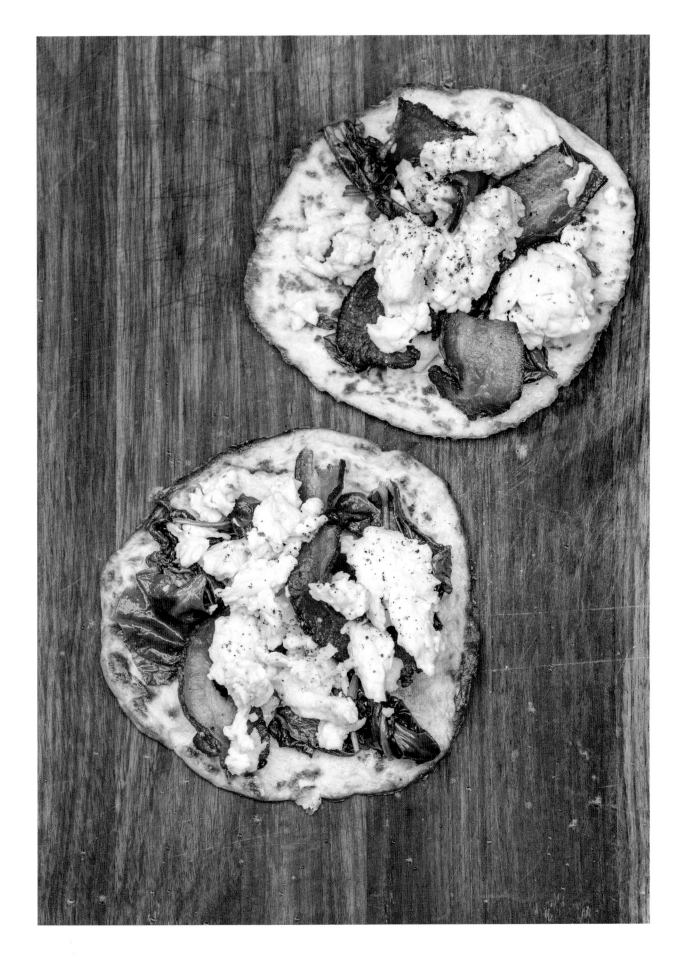

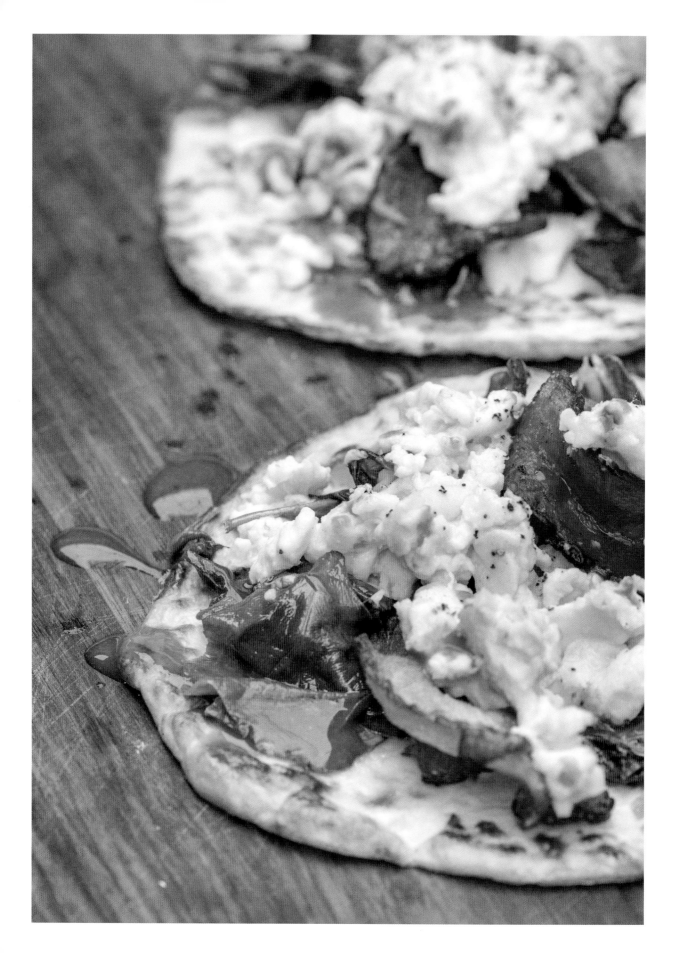

the wraps and increase the oven temperature to 400°F. (*Note:* You can toast the wraps in a dry skillet over high heat for a few minutes to brown and crisp them before serving, if desired.)

6. Make the filling: Line a rimmed baking sheet with parchment paper, then place a cooling rack inside the lined baking sheet. Lay the bacon strips on the rack. Bake the bacon for 12 to 15 minutes, or until it reaches your desired level of doneness.

7. Meanwhile, cook the eggs and spinach: Melt 1 teaspoon of the butter in a medium nonstick skillet over medium-low heat. Add the onion, sprinkle with salt, and cook, stirring occasionally, until tender and translucent, about 5 minutes.

8. Season the beaten eggs with salt and pepper, give them a quick whisk, and pour into the skillet. Use a silicone spatula to continuously swirl the eggs in small circles around the pan, until they have thickened slightly and very small curds have begun to form, 30 seconds to 1 minute. When the eggs are softly set and slightly runny in places, remove the pan from the heat and let stand for a few seconds to finish cooking the eggs. Remove the eggs from the pan.

9. Add the remaining teaspoon of butter to the skillet, then add the spinach, sprinkle with salt, and cook, stirring, until wilted, 3 to 4 minutes.

10. Place the wraps on two plates. Top each with half of the spinach, bacon, and eggs. Sprinkle with hot sauce, if desired.

CREAMY SCRAMBLED EGGS
WITH SMOKED SALMON

SERVES: 2 | **PREP TIME:** 15 minutes | **COOK TIME:** 7 minutes

Ashleigh is from Nova Scotia and Beth is from New York—we couldn't *not* include a smoked salmon recipe. This one is classic, simple, and approved by the most discerning smoked salmon lovers (us).

4 large eggs

1 tablespoon milk, heavy cream, or unsweetened full-fat coconut milk

1 tablespoon (½ ounce) unsalted butter

2 small leeks, white and light green parts only, trimmed, thoroughly cleaned, and diced (about ½ cup)

½ cup crumbled fresh (soft) goat cheese (about 3 ounces)

Flaky sea salt and freshly ground black pepper

4 ounces smoked salmon

1.   In a large bowl, whisk together the eggs and milk. Melt the butter in a medium nonstick skillet over medium-low heat. When the butter begins to bubble, add the leeks and cook, stirring often, until softened and translucent, about 3 minutes.

2.   Pour the egg mixture into the skillet and use a silicone spatula to continuously swirl the eggs in small circles around the pan until they have thickened slightly and very small curds have begun to form, 30 seconds to 1 minute. Change from making circles to making long sweeps across the pan with the spatula until you see larger, creamy curds, about 20 seconds.

3.   When the eggs are softly set and slightly runny in places, remove the pan from the heat and let stand for about 30 seconds to finish cooking the eggs (this keeps them from overcooking and becoming rubbery).

4.   Divide the eggs between two plates, top with the goat cheese, and sprinkle lightly with salt and pepper. Serve the salmon alongside the eggs.

NOTE: ─────────────────────────

> *Swap in the green parts of 2 scallions for the leeks if you prefer.*

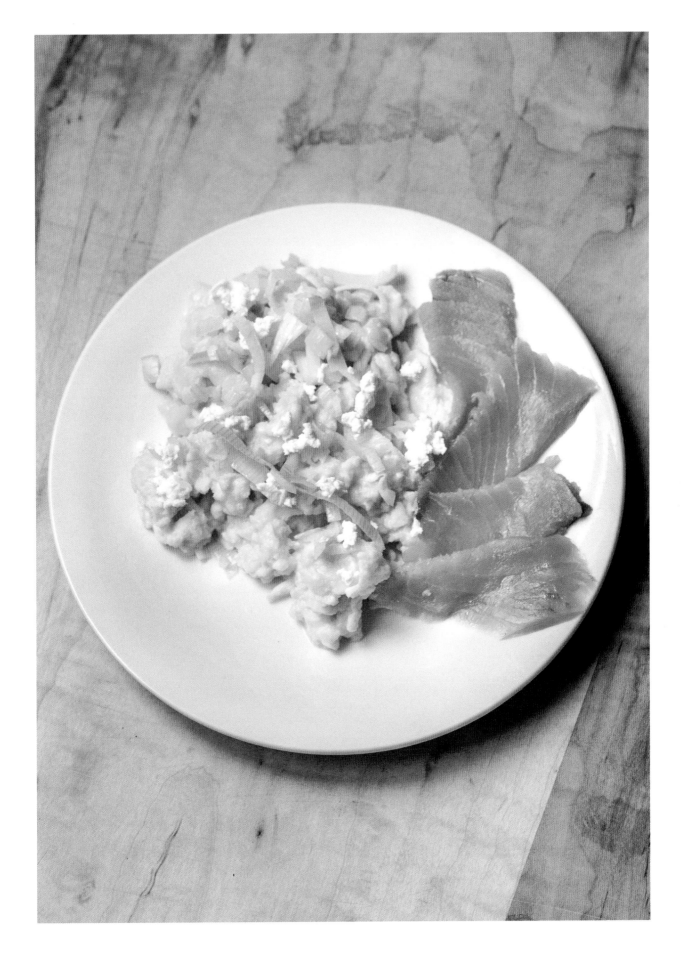

CARNIVORE BAKED SCOTCH EGGS

MAKES: 6 eggs | **PREP TIME:** 15 minutes | **COOK TIME:** 20 minutes

Scotch eggs, a popular picnic snack in the UK, are a meat lover's dream: hard- or soft-boiled eggs wrapped in sausage. It's portable protein at its most delicious. We made this traditional dish our own by using pork panko rather than breadcrumbs in the meat coating and baking rather than deep-frying the eggs. In our experience, a couple of these for lunch will keep you full and energized for quite a while.

1 pound ground pork (can substitute chicken, turkey, or beef)

1 raw large egg

½ cup pork panko, plus more for topping if desired

6 hard-cooked or soft-boiled large eggs, peeled

1. Preheat the oven to 350°F. Line a rimmed baking sheet with parchment paper.

2. Combine the ground pork, raw egg, and panko in a large bowl. Using wet hands, form the mixture into 6 equal portions; roll into balls. Place the meatballs on the baking sheet and press flat with your hand to a ¼-inch thickness.

3. Place a boiled egg in the middle of each flattened meatball and mold the meat around the egg, leaving no gaps. Sprinkle the wrapped eggs with panko, if desired.

4. Bake until the outsides begin to turn brown, about 10 minutes. Carefully flip over with tongs and bake until the meat is cooked through and browned, about 10 minutes longer. Serve right away, or let cool to room temperature before storing in an airtight container in the fridge. They taste great cold or hot.

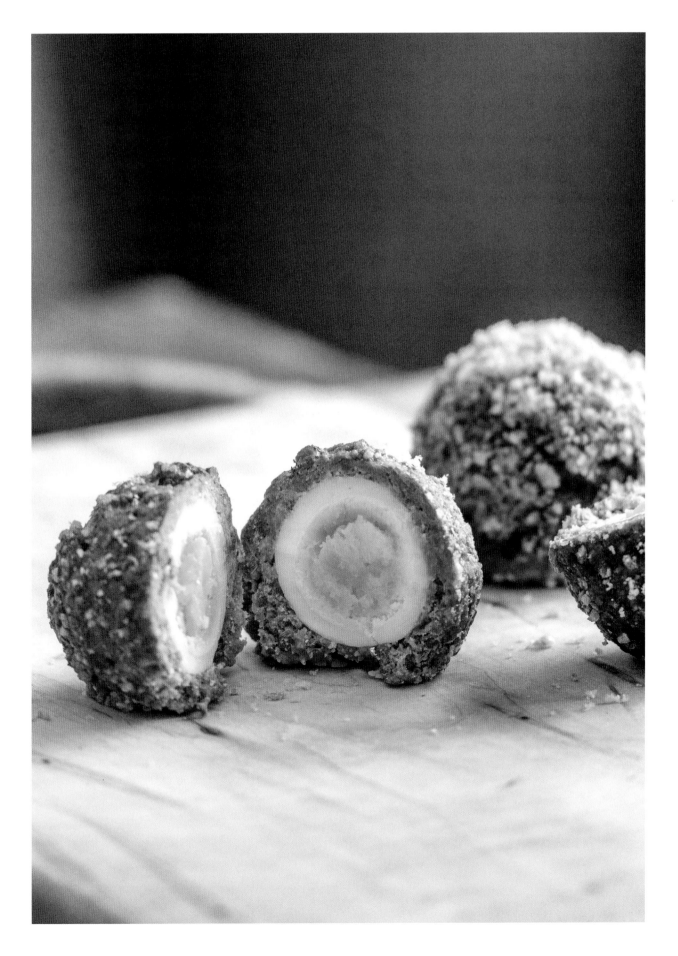

STEAK AND EGGS WITH LEMON "HOLLANDAISE" SAUCE

SERVES: 4 | **PREP TIME:** 10 minutes | **COOK TIME:** 20 minutes

Steak and eggs are a staple in any protein-forward diet, and we have added a little zing with our bright, lemon-forward take on traditional hollandaise. Have it for brunch, for dinner—it's hearty and satisfying any time of day.

STEAK AND EGGS:

1 pound hanger or sirloin steak (about 1 inch thick)

Fine sea salt and freshly ground black pepper

4 tablespoons (2 ounces) unsalted butter, divided

8 large eggs

SAUCE:

¼ cup extra-virgin olive oil

2 teaspoons fresh lemon juice

½ teaspoon flaky sea salt

2 large egg yolks

⅛ teaspoon turmeric powder (optional, for color)

1. Remove the steak from the fridge and let it come to room temperature, about 30 minutes. Preheat the oven to 350°F. Rub the steak with 1½ teaspoons of salt and 1 teaspoon of pepper.

2. Make the sauce: In the top of a double boiler over medium heat, whisk together the olive oil, lemon juice, salt, egg yolks, and turmeric, if using. Continue whisking vigorously until the sauce is hot and thickened enough to coat the back of a wooden spoon, about 5 minutes. Make sure to whisk continuously so the yolks don't cook. Pull the pan off the heat and transfer the sauce to the top of the double boiler, allowing the hot water to keep it warm, stirring every few minutes to keep the sauce from separating.

3. Preheat a large cast-iron skillet over medium heat until hot. Raise the heat to high and melt 2 tablespoons of the butter. Put the steak in the skillet and cook, turning once, until well browned yet medium-rare on the inside, about 2 minutes per side.

4. Transfer the steak to a cutting board. Cover loosely with foil and let rest for 10 minutes before carving.

5. While the steak is resting, cook the eggs. Preheat 2 large skillets over medium-low heat. Melt 1 tablespoon of the remaining butter in each pan, then crack 4 eggs into each pan. Season the eggs lightly with salt and pepper and cook until the whites are just set, about 3½ minutes. (If you want the yolks to be cooked through, cover and continue cooking for 1 to 2 minutes longer.) Divide the eggs among four plates.

6. Cut the steak against the grain into 1-inch thick slices. Divide among the plates, drizzle with the sauce, and serve.

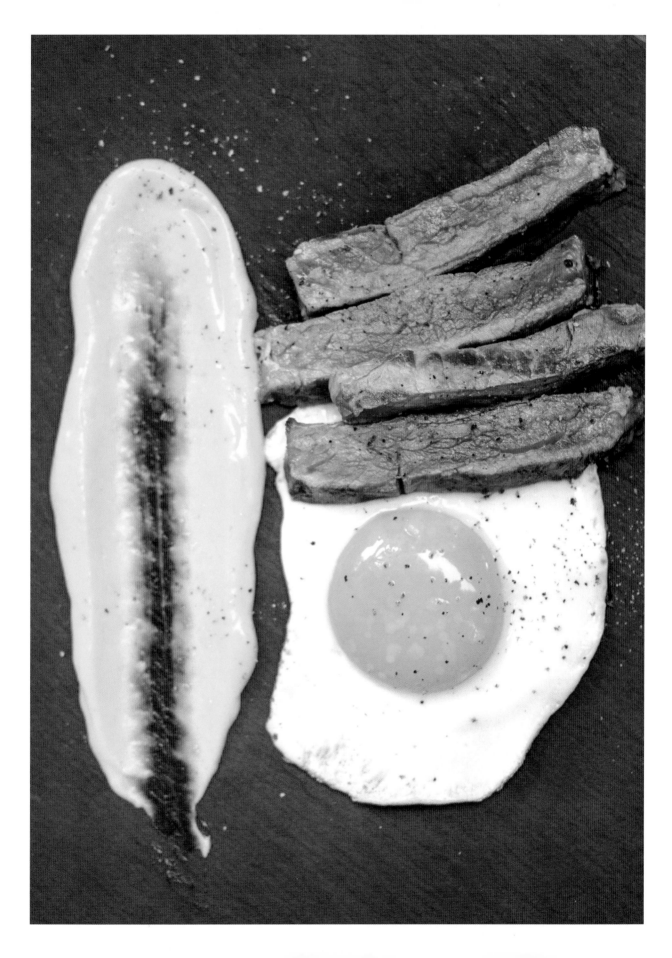

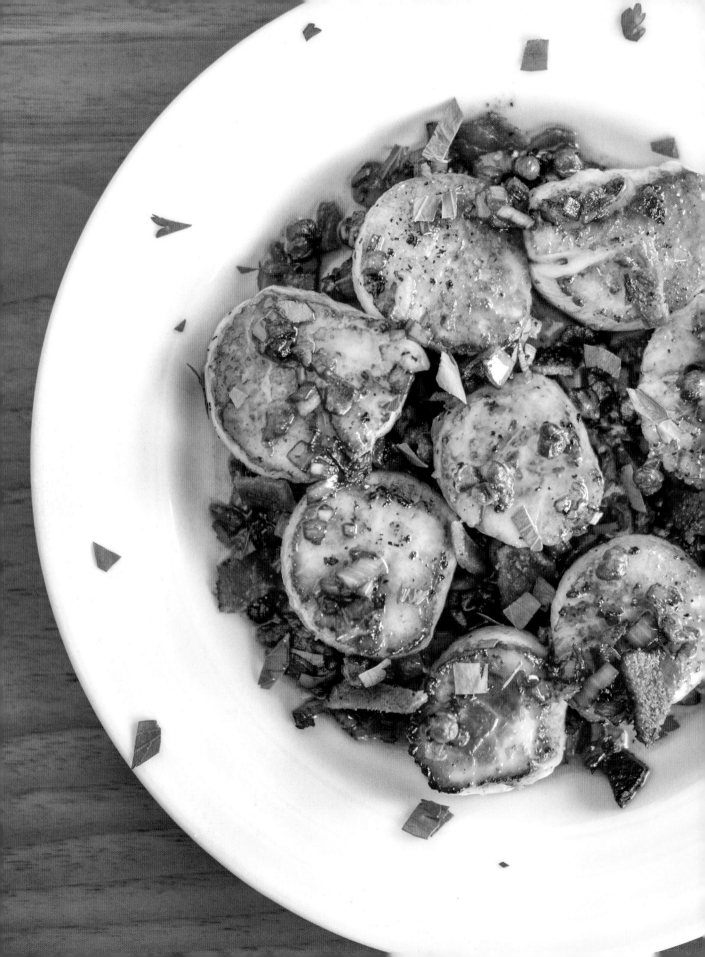

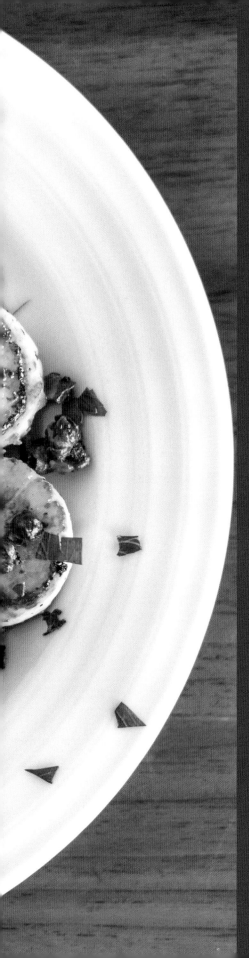

CHAPTER 8:
SEAFOOD

LEMON-TARRAGON LOBSTER SALAD

SERVES: 2 (4 as an appetizer) | **PREP TIME:** 25 minutes | **COOK TIME:** 2 minutes

Bright, aromatic tarragon is a great match with lobster, which is mildly flavored but meaty enough to stand up for itself. A little tarragon goes a long way. If you don't care for it, leave it out, or swap in an equal amount of chopped fresh dill.

1½ tablespoons extra-virgin olive oil

1 small shallot, minced (about 2 tablespoons)

1 pound cooked lobster meat, patted dry and torn or chopped

2 tablespoons avocado oil mayonnaise

1 medium rib celery, minced (about ¼ cup)

2 tablespoons fresh lemon juice

1½ teaspoons finely chopped fresh tarragon

¼ teaspoon coconut aminos

Fine sea salt and freshly ground black pepper

Endive spears, grain-free crackers, homemade (page 308) or store-bought, or Boston lettuce cups, for serving (optional)

1. Combine the olive oil and shallot in a small unheated skillet. Place over low heat and cook until the mixture begins to sizzle. Allow to sizzle for 1 minute more, then transfer the mixture to a small bowl to cool.

2. Put the lobster, mayonnaise, celery, lemon juice, tarragon, and coconut aminos in a large bowl. Add the cooled shallot and fold together until all of the ingredients are combined and the lobster is lightly coated. Taste and season with salt and pepper. (You can make the salad up to 1 day ahead; keep it covered in the fridge. Stir gently before serving.)

3. Serve the salad with endive spears or crackers or spooned into lettuce cups, if desired.

NOTE:

You can buy precooked lobster meat, usually frozen, at fishmongers and high-end supermarkets. In general, if you take apart a whole lobster, 20 to 25 percent will be meat. To get the 1 pound of meat needed for this recipe, you would need to cook 4 to 4½ pounds of fresh whole lobster.

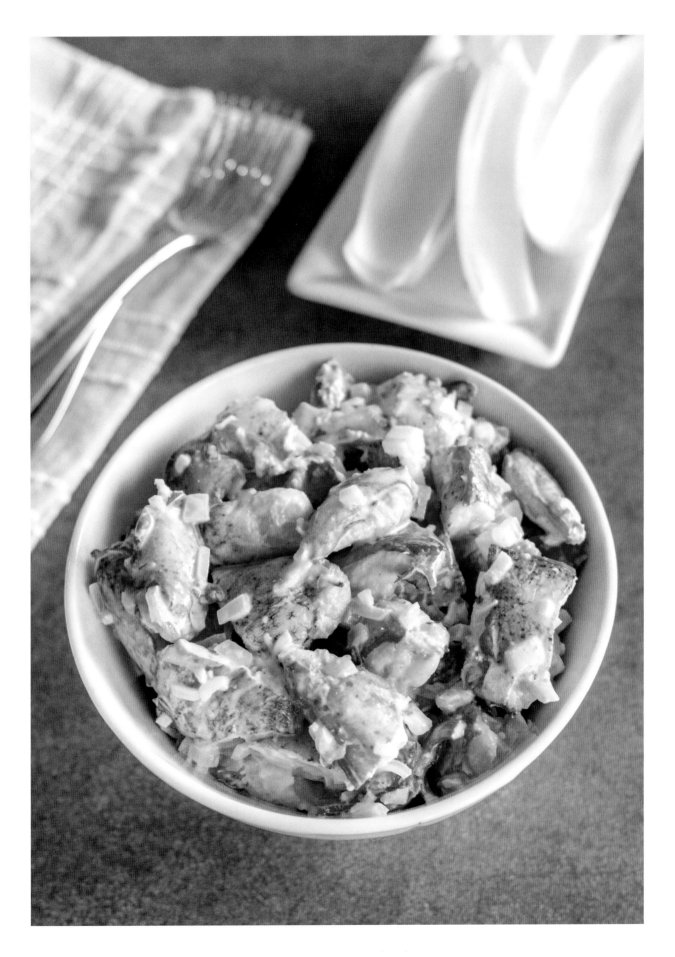

LEMON-GARLIC BUTTER ROASTED COD

SERVES: 4 | **PREP TIME:** 15 minutes | **COOK TIME:** 12 minutes

When you make this recipe, it's going to seem like a lot of butter. That's because it *is* a lot of butter. Just go with it; trust us on this one. Don't skip the capers, either. Though the dish doesn't taste caper-y, they add a hint of brine that really elevates the meal.

4 tablespoons (2 ounces) unsalted butter, at room temperature

4 cloves garlic, minced (about 1 tablespoon plus 1 teaspoon)

2 tablespoons chopped fresh flat-leaf parsley

1 teaspoon drained capers, chopped

1 lemon, scrubbed and dried

Fine sea salt and freshly ground black pepper

4 (6-ounce) skinless cod fillets, patted dry

1. Preheat the oven to 400°F. Oil a 9 by 13-inch baking dish.

2. In a small bowl, mash the butter, garlic, parsley, and capers with a fork (alternatively, if you have a small food processor, you can blend the ingredients). Grate 1 teaspoon of zest off the lemon; stir the zest into the mixture. Taste and season with salt and pepper.

3. Thinly slice the lemon and remove any seeds. Put the fish fillets in the prepared baking dish, then season all over with salt and pepper. Spread about 1 tablespoon of the garlic butter over each piece of fish. Top each with 2 or 3 lemon slices. Roast until the fish is just cooked through and flakes easily with a fork, 10 to 12 minutes. Serve hot.

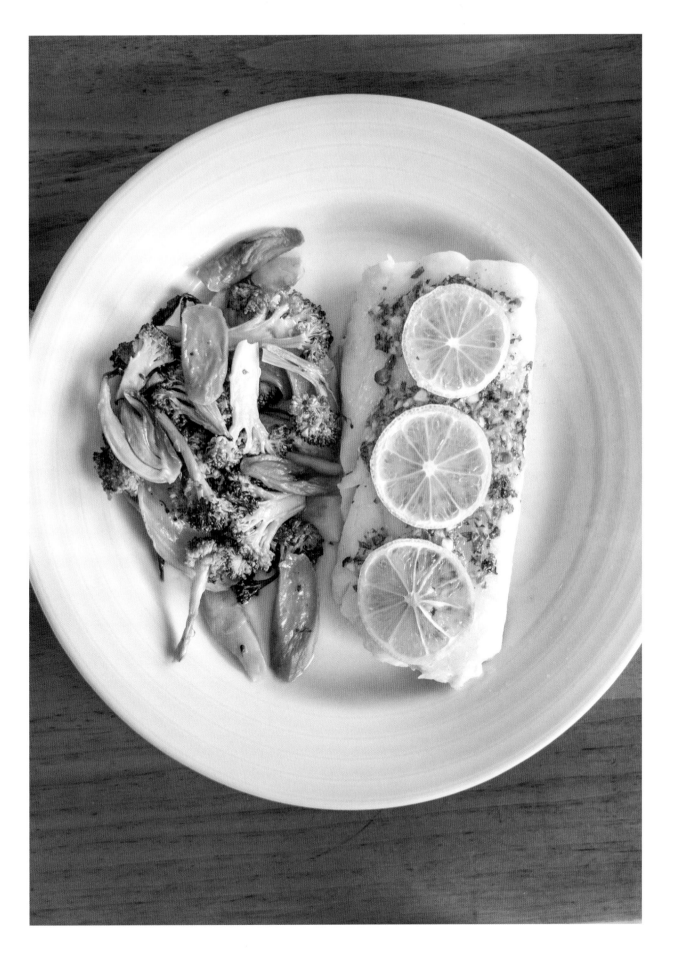

SEARED SCALLOPS WITH BACON, FRIED CAPERS, AND SHALLOT BUTTER

SERVES: 4 | **PREP TIME:** 15 minutes | **COOK TIME:** 20 minutes

Bacon-wrapped scallops always sound good, but it can be tricky to get it just right so the bacon is crisp and the scallops aren't overcooked. So we decided to deconstruct it: you cook the bacon and the scallops exactly right and *then* put them together. As for the shallot butter, we basically want to drizzle it over our whole lives. Make sure you have all of the ingredients ready to go before you start cooking; everything happens really quickly.

4 ounces bacon (about 4 slices)

2 tablespoons drained capers, patted dry

1½ pounds sea scallops, muscle removed (see opposite) and thoroughly patted dry

Fine sea salt and freshly ground black pepper

¼ cup dry white wine

4 tablespoons (2 ounces) unsalted butter

1 medium shallot, minced (about ⅓ cup)

3 cloves garlic, minced (about 1 tablespoon)

1 to 2 tablespoons chopped fresh flat-leaf parsley

Lemon wedges, for serving

1. Put the bacon in a large unheated cast-iron skillet over medium-low heat. Cook until the fat has rendered and the bacon is crisp, about 10 minutes. Transfer the bacon to a cutting board and crumble or chop. Drain all but 1 tablespoon of the bacon fat; reserve the extra fat. (*Note:* If your bacon doesn't render much fat, top it up as needed with avocado oil.)

2. Raise the heat to medium-high. Add the capers to the skillet and cook, stirring, until golden, about 2 minutes. Transfer to a small plate. Swirl 1 tablespoon of the reserved bacon fat in the skillet. Season the scallops with salt and pepper and cook, flipping once, until well seared on both sides, 1 to 2 minutes per side. Transfer to a plate and keep warm.

3. Lower the heat to medium. Add the wine to the skillet; cook, stirring, until reduced to 1 tablespoon, about 1 minute. Melt the butter in the skillet. Add the shallot and garlic, season with a pinch of salt, and cook, stirring, until tender, 1 to 2 minutes.

4. Divide the scallops among four plates. Top with the garlic butter sauce. Sprinkle the bacon, capers, and parsley over the scallops. Serve hot, with lemon wedges.

A muscle you don't want

When prepping scallops, you'll notice most have a side muscle—that is, a flap of flesh on one side that sticks out a little and feels a bit tougher than the rest of the scallop. All you have to do is grasp it with your fingers and pull it off. Don't worry if you find some scallops without the side muscle; most likely it came off when the scallop was harvested or in transit.

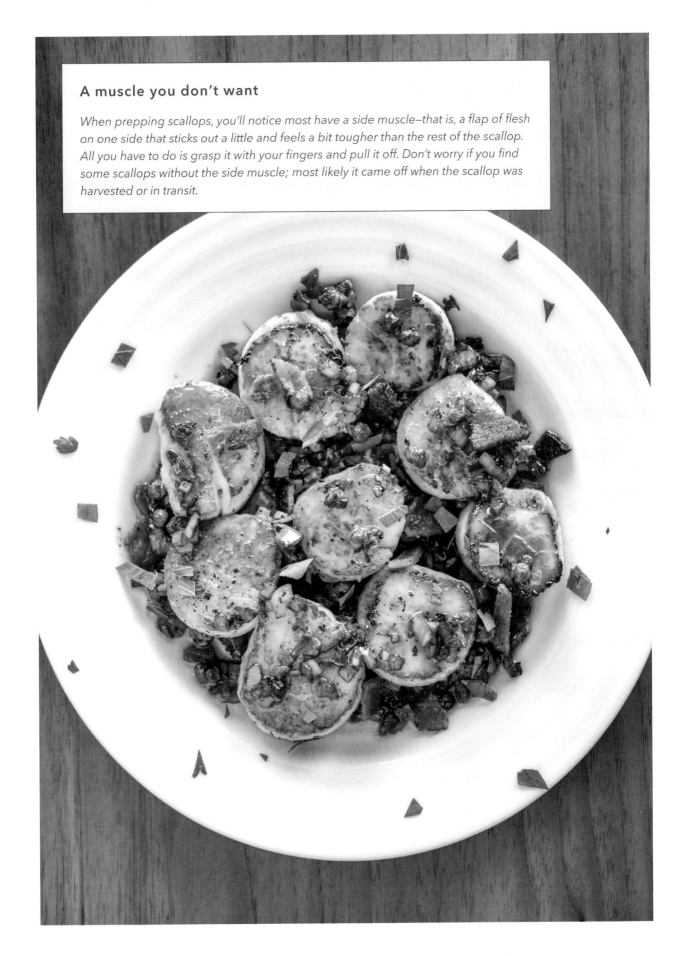

EVERYTHING BAGEL SALMON

SERVES: 4 | **PREP TIME:** 10 minutes | **COOK TIME:** 7 minutes

You may already love salmon and everything bagel seasoning together after years of bagel breakfasts with lox; why not put them together for a fun spin on lunch or dinner? Bonus: this delicious, family-pleasing meal is on the table in 20 minutes.

1½ teaspoons grated lemon zest

1½ teaspoons fresh lemon juice

3 tablespoons avocado oil mayonnaise

4 (6-ounce) wild-caught salmon fillets, skin on

2 tablespoons avocado oil, divided

3 to 4 tablespoons everything bagel seasoning

1. Preheat the oven to 450°F; place a large cast-iron skillet in the oven as it preheats.

2. In a small bowl, combine the lemon zest and juice with the mayonnaise. Pat the salmon thoroughly dry. Brush the fish all over with 1 tablespoon of the avocado oil and place on a cutting board or platter. Spread the mayo mixture over the top of the salmon; sprinkle with 3 tablespoons of the everything bagel seasoning and lightly pat to adhere. You want the mayo mixture completely covered with the seasoning; sprinkle on the remaining tablespoon of seasoning, if needed.

3. Carefully remove the skillet from the oven, place over high heat, and swirl in the remaining 1 tablespoon of oil. Add the salmon skin side down and cook for 2 minutes; this helps crisp the skin. Transfer to the oven and roast until the fish is medium-rare in the center, 2 to 5 minutes (depending on thickness). You can also cut it open to check for doneness; the center should be moist and slightly darker. Serve hot.

NOTE:

In general, salmon needs 4 to 6 minutes of total cooking time per half inch of thickness to reach medium-rare. Use that as a guide, and don't forget to factor in the 2 minutes of cooking time when searing the skin. When in doubt, it's better to undercook it than overcook it; you can always give it another minute or two of heat if it's too rare for you.

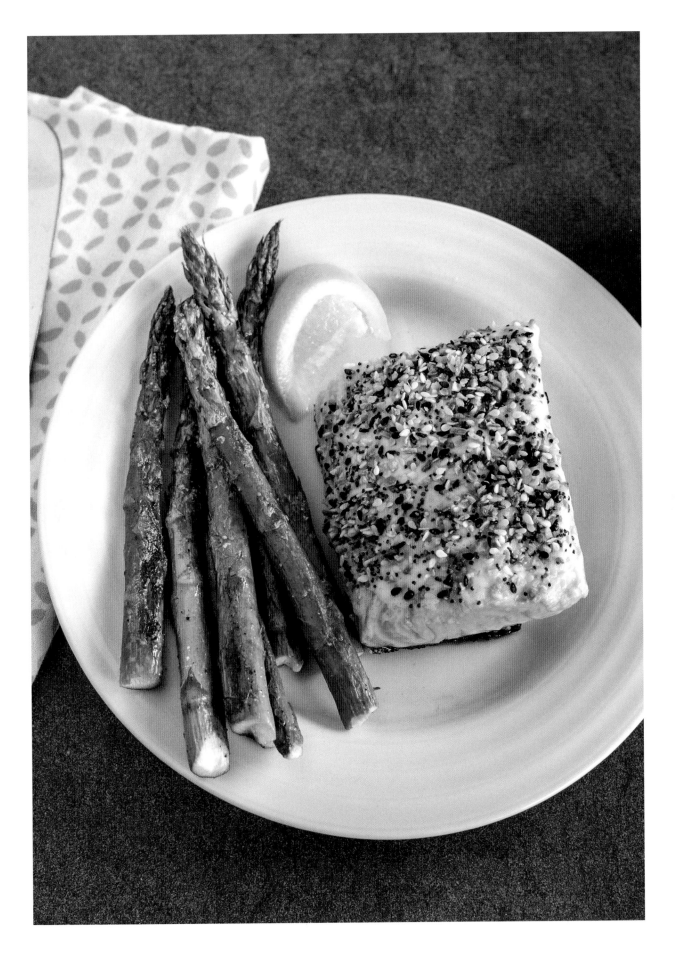

ROASTED WHOLE RED SNAPPER

SERVES: 4 | **PREP TIME:** 10 minutes | **COOK TIME:** 25 minutes

There's something so satisfyingly primal about cooking a whole fish, similar to a whole chicken or a larger bone-in cut of meat. Plus, the end result looks fancy but is actually really simple, and you get to sample parts of the fish other than the fillets, such as the cheeks. The fish you buy will likely be gutted and scaled, but ask your fishmonger if you aren't sure (they'll do it for you). Yes, carving the fish at the table is a little extra work, and you'll get a few little bones in your mouth, but that amazing flavor is 100 percent worth it.

2 (2-pound) whole red snappers, cleaned, scaled, and patted dry

3 tablespoons extra-virgin olive oil

Fine sea salt and freshly ground black pepper

2 cloves garlic, sliced

6 sprigs fresh thyme

1 lemon, scrubbed, thinly sliced and seeded, plus extra wedges for serving

Lemon-Caper Aioli (page 346), for serving (optional)

1. Preheat the oven to 450°F. Line a rimmed baking sheet with parchment paper.

2. Brush the fish inside and out with the olive oil and season generously with salt and pepper. Fill the cavities with the garlic, thyme, and lemon slices. Place the fish on the lined baking sheet and roast until the fish is crisp on the outside and the flesh flakes easily with a fork, 20 to 25 minutes.

3. Serve hot with lemon wedges and aioli, if desired.

NOTES:

For crispier skin, you can broil the fish for a minute or two at the end. Remove the parchment from under the fish first (it can catch fire under the broiler). Watch the fish carefully to prevent it from burning.

While you're roasting the fish, roast a lemon as well for flavor (and because it looks pretty). Halve a lemon and rub the cut sides with a little oil. Place on the baking sheet cut side down and roast along with the fish; the lemon flesh will get tender and turn golden.

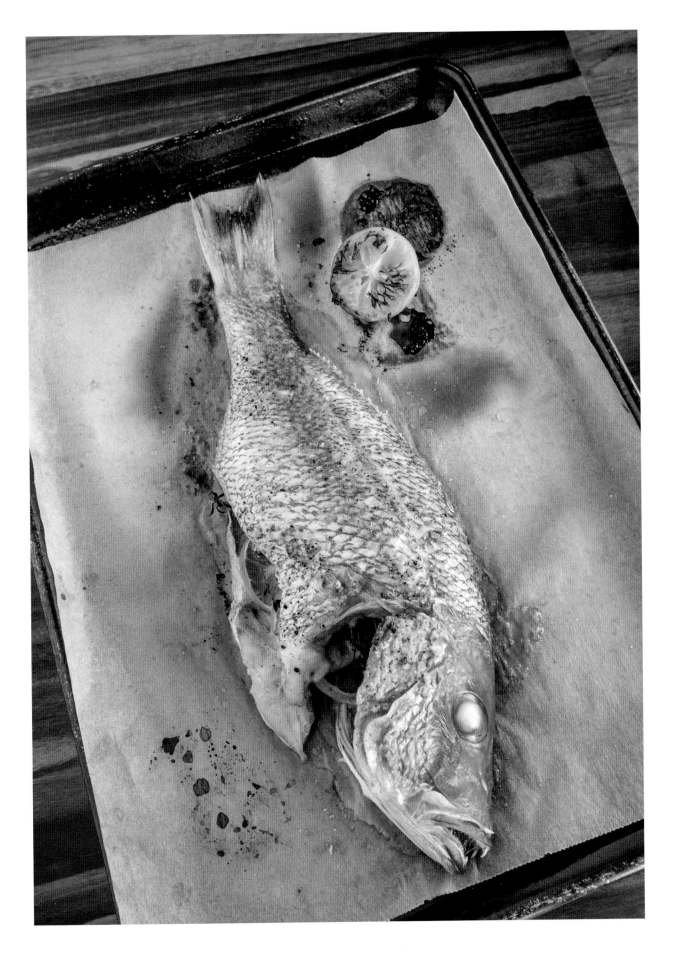

GRILLED MUSSELS

SERVES: 4 (8 to 10 as an appetizer) | **COOK TIME:** 10 minutes

Mussels are amazing: they're delicious, cheap, and easy to cook, and they're loaded with good nutrition. They're chock-full of vitamins B_{12} and C, along with tons of iron, selenium, manganese, and other minerals. Grilling is a fun and different way to cook them, and it's almost too simple. They make a perfect carnivore-ish appetizer at a cookout or a quick weeknight dinner. Our compound butter is great with these mussels, but honestly, they're fantastic straight off the grill, nothing added.

4 pounds scrubbed and debearded mussels (see Note)

Parsley-Chive Butter (page 350), for serving (optional)

1. Preheat a grill to medium heat.

2. Place the mussels on the grill in a single layer (work in batches if necessary). Cover and cook until the shells open, 5 to 7 minutes. If any of the mussels don't open, cover and cook for 2 minutes longer. Discard any mussels that don't open after that.

3. Transfer the mussels to four bowls, top with slices of the parsley-chive butter, if using, and serve.

NOTE:

Ask your fishmonger (or at your supermarket's fish counter) if the mussels are already scrubbed and debearded. If not, ask them to do those tasks for you.

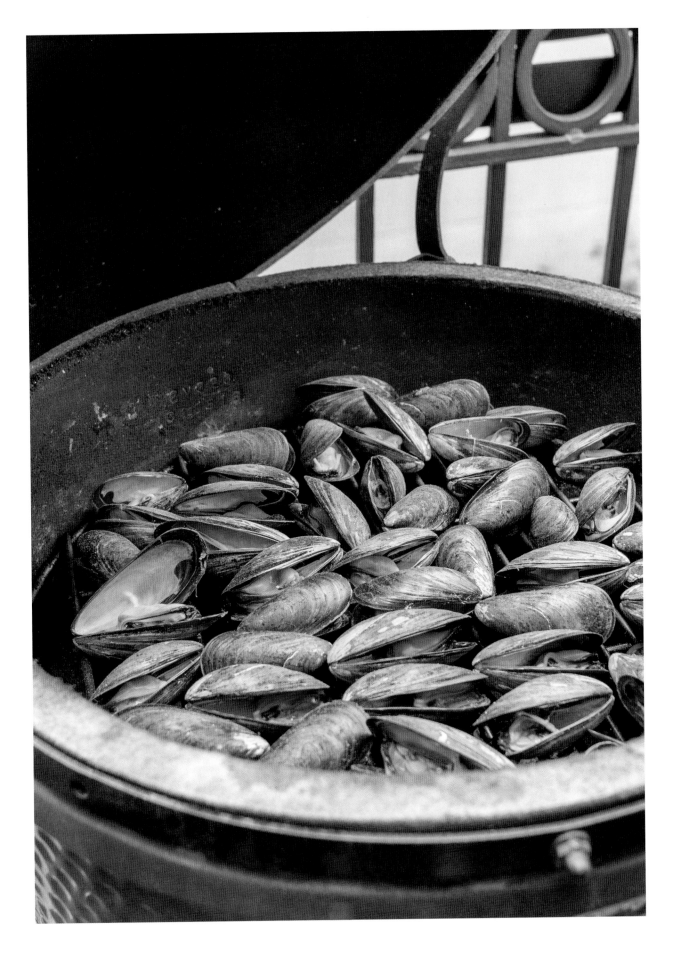

TRADITIONAL NOVA SCOTIA CHOWDER

MAKES: 5 quarts (10 large servings) | **PREP TIME:** 10 minutes | **COOK TIME:** 35 minutes

You can thank Ashleigh's mother-in-law for this simple, traditional, and well-loved maritime staple. Omit the potatoes if you're looking to go low-carb, and feel free to throw in mussels or other seafood of your choice. Whichever way you go, this is a comforting and hearty chowder that brings out the Nova Scotian in everyone.

4 tablespoons (2 ounces) unsalted butter

1 medium white onion, diced (about 1 cup)

4 medium starchy white potatoes, peeled and chopped

1 pound skinless haddock or cod fillets, chopped

12 sea scallops, thawed if frozen

12 raw medium shrimp, thawed if frozen, peeled and deveined

10 ounces chopped cooked lobster meat

1 cup heavy cream, at room temperature

Fine sea salt and freshly ground black pepper

½ teaspoon dried dill weed, for finishing

1. Melt the butter in a large soup pot over medium heat. Add the onion and cook until softened, about 5 minutes. Add the potatoes and enough water to just cover the potatoes. Bring to a low boil, then lower the heat and boil gently until the potatoes are just softened, about 10 minutes.

2. Add the fish fillets, scallops, and shrimp; continue to simmer, stirring occasionally, until cooked through (the fish will be white and flaky, the shrimp and scallops no longer translucent), 5 to 7 minutes longer. In the last minute, add the cooked lobster.

3. Pour in the cream; cook, stirring continually, until thickened, about 5 minutes. Taste and season with salt and pepper. Serve hot, finished with a sprinkle of dill weed.

NOTE:

For the cooked lobster meat, you can usually find canned pretty easily, or you can use freshly cooked lobster removed from the shell; you'd need about 3 pounds of lobster to get 10 ounces of meat.

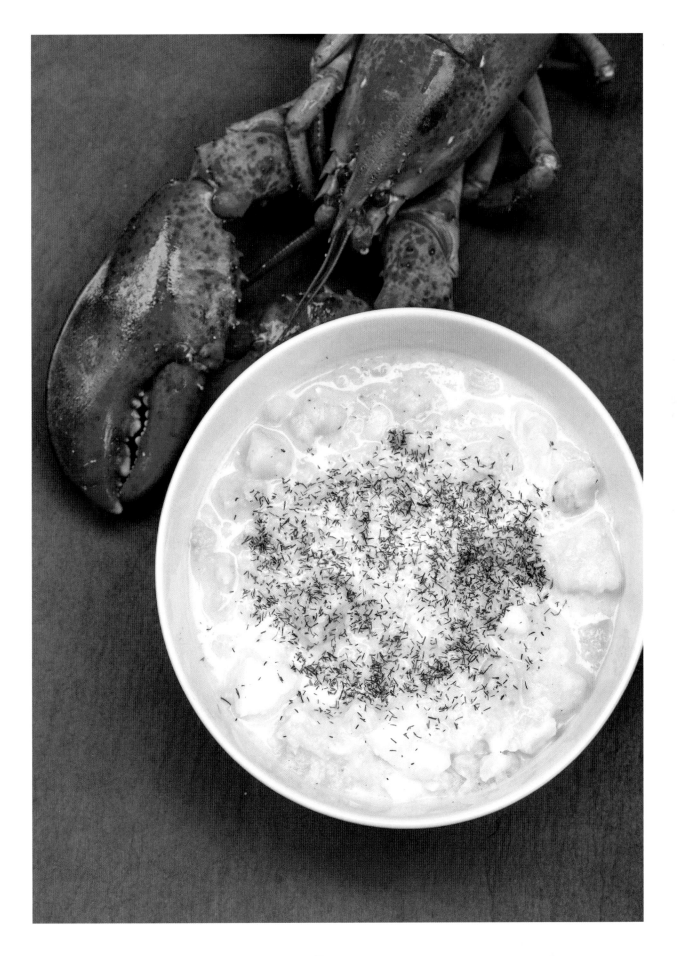

TROUT CEVICHE

SERVES: 2 | **PREP TIME:** 10 minutes, plus 2 hours to cure

As far as we're concerned, trout is an underrated fish—it's packed with protein, omega-3 fatty acids, and potassium and has a mild, delicate flavor that works well in a zesty ceviche. Ceviche, a Peruvian dish, involves "cooking" fish without heat in a citrus-based marinade. It still retains a bit of that fresh, sushi-like quality without technically being raw, but of course, you want the freshest and best-quality fish for this preparation. Use our sweet potato chips (page 276) or tostones (page 282) to scoop up the ceviche. Lettuce wraps are a nice option, too.

8 ounces boneless, skinless trout (we used rainbow), cut into 1-inch chunks

½ cup cooked corn kernels (canned or fresh)

Juice of 2 limes

3 tablespoons fresh grapefruit juice

½ red onion, finely diced (about 1 cup)

½ red bell pepper, seeded and finely diced (about ½ cup)

½ green bell pepper, seeded and finely diced (about ½ cup)

½ habanero pepper, seeded and minced (about 2 tablespoons)

1 medium tomato, chopped (about 1 cup)

2 tablespoons chopped fresh cilantro (optional)

Fine sea salt and freshly ground black pepper

1. In a medium bowl, combine the trout, corn, lime juice, grapefruit juice, onion, red and green bell peppers, and habanero. Cover and refrigerate for 2 hours.

2. Remove the ceviche from the fridge and drain the liquid. Add the tomato and cilantro, if using, and toss to combine. Season with salt and pepper to taste and serve.

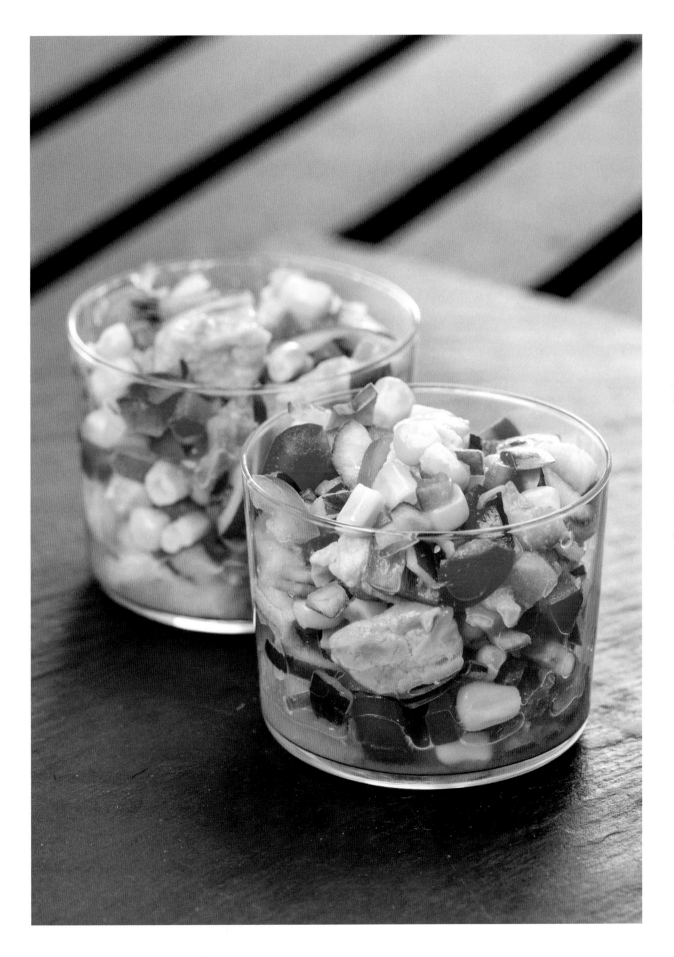

SHRIMP, AVOCADO, AND CITRUS SALAD

SERVES: 4 | **PREP TIME:** 10 minutes | **COOK TIME:** 5 minutes

What's better than a bright, refreshing salad on a hot day? This one has protein-packed shrimp, creamy avocado for healthy fats, and our favorite citrus. We can picture ourselves enjoying this one poolside.

1 grapefruit

1 ripe avocado

1 pound raw large shrimp, thawed if frozen, peeled and deveined

¾ teaspoon fine sea salt, divided

3 tablespoons avocado oil, divided

¼ teaspoon freshly ground black pepper

1 (5-ounce) package mixed salad greens (about 6 cups)

½ cup raw walnuts or pecans, chopped

1. Slice the top and bottom off the grapefruit. Cutting top to bottom, slice the peel and white pith off the fruit, taking care to cut off as little of the flesh as possible. Working over a bowl to catch the juices, segment the grapefruit sections, then cut them into 1-inch pieces. Set the grapefruit pieces and juice aside in separate bowls. Halve, pit, and slice the avocado.

2. Pat the shrimp dry and season with ¼ teaspoon of the salt. Heat 1 tablespoon of the avocado oil in a large skillet over medium-high heat. Add the shrimp and sauté until cooked through and opaque, about 5 minutes. Transfer the shrimp to a medium bowl.

3. Make the dressing: Transfer 2 tablespoons of the reserved grapefruit juice to a large bowl. Add the remaining 2 tablespoons of oil, remaining ½ teaspoon of salt, and the pepper and whisk to combine. Put the mixed greens in the bowl and toss to coat.

4. Divide the dressed greens among four serving bowls. Top with the shrimp, grapefruit pieces, avocado, and nuts and serve.

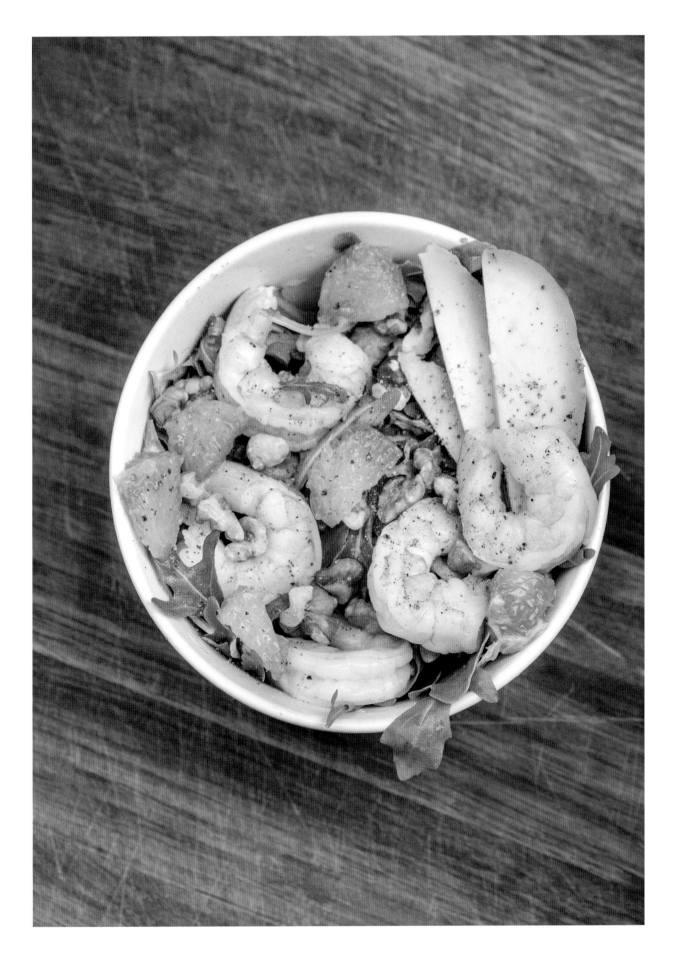

SALMON POKE BOWL

SERVES: 2 | **PREP TIME:** 15 minutes, plus 30 minutes to marinate

Raw fish is one of those foods many people find intimidating to try at home, but it's all about quality and freshness. (This is where having a good fishmonger is key.) With a little attention to detail, you'll enjoy a fresh, light, nutrient-packed salad with so much texture and flavor. You can always sear the salmon if raw seems too scary.

MARINADE:

2 tablespoons coconut aminos

2 tablespoons apple cider vinegar

2 tablespoons extra-virgin olive oil

1 tablespoon maple syrup, raw honey, or liquid monk fruit (optional)

BOWL:

8 to 10 ounces sushi-grade salmon fillet

1 cup cooked white rice or Cauliflower Rice (That Doesn't Suck) (page 268)

½ cup julienned or shredded carrots

½ cup sliced English cucumber

1 avocado, pitted and sliced

FOR GARNISH (OPTIONAL):

2 tablespoons shredded nori

2 teaspoons sesame seeds

2 teaspoons grated fresh ginger

1. Make the marinade: In a small bowl, whisk together the coconut aminos, vinegar, olive oil, and maple syrup, if using. Set aside
2 tablespoons in a cup.

2. With a sharp knife, slice the salmon fillet against the grain into 1-inch cubes and place in a medium glass container. Pour the remaining marinade over the salmon, cover, and refrigerate for at least 30 minutes or up to 2 hours.

3. Divide the rice and salmon between two bowls. Top with the carrots, cucumber, and avocado; drizzle with the reserved marinade. Garnish with the shredded nori, sesame seeds, and/or grated ginger, if desired, and serve.

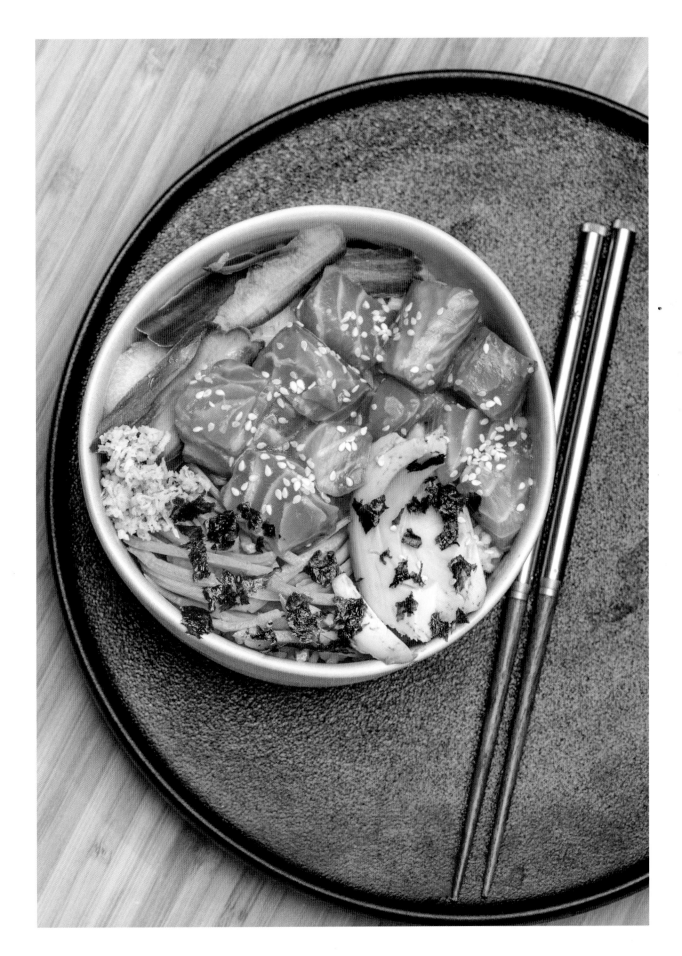

BERMUDA-STYLE CODFISH CAKES

SERVES: 4 | **PREP TIME:** 20 minutes, plus overnight to soak and 1 hour to cool | **COOK TIME:** 35 minutes

Codfish cakes are a traditional Easter dish in Bermuda, where Ashleigh's mother grew up and where Ashleigh herself lived for a few years after she graduated university. This recipe is adapted from longtime friends, the Gibbons family, who often incorporate crumbled chorizo for an added kick. We kept it classic for this version and omitted the onion that often comes with it. Simple yet satisfying, this is the perfect comfort dish. Keeping with the Easter theme, these patties are usually served with hot cross buns, but our favorite way to enjoy them, besides as-is with a squeeze of lemon, is topped with a runny egg and some hollandaise sauce for a different take on eggs Benedict.

1 (1-pound) package dry salt cod (boneless and skinless)

½ pound white potatoes, peeled

2 tablespoons chopped fresh flat-leaf parsley

1 teaspoon curry powder

½ teaspoon freshly ground black pepper

¼ teaspoon ground dried thyme

¼ cup gluten-free flour of choice

4 tablespoons (2 ounces) unsalted butter or avocado oil

Flaky sea salt, for finishing (optional)

Lemon wedges, for serving (optional)

1. Submerge the salt cod in water, cover, and place in the fridge. Let soak overnight.

2. Put the potatoes in a large soup pot and cover with water by 1 inch. Bring to a boil over high heat. Lower the heat to medium and boil until the potatoes are nearly cooked but not fully soft, about 15 minutes.

3. Drain the fish and add it to the potatoes. Add enough water just to cover and continue to simmer until the potatoes are fully cooked, about 10 minutes longer. Drain the fish and potatoes and let cool, then transfer to a bowl and place in the fridge until chilled, about 1 hour.

4. Use a potato masher or fork to mash and blend the fish and potatoes; you may leave some texture and chunkiness or aim to get it as smooth as possible, depending on your preference. Fold in the parsley, curry powder, pepper, and thyme.

5. With wet hands, form the mixture into palm-sized patties, about 1½ inches thick.

6. Melt the butter in a large skillet over medium-high heat. Coat the cakes liberally in the flour and fry until golden brown, 3 to 4 minutes per side. Transfer the cakes to a paper towel-lined platter to drain before serving. Sprinkle with flaky salt and serve with lemon wedges, if desired.

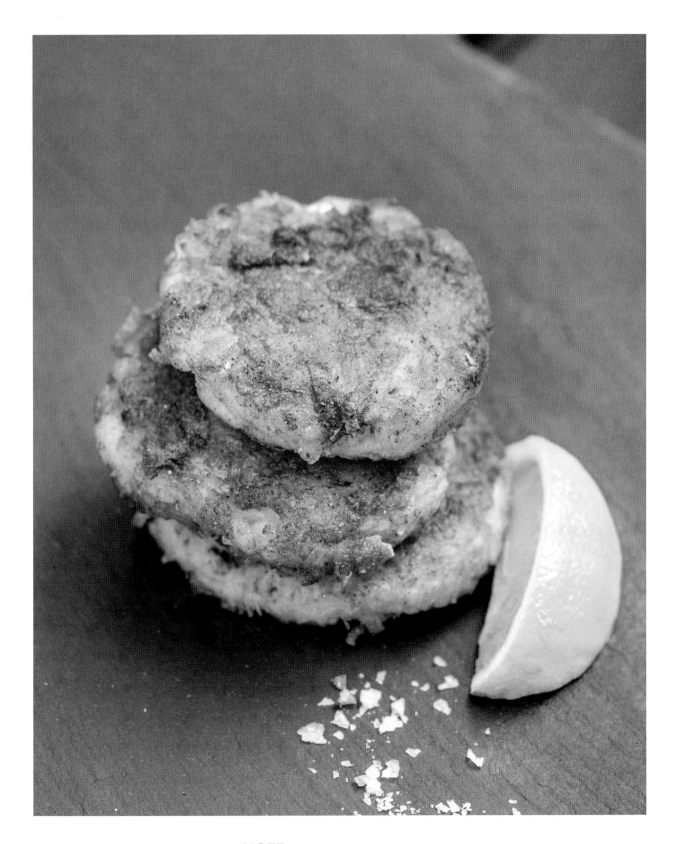

NOTE:

These cakes are best when freshly cooked.

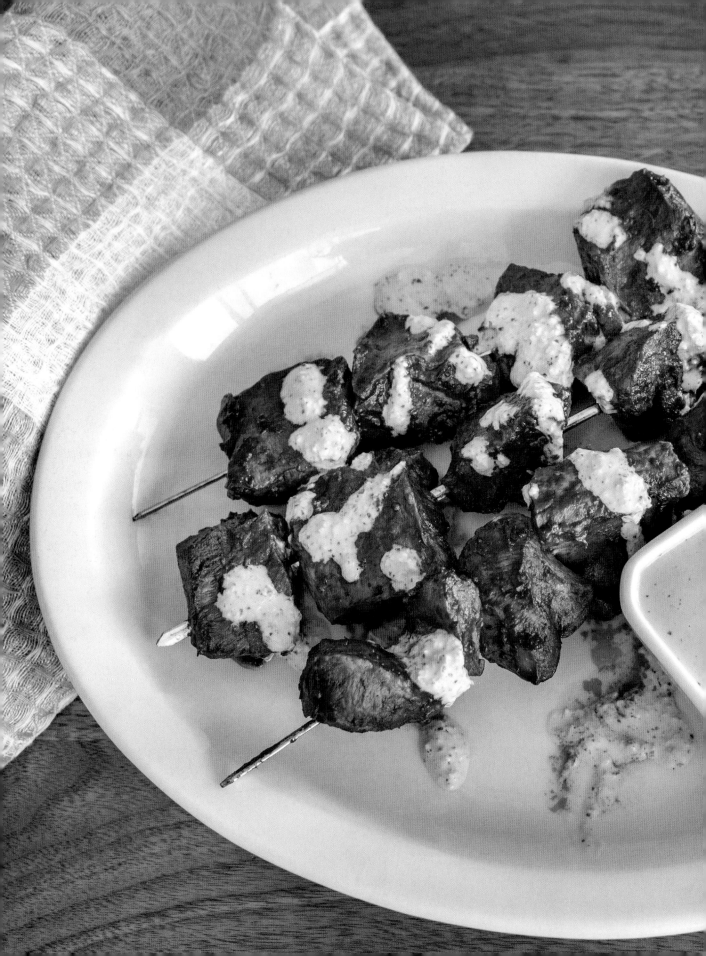

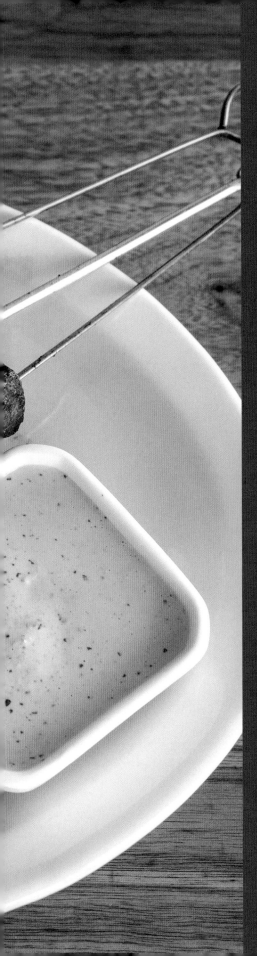

CHAPTER 9:
OFFAL

ROASTED MARROW BONES

SERVES: 4 | **PREP TIME:** 5 minutes | **COOK TIME:** 20 minutes

There's something so primal and satisfying about bone marrow. It's rich and luscious and just so good—and it's also good for you, full of vitamins, minerals, and healthy fat. Research has pointed to its gut health and disease-fighting benefits, too. Different bones will yield different amounts of marrow; don't be surprised if some have a lot and others not that much. The warm marrow is delicious spread on crusty bread or crackers or just licked off a spoon (uh, not that we've done that…).

3 to 4 pounds canoed beef marrow bones (see Note)

Fine sea salt

1 teaspoon chopped fresh thyme leaves

Grain-free bread slices, toasted

1. Let the bones stand at room temperature for 20 minutes. Preheat the oven to 425°F; line a rimmed baking sheet with parchment paper.

2. Place the bones marrow side up on the lined baking sheet. Season generously with salt and sprinkle with the thyme. Roast until the marrow is softened (but not melted), has started to bubble and brown, and has begun to pull away from the bone, 15 to 20 minutes. To test the softness of the marrow, stick a toothpick or fork in it; it will be gelatinous and soft all the way through.

3. Scoop the marrow out of the bones, taste and season with additional salt, if needed, and serve with toasted bread.

NOTES:

Call your butcher ahead to order the bones; some places only keep them frozen.

Ask your butcher to cut the bones lengthwise (aka "canoed" or "canoe-cut"); this makes it easier to scoop out the marrow.

You can lay a sprig of thyme over the bone instead of picking off the leaves and chopping them if you like. Remove it before serving.

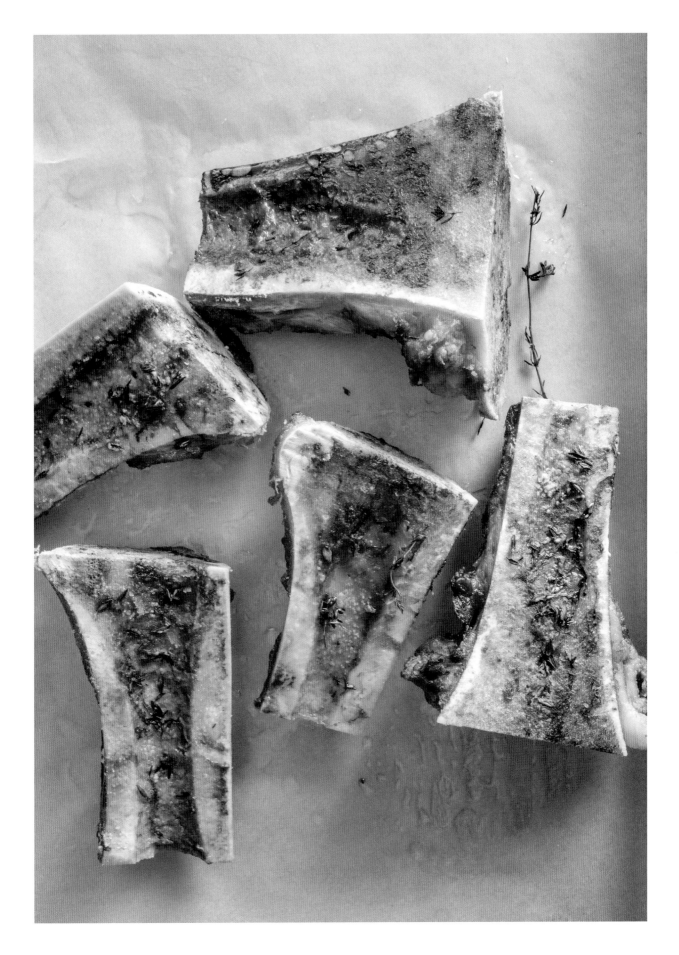

PERUVIAN-STYLE GRILLED BEEF HEART

SERVES: 4 | **PREP TIME:** 25 minutes, plus 3½ hours to marinate |
COOK TIME: 10 minutes

This recipe is inspired by the popular Peruvian street food anticuchos. Its deep flavor comes from the aji panca, a smoky, fruity pepper found in Peru. It is sold dried or prepared as a paste, which is what we use here. You can buy the paste in jars from ethnic markets and online. It's worth buying; you'll use quite a bit in the marinade as well as some in the green sauce, and there really isn't a swap that will give you the same flavor. (If you don't care about that, feel free to blend up some seeded chipotles in adobo and use that instead.) Slather leftover aji panca on chicken or ribs, or add it to your favorite homemade barbecue sauce. We took liberties with the green sauce and used jalapeños instead of aji amarillo, another Peruvian pepper.

BEEF HEART:

⅓ cup extra-virgin olive oil, divided

3 cloves garlic, grated (about 1 tablespoon)

½ cup aji panca paste

¼ cup apple cider vinegar

1 tablespoon dried oregano leaves

½ teaspoon ground cumin

½ teaspoon fine sea salt

¼ teaspoon freshly ground black pepper

1 beef heart (2 to 3 pounds), cleaned (see Note, page 257) and cut into 1½- to 2-inch pieces

GREEN SAUCE:

2 tablespoons extra-virgin olive oil

3 cloves garlic, minced (about 1 tablespoon)

3 medium jalapeño peppers, seeds and ribs removed, chopped (about 1 scant cup)

½ teaspoon grated lime zest

2 tablespoons fresh lime juice

1 cup fresh cilantro leaves

½ cup avocado oil mayonnaise

¼ cup sour cream

1 teaspoon apple cider vinegar

¼ teaspoon aji panca paste

Fine sea salt and freshly ground black pepper

Special equipment:
8 (14-inch) metal skewers

1.   Marinate the beef heart: Combine 2 tablespoons of the olive oil and the garlic in a small unheated skillet. Place over low heat and cook undisturbed until it begins to sizzle. Let it sizzle for 30 seconds more, then transfer to a large bowl. Whisk in the remaining oil, aji panca, vinegar, oregano, cumin, salt, and pepper. Add the beef heart cubes; stir to coat them with the marinade. Cover and refrigerate for at least 3½ hours or up to overnight. Let stand in the marinade at room temperature for 30 minutes before cooking.

(continues on page 257)

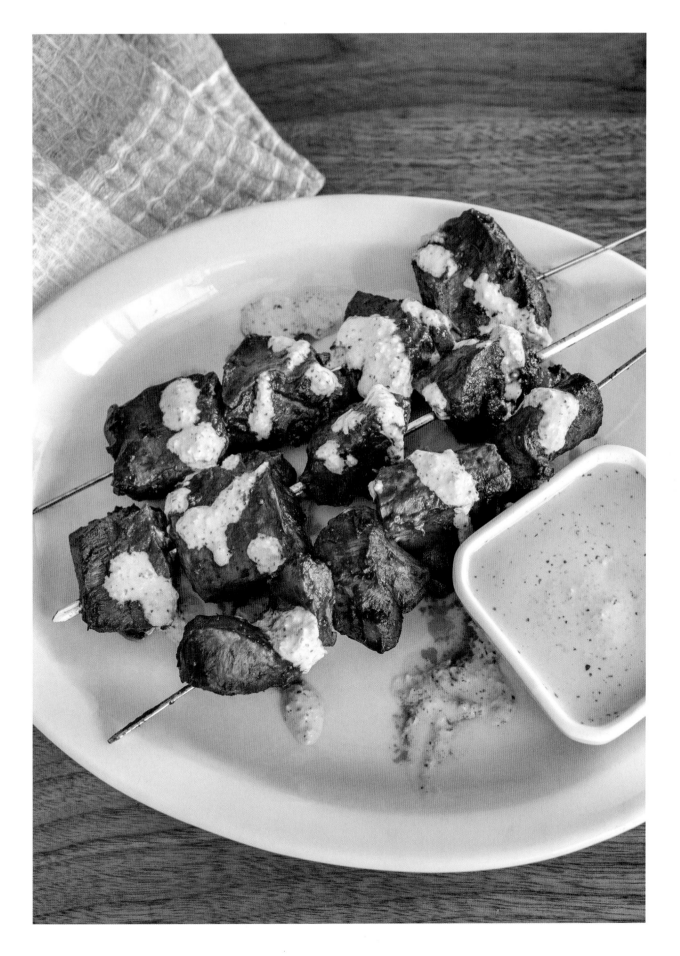

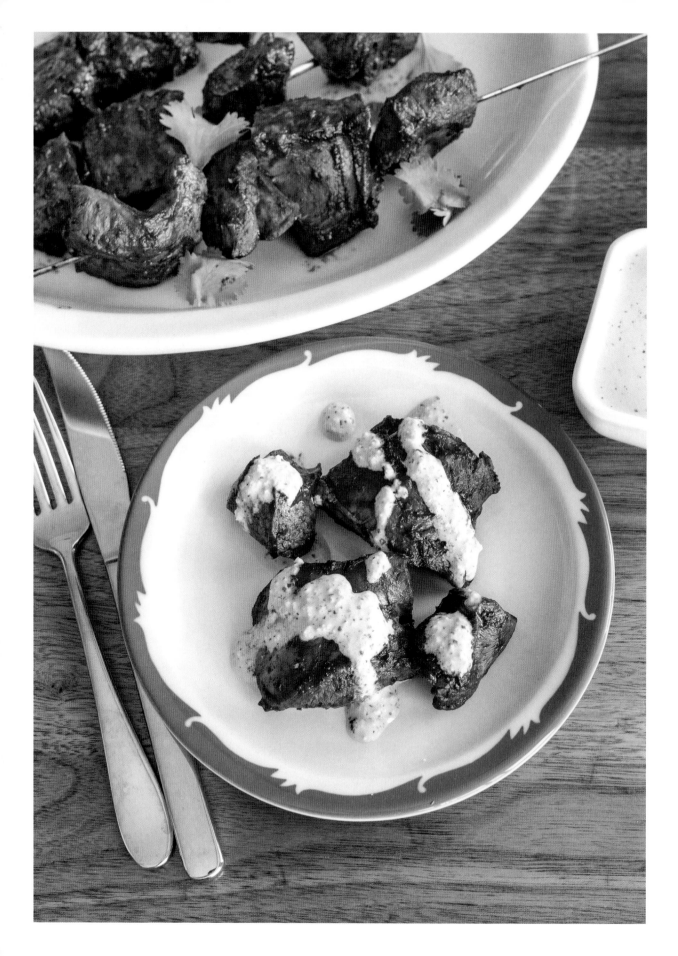

2. Make the green sauce: Combine the olive oil and garlic in a small unheated skillet. Place over low heat and cook undisturbed until it begins to sizzle. Let it sizzle for 30 seconds more, then transfer to a small bowl to cool. In a food processor, combine the jalapeños, lime zest and juice, cilantro, mayonnaise, sour cream, vinegar, and aji panca. Add the garlic mixture and process until smooth, stopping to scrape down the sides and bottom of the bowl as needed. Taste and season with salt and pepper. (You can make the sauce up to 2 days ahead; keep it covered and refrigerated.)

3. When you're ready to cook the beef heart, preheat a grill to medium heat. Remove the beef heart pieces from the marinade and thread them onto metal skewers (discard the leftover marinade). Grill, turning once, until the meat is cooked to medium-rare, 3 to 5 minutes per side (cut open a piece to check; it will look pink in the center, similar to steak). Transfer to a platter, tent with foil, and let rest for at least 5 minutes. Serve hot with the sauce.

NOTE: ———————————————————————————

Cleaning the beef heart is the most challenging part of this recipe. It just takes a little patience and a sharp knife. Cut away any hard, white exterior fat and membranes as well as any valves from the top of the heart, or anything that feels tough. Depending on the heart, you may need to trim away quite a bit; that's OK. You definitely want the tender meat, not any of the tough parts, which won't hurt you but just aren't as pleasant to eat. Especially if you're making this dish for people who are squeamish or skeptical, you want the experience to be seamless.

SAVORY MEAT "MUFFINS"

MAKES: 12 muffins | **PREP TIME:** 15 minutes | **COOK TIME:** 25 minutes

This is one of the more strict carnivore recipes in this book. The "muffins" may not look like much, but they bring together simple, nourishing ingredients to create a surprisingly savory and satisfying snack (or you could have two or three and call it dinner). The liver adds a mineral richness, while the tallow adds a depth of flavor. On-the-go carnivore snacks can be tricky or tedious to find, and this recipe solves that problem.

1 pound ground beef and beef liver mixture (see Notes)

4 large eggs, beaten

1 tablespoon beef tallow or duck fat, melted, plus more for greasing

1 teaspoon fine sea salt

1½ teaspoons spice(s) of choice (optional; see Notes)

Flaky sea salt, for finishing (optional)

1.   Preheat the oven to 350°F. Grease a 12-cup muffin tin with melted fat or line it with foil liners.

2.   Put the meat mixture in a large bowl. Pour in the eggs and use your hands to combine. Add the tallow, salt, and spices, if using; mix until all of the ingredients are incorporated. Divide the mixture evenly among the muffin cups, filling them about three-quarters full.

3.   Bake until a toothpick inserted in the middle of a muffin comes out clean, about 25 minutes. Let cool for 10 minutes before serving. Sprinkle with flaky sea salt, if desired.

NOTES:

You can purchase the ground beef and liver mixture online from a quality meat purveyor (see page 364). Alternatively, most butcher shops will be able to prepare it for you; generally they use (or you can request) a 4:1 ratio of ground beef to ground liver. This ratio ensures the organ meat won't really make a difference in how you use or cook the meat mixture and won't significantly affect its taste, either.

Feel free to use whatever ground meat/offal mix you like best; for example, if you prefer ground pork or turkey and you like the flavor and texture of heart more than liver, you can use those instead of the more typical option of ground beef mixed with beef liver.

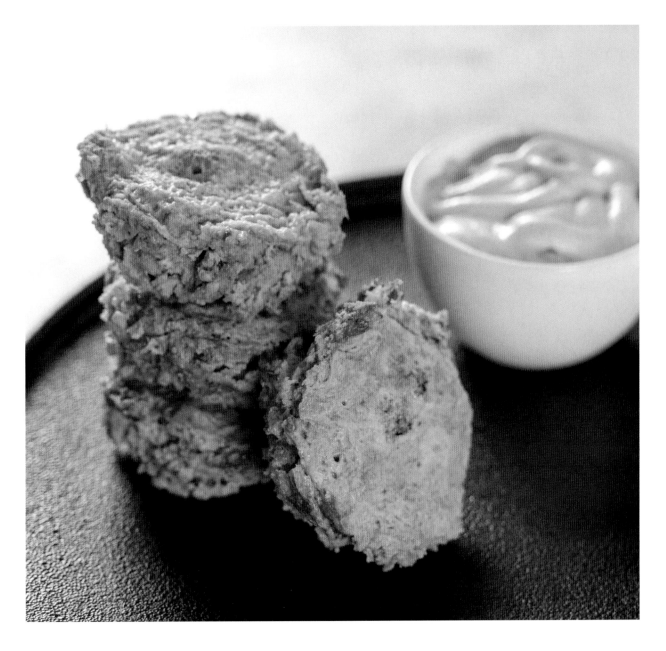

NOTES:

For the spices, we suggest ½ teaspoon each of garlic powder, ground black pepper, and onion powder. But feel free to experiment with dried herbs such as rosemary or thyme.

If you have a silicone muffin tin, it will work well here, as items tend to pop out easily.

Store leftovers in an airtight container in the fridge for up to 5 days; we think these muffins taste pretty good cold too, for when you need a quick snack on the go.

BONE MARROW BURGERS

SERVES: 4 | **PREP TIME:** 10 minutes | **COOK TIME:** 10 minutes

This recipe may ruin you for regular burgers forever. The bone marrow adds richness, luscious fat, and a hit of umami that, when balanced correctly, is deeply satisfying without being over-the-top decadent. We like stone-ground mustard and pickles to cut the meatiness, but add whatever condiments you like. Your keto-carnivore friends will love this one.

1 or 2 frozen canoed beef marrow bones

1¼ pounds ground beef

½ teaspoon flaky sea salt, plus more for finishing

¼ teaspoon freshly ground black pepper

FOR SERVING:

Grain-free buns or lettuce wraps

Stone-ground mustard (optional)

Pickles (optional)

1. Put the frozen marrow bones in the fridge until just defrosted, no longer than 20 minutes. Use a spoon to scoop out the marrow. Place the marrow on a cutting board and coarsely chop it. Transfer to a large bowl.

2. Add the ground beef, salt, and pepper to the bone marrow and mix gently with your hands until just incorporated (don't overmix; as you don't want the marrow to melt). Divide the mixture into four equal portions, then form into 2-inch-thick patties.

3. Preheat a large cast-iron skillet over medium heat. Cook the patties until an instant-read thermometer stuck into the center reads 145°F for medium-rare, about 5 minutes per side.

4. Finish with flaky sea salt and serve in buns or lettuce wraps with mustard and pickles, if desired.

NOTE:

If your skillet is well seasoned, you won't need to add fat to it before placing the patties in it. If yours isn't well seasoned, or you aren't sure, swirl a tablespoon of avocado oil in the skillet when it's hot.

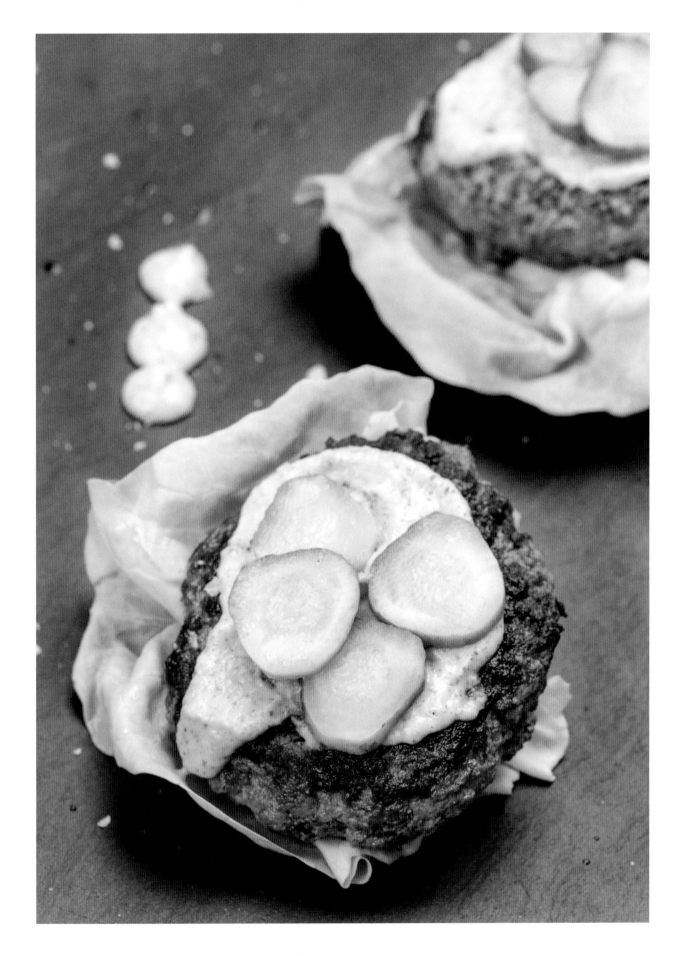

GRILLED CHICKEN HEART COBB SALAD

SERVES: 2 | **PREP TIME:** 10 minutes | **COOK TIME:** 7 minutes

We've all had Cobb salads—and they're full of color and healthy ingredients. But we think it's time to switch it up a bit. Here, we have swapped out chopped chicken breast for a much more interesting (and nutrient-dense) part of the bird: hearts. Chicken hearts have a delightfully chewy dark meat flavor and are packed with protein, vitamin B_{12}, zinc, and other important micronutrients. They also take less time to prepare than chicken breasts, so it's a win-win.

1 tablespoon (½ ounce) unsalted butter or ghee

8 ounces chicken hearts, rinsed (see Note)

Fine sea salt and freshly ground black pepper

1 medium head romaine lettuce, coarsely chopped (about 6 cups)

2 to 4 tablespoons Warm Bacon Vinaigrette (page 358)

4 large eggs, hard-cooked, peeled, and sliced

1 large avocado, pitted and chopped

2 small vine tomatoes, such as Campari, quartered, or 1 cup halved cherry tomatoes

¼ cup crumbled blue cheese (about 1½ ounces)

1. Melt the butter in a medium skillet over medium heat. Add the chicken hearts and cook, turning a few times, until just cooked through (they will be brown throughout when sliced open), about 7 minutes. Add a pinch each of salt and pepper and remove the pan from the heat.

2. Divide the lettuce between two bowls and toss with 1 to 2 tablespoons of vinaigrette per bowl. Top with the chicken hearts, eggs, avocado, tomatoes, and blue cheese and serve.

NOTE: —————————

You can buy chicken hearts at many grocery stores. They tend to be already cleaned and are generally ready to cook after rinsing thoroughly in cold water. (Pro tip: Squeeze the hearts while rinsing to ensure you get rid of trace amounts of blood inside them.)

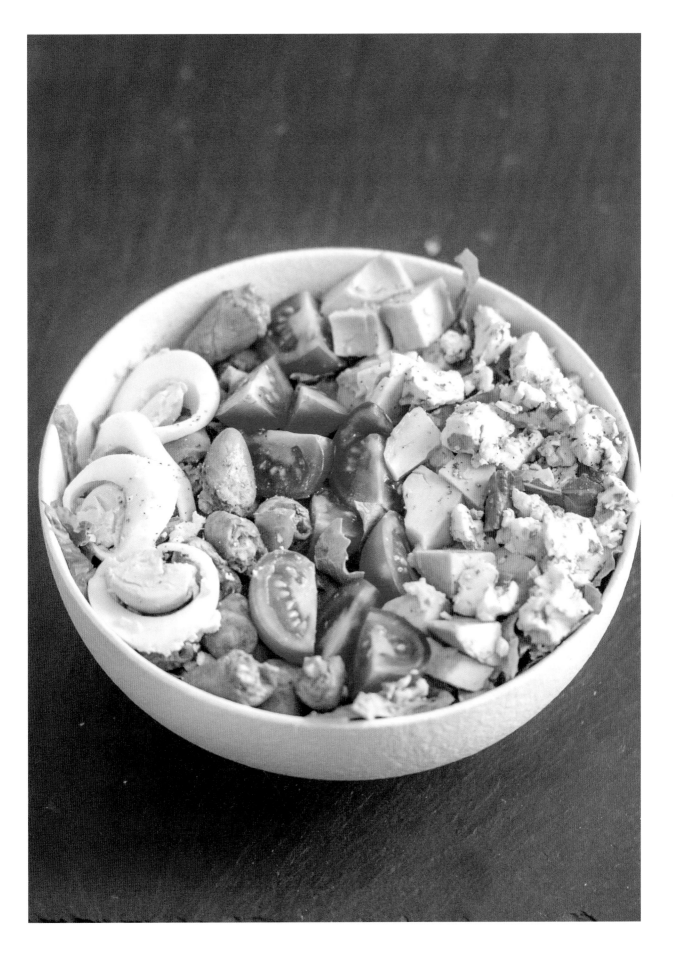

TONGUE SLIDERS

SERVES: 8 | **PREP TIME:** 15 minutes | **COOK TIME:** 3 hours

These sliders are a great starter for a dinner party and cover every base: salty crunch from the tostones, creamy fat from the avocado, rich flavor from the juicy pulled tongue, and a bit of acid and sweetness from the pickled onions. They look pretty and taste even better. Shredded lengua (tongue) is a pretty common taco ingredient these days, but even if you're usually less adventurous, this recipe might win you over.

1 beef, buffalo, or bison tongue (about 2 pounds)

3 cloves garlic, peeled and smashed with the side of a knife

1 tablespoon ground dried oregano

1 teaspoon fine sea salt

1 teaspoon freshly ground black pepper

1 batch Tostones (page 282)

2 large avocados, pitted and sliced

½ cup pickled onions (below)

Lime wedges, for serving (optional)

1. Put the tongue, garlic, and oregano in a large soup pot and cover with water. Cover the pot, place over medium-low heat, and simmer until the tongue is tender and easily pierced with a fork, about 3 hours. (Check every 30 minutes to make sure the tongue remains covered with water; add more if the level is getting too low.)

2. Remove the tongue from the pot and transfer it to a cutting board. Let stand until cool enough to handle, about 15 minutes. Use a sharp knife to slice across the base (wider end) of the tongue and peel off the thick outer layer of skin. With a fork, shred the meat. Season with the salt and pepper.

3. Top the tostones with avocado slices, shredded meat, and pickled onions. Serve with lime wedges, if desired.

DIY Pickled Onions

These easy pickled onions add a zesty crunch to most any meat dish.

¼ cup distilled white vinegar

¼ cup apple cider vinegar

1 tablespoon granulated sugar

1 tablespoon kosher salt

1 red onion, thinly sliced

1 clove garlic, peeled

Special equipment:
Air release valve and jar weight for mason jar

1. Combine the vinegars, sugar, and salt in a wide-mouth pint-sized mason jar. Cover and shake until the sugar and salt have dissolved. Stuff the onion slices and garlic clove into the jar, cover with an air release valve and jar weight, and put the jar in a dark cupboard for 24 hours.

2. Replace the air release valve with a regular jar lid and put the jar in the fridge for up to a week before opening. Alternatively, let sit at room temperature, loosely covered, for 2 hours, then cover tightly and refrigerate. The pickled onions will keep for up to 2 weeks in the fridge. *Makes about 2 cups.*

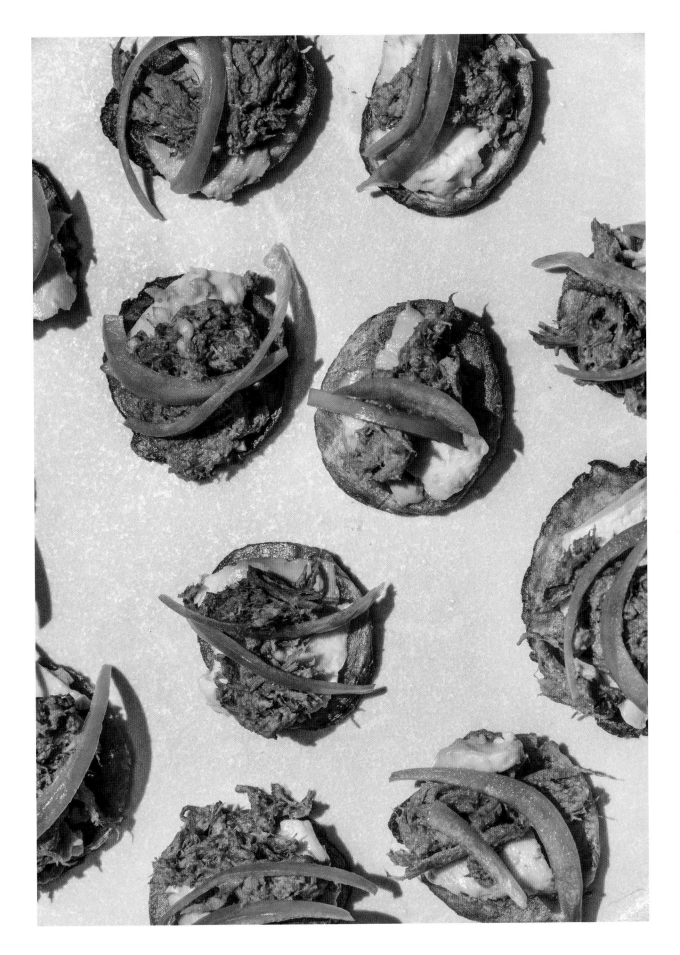

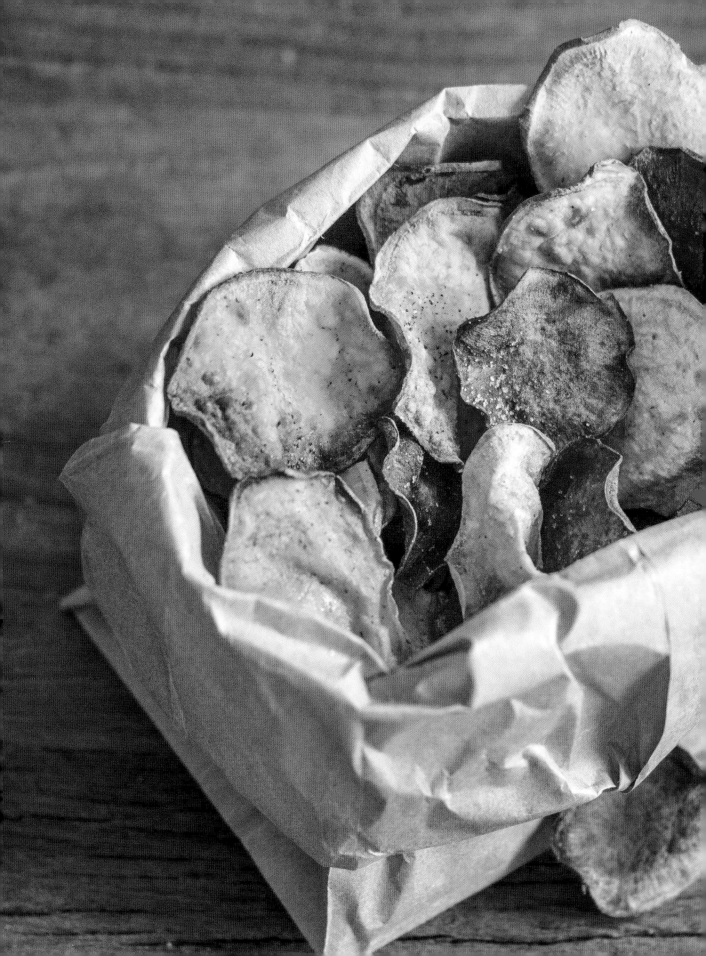

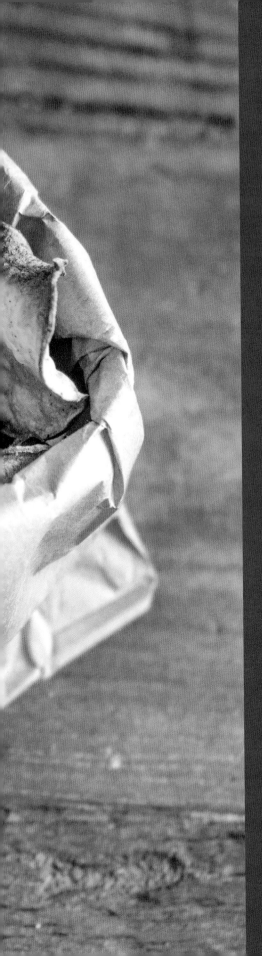

CHAPTER 10:

SIDES

CAULIFLOWER RICE
(THAT DOESN'T SUCK)

MAKES: 1¼ cups (2 to 4 servings) | **PREP TIME:** 5 minutes | **COOK TIME:** 25 minutes

When we need riced cauliflower, we always buy it prericed and frozen. Sure, you can make it yourself, but why? It's a pain to DIY and readily available premade. Frozen is more convenient because the fresh stuff can turn pretty quickly. With frozen, it's always there, quick and easy to cook, no need to defrost, and you can grab just the amount you need. You can cook cauliflower rice on the stove, but we prefer to roast it, which is simpler and more hands-off and yields a better taste and texture.

1 (12-ounce) package frozen riced cauliflower

1 tablespoon avocado oil or extra-virgin olive oil

Fine sea salt and freshly ground black pepper

1. Preheat the oven to 400°F. Line a rimmed baking sheet with parchment paper.

2. Spread the frozen cauliflower on the lined baking sheet; press out any clumps. Drizzle with the oil and season lightly with salt and pepper. Roast for 15 minutes, until the rice has thawed and begun to cook. Stir the rice, spread in an even layer, and continue to roast until it's cooked through, fluffy, and light golden in spots, about 10 minutes longer.

3. Taste and season with additional salt and pepper, if needed. Serve hot, or let cool to serve at room temperature or to use cold in a rice salad.

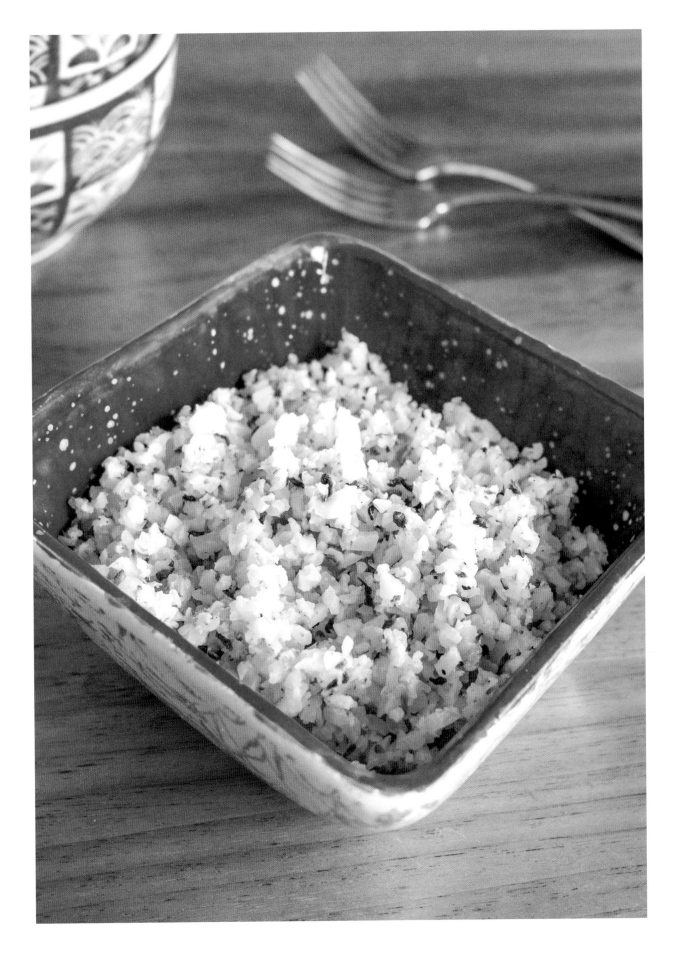

ZUCCHINI NOODLES
(THAT DON'T SUCK)

MAKES: About 2 cups (2 servings) | **PREP TIME:** 10 minutes | **COOK TIME:** 2 minutes

Zucchini noodles are a low-carb eater's BFF. You get the twirl-it-up-on-your-fork fun of eating noodles with none of the gluten or excess carbs in pasta, plus a shot of added fiber and vitamins A and C. They're neutrally flavored, so you can top them with Bolognese (see our recipe on page 188) or put them in a pad Thai. To manage your expectations: no, it's not the same as eating noodles, and it never will be. But once you accept that and learn to love them for what they are, you're in business. In general, one medium zucchini will make enough noodles for one person, so plan for that when you're shopping.

2 medium zucchini, trimmed

1 tablespoon extra-virgin olive oil or avocado oil

Fine sea salt and freshly ground black pepper

Red pepper flakes (optional)

1. Use a spiralizer, julienne peeler, or mandoline slicer to cut the zucchini into noodles.

2. Warm the oil in a large skillet over medium heat. Add the zucchini noodles, season lightly with salt and pepper (and a pinch of red pepper flakes, if you like a little heat), and cook, tossing with tongs, until tender, 1 to 2 minutes. Lift the noodles out of the pan with the tongs and transfer to a colander to drain.

3. Pat the noodles dry with paper towels, then divide between two plates or bowls and serve.

NOTES: ───────────────

If you don't have one of those gadgets needed to spiralize, or you just want to save a step, you can buy zucchini noodles already made. Look for them in the produce section of your supermarket. If you're curious about spiralizers but don't want to spend a lot, we love the OXO Good Grips Hand-Held Spiralizer, which you can get for around $15.

There's no need to peel the zucchini. The peel adds a pop of color and can help keep the noodles from getting too soft.

Draining the zucchini noodles and patting them dry will keep your sauce from getting watered down. But if you prefer, you can also make your sauce thicker than normal, transfer the cooked noodles directly from the skillet to the sauce, and toss the noodles in it to thin it out.

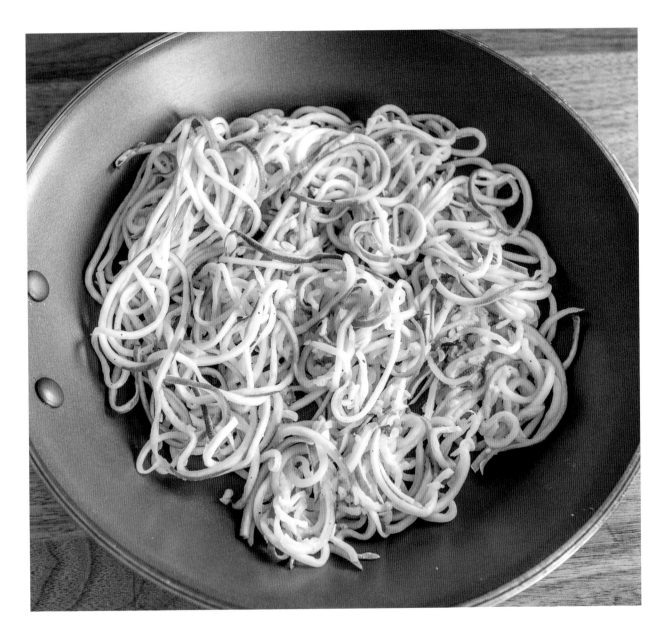

NOTES:

Zucchini noodles make a great side dish, even without sauce. Cook some chopped garlic in the oil before you add the noodles, then toss them with lots of grated Parmesan cheese just before serving. (Add a pinch of red pepper flakes if you like.)

If you're adding zucchini noodles to a soup, you can skip precooking and add them directly to the soup. Allow to simmer until softened. Be sure to check the seasoning of the soup after they've softened, since the zucchini will add a bit of water. Only do this with soup you're eating right away; if the zucchini sits in the soup overnight or longer, it may get mushy.

PARSNIP MASH

MAKES: About 3½ cups (4 servings) | **PREP TIME:** 15 minutes |
COOK TIME: 20 minutes

Confession time: Beth is not a fan of potatoes. Weird, right? But the
thing is, lots of other vegetables make a good mash. Parsnips do the
job here, and this dish is carnivore-ish thanks to the addition of bone
broth, cream cheese, and butter.

2 pounds parsnips, peeled and
sliced ¼ inch thick

4 cloves garlic, peeled and
smashed with the side of a
knife

6 sprigs fresh thyme

1 dried bay leaf

2 cups chicken or beef bone
broth

3 tablespoons whipped cream
cheese

2 tablespoons (1 ounce)
unsalted butter

Fine sea salt and freshly
ground black pepper

Extra-virgin olive oil, for
drizzling

1. Put the parsnips, garlic, thyme, and bay leaf in a medium
saucepan. Pour in the broth and bring to a boil over medium-high
heat. Lower the heat to medium-low, cover, and simmer until the
parsnips are very tender and easily pierced with a knife, 10 to
15 minutes. Drain, reserving the cooking liquid.

2. Remove the bay leaf and thyme stems and discard (don't worry
about the thyme leaves). Transfer the parsnips and garlic to a food
processor. Add the cream cheese and butter and process until
smooth. If the mash is too thick, add the reserved cooking liquid a
tablespoon or two at a time and continue to process until the puree
is smooth and velvety. Taste and season with salt and pepper.

3. Transfer the puree to a serving bowl, drizzle with olive oil, and
serve.

NOTES:

*You can make the puree up to 1 day ahead. Let cool, cover,
and refrigerate. To rewarm, place it in a heatproof bowl
set over a pan of lightly boiling water and cook, stirring
occasionally, until warmed through.*

*If you have block cream cheese, you can use it instead of
whipped. Use 1¼ ounces, a little over 2 tablespoons.*

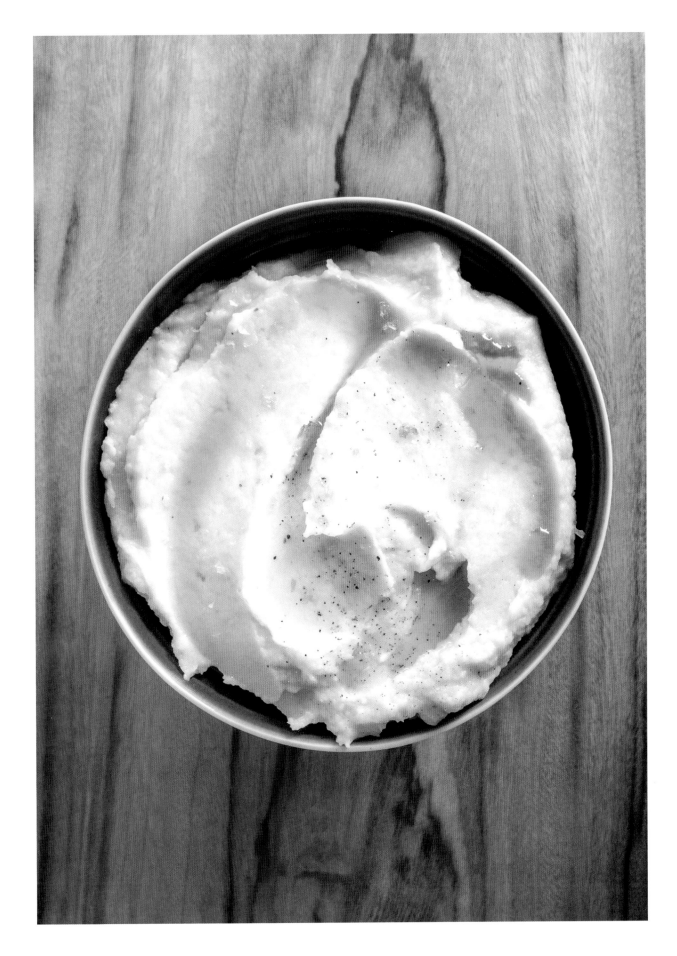

CAESAR SALAD WITH PORK BELLY "CROUTONS"

SERVES: 4 | **PREP TIME:** 20 minutes | **COOK TIME:** 1 hour 10 minutes

Pork belly chunks take the place of traditional croutons to make this salad so satisfying. Most butchers carry pork belly, but if you have trouble finding it, get some thickly cut bacon, cut it into chunks, and fry that up instead.

DRESSING:

3 jarred anchovy fillets, chopped

3 cloves garlic, minced (about 1 tablespoon)

4 tablespoons extra-virgin olive oil, divided

½ teaspoon grated lemon zest

2 tablespoons fresh lemon juice

¼ cup freshly grated Parmesan cheese (about ¾ ounce)

1 tablespoon chopped fresh flat-leaf parsley

1 large egg yolk (see Note)

Freshly ground black pepper

SALAD:

1 pound pork belly, patted dry and cut into 1-inch cubes

Fine sea salt and freshly ground black pepper

1 large or 2 medium heads romaine lettuce, chopped (about 8 cups)

3 tablespoons freshly grated Parmesan cheese, plus more if desired

1. Make the dressing: Put the anchovies, garlic, and 2 tablespoons of the olive oil in a small unheated skillet. Place over low heat and cook until the mixture sizzles. Allow to sizzle undisturbed for 30 seconds, then transfer to a small bowl to cool.

2. In a small food processor, combine the lemon zest and juice, Parmesan, parsley, and egg yolk. Add the cooled anchovy mixture and blend well. With the machine running, blend in the remaining 2 tablespoons of oil until the dressing has thickened and emulsified. Taste and season with pepper. (You can make the dressing up to 1 day ahead; keep it covered and refrigerated. Whisk before using.)

3. Prepare the pork belly: Preheat the oven to 300°F. Warm a large ovenproof skillet over medium heat. Season the pork belly with salt and pepper. Cook the pork belly in the skillet, turning occasionally, until golden all over, 10 to 12 minutes. Transfer the skillet to the oven and bake the pork belly, stirring occasionally, until browned and crisp, 45 to 60 minutes, stirring every 15 minutes. Transfer to a plate.

4. Make the salad: Just before serving, toss the lettuce with ¼ cup of the dressing. Divide among four plates. Sprinkle with the Parmesan (add more if you prefer it cheesier). Divide the pork croutons among the salads and serve, passing the remaining dressing on the side.

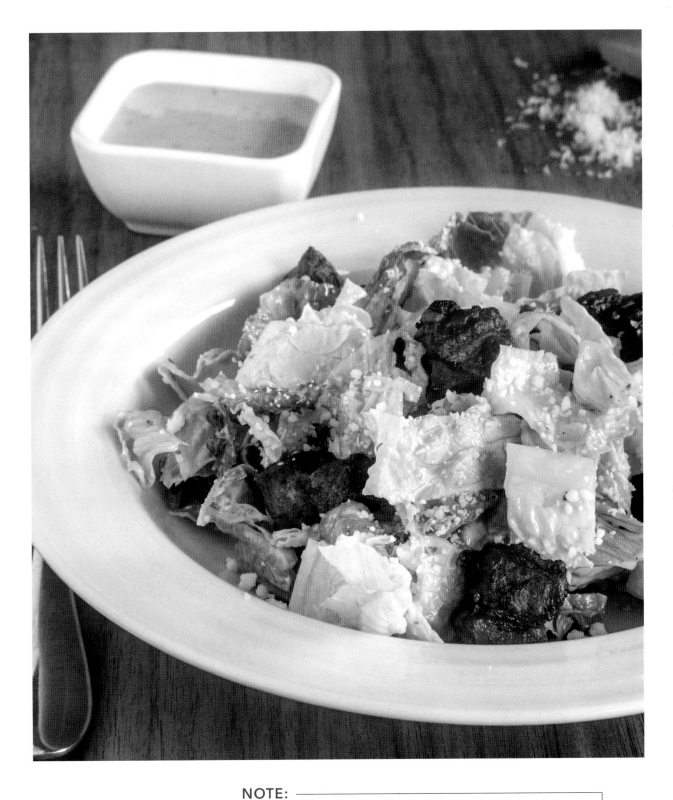

AIR FRYER MIXED SWEET POTATO CHIPS

SERVES: 4 | **PREP TIME:** 15 minutes | **COOK TIME:** 24 minutes

Who doesn't love light, crisp, salty chips? And when you make them yourself, you know exactly what ingredients are in them. We love this combination of orange and purple sweet potatoes, both for the color and the slight flavor differences—Ube potatoes tend to be a bit starchier and just a tad sweeter. Work in batches so you don't overcrowd the fryer, or you won't get the crisp texture you want.

2 large sweet potatoes, scrubbed and dried

2 large Ube potatoes, scrubbed and dried

1 tablespoon extra-virgin olive oil

Fine sea salt and freshly ground black pepper

Special equipment:
Mandoline slicer

1.   Using a mandoline slicer, thinly slice all of the potatoes (think potato chip thickness, not translucent). Place in a large bowl; drizzle with the olive oil and season with 1 tablespoon of salt, then toss to coat.

2.   Preheat an air fryer to 300°F for 5 minutes. Mist the basket with cooking spray.

3.   Working in batches, add the potato slices to the basket in a single layer and air-fry at 300°F until they begin to crisp, about 5 minutes. Open the basket, toss the potatoes, spread in a single layer again, and cook until crisp and beginning to brown, 2 to 3 minutes longer. Repeat until all of the chips have been fried, placing the finished chips on a rimmed baking sheet. Toss with more salt and pepper to taste and serve right away.

NOTES: ——————————

You can peel the potatoes or leave the skins on, depending on your preference. If you peel them, you don't have to scrub them; just a rinse will do.

Eat these chips as soon as possible, and definitely the same day you make them. After that, they lose their crispness.

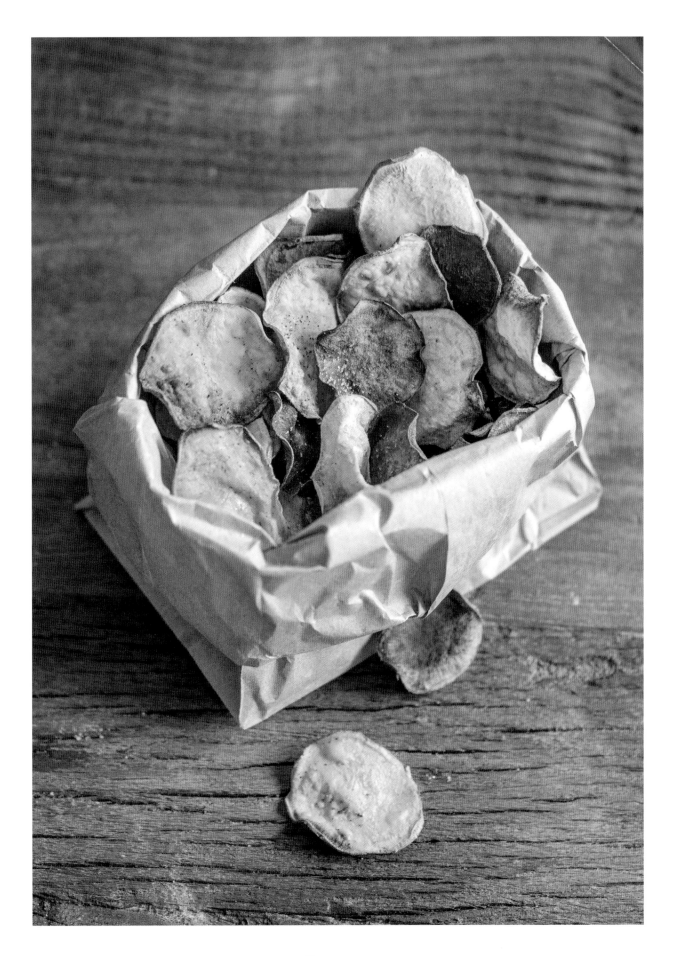

GARLICKY SPAGHETTI SQUASH

SERVES: 8 | **PREP TIME:** 15 minutes | **COOK TIME:** 45 minutes

You don't have to be a chef to know that plenty of butter and garlic will make anything taste better. This holds especially true with spaghetti squash, which is versatile and nutritious but rather bland on its own. This recipe elevates it to a flavorful side dish worthy of your favorite meals, and it's a fantastic base for our Wild Boar Meatballs (page 192).

1 medium spaghetti squash (about 4 pounds)

4 cloves garlic, chopped (about 1 tablespoon plus 1 teaspoon)

2 tablespoons (1 ounce) unsalted butter

Fine sea salt and freshly ground black pepper

1. Preheat the oven to 400°F. Grease a 3-quart glass baking dish.

2. Cut the squash crosswise into 1½-inch-thick slices; scoop out the seeds. Lay the squash rings in a single layer in the baking dish. Sprinkle the garlic on top of the squash.

3. Bake until the squash is soft and stringy and easily pierced with a knife, and the edges have begun to brown, about 45 minutes.

4. Let the squash stand until cool enough to handle. Rake a fork through the squash so the flesh comes apart in "noodles" and scrape it off the skin. Transfer the squash to a large bowl. Add the butter and toss until coated and the butter has melted. Season generously with salt and pepper and serve.

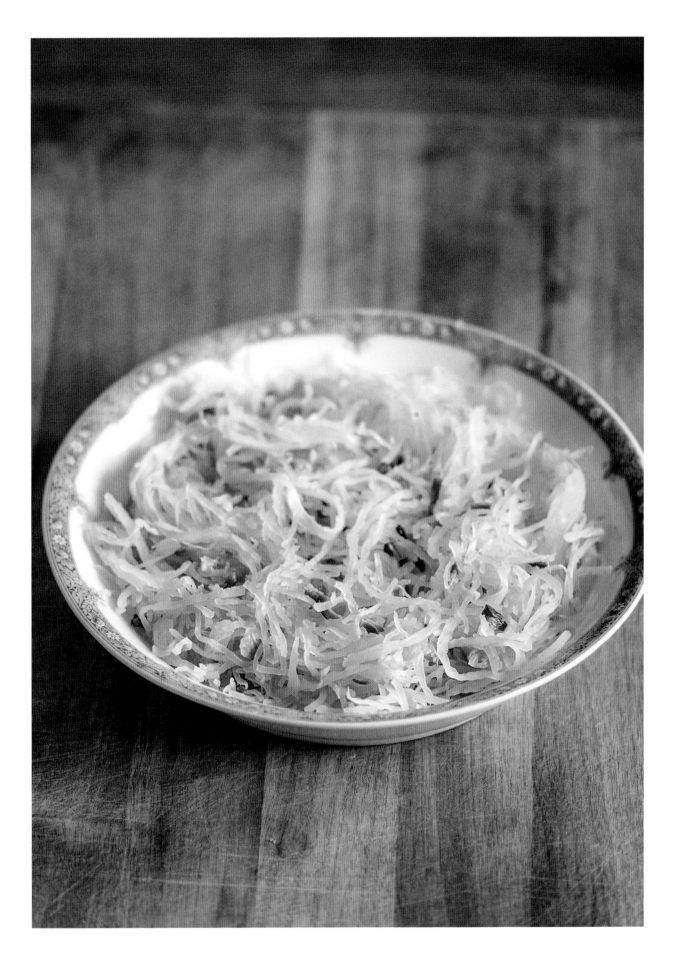

PORK PANKO ONION RINGS

SERVES: 2 to 4 | **PREP TIME:** 30 minutes, plus 1 hour to soak |
COOK TIME: 20 minutes

Full disclosure: this recipe is a bit messy and chaotic, and it's best done as a team, with one person battering and the other frying. If you read "messy and chaotic" and think, "Fun!" then this one's for you (and no judgment if not; we get it). First you dredge the rings in a seasoned cassava flour mixture, then you coat them in a buttermilk batter, and then you toss them in pork panko. It's definitely worth it; these onion rings are crisp on the outside, tender inside, and loaded with savory flavor.

1 large sweet onion, such as Vidalia or Walla Walla, cut into ¼-inch slices, rings separated

2 cups buttermilk

1 to 2 cups avocado oil, for frying

1¼ cups (175 grams) cassava flour

1¼ teaspoons baking powder

1 teaspoon garlic powder

1 teaspoon fine sea salt

½ teaspoon freshly ground black pepper

¼ teaspoon chili powder

2 to 3 cups pork panko

1 large egg, beaten

Ketchup, mayo, or Cheeseburger Salad dressing (page 84), for serving (optional)

1. Put the onion slices in a large bowl. Pour in the buttermilk. Let soak for 1 hour, stirring occasionally.

2. Pour 1 inch of avocado oil into a large, deep skillet (with sides at least 2 inches high) or Dutch oven and warm over medium heat to 365°F. (Don't have a deep-fry thermometer? Flick a little bit of water into the skillet; if the oil sizzles, it is hot enough.) Preheat the oven to 225°F. Put a cooling rack inside a rimmed baking sheet and place it in the oven. Put a separate cooling rack inside another rimmed baking sheet or on newspaper and set on the counter.

3. In a large bowl, whisk together the cassava flour, baking powder, garlic powder, salt, pepper, and chili powder. Put 2 cups of panko in a separate large bowl. Remove the onion slices from the buttermilk, shaking off the excess, and place on a large plate. Working with a few at a time, put the onion pieces in the bowl with the cassava flour mixture and toss to coat. Remove one at a time, shaking off the excess flour mixture, and place on the cooling rack on the counter. Reserve the leftover buttermilk. Wipe off the plate.

4. Add the reserved buttermilk, egg, and ½ cup water to the cassava flour mixture; whisk until smooth (the batter will be thin, like pancake batter). Working with a few at a time, add the floured onions to the bowl with the batter; turn to coat the slices with the batter. Place on the plate.

5. Working with a few at a time, add the battered onion slices to the panko and toss to coat. (Add the additional cup of panko if needed.)

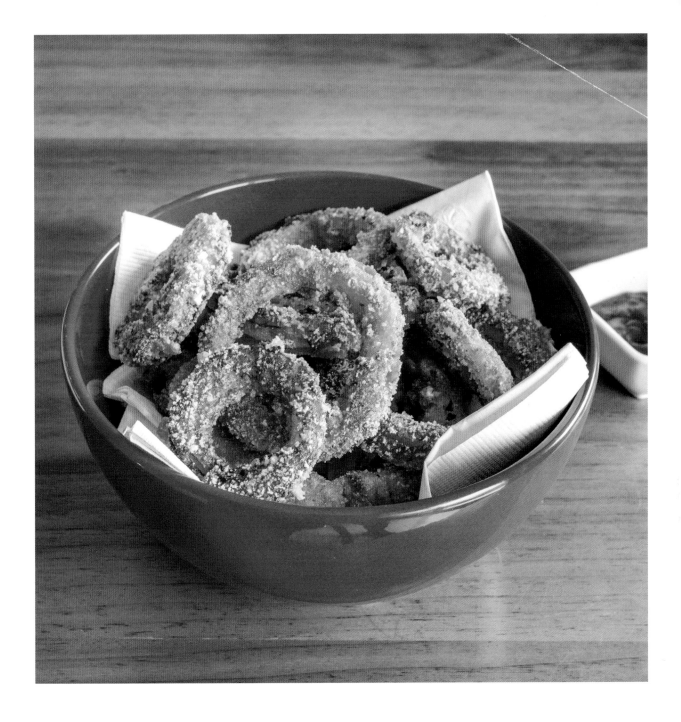

6. Place a few of the panko-coated onion slices in the hot oil. Fry until golden, turning once, about 2 minutes. Transfer the cooked onion rings to the rack in the oven and keep warm while you coat the remaining onion rings in panko and fry them. (You can see why it's useful to have more than one person working on this.) Adjust the heat under the oil as needed to keep the temperature steady at 365°F.

7. Serve the onion rings hot, with condiments for dipping, if desired.

TOSTONES

SERVES: 4 | **PREP TIME:** 3 minutes | **COOK TIME:** 15 minutes

These fried green plantains not only taste great and work beautifully to scoop up chili or guac, but they're also good for you. Green plantains are loaded with resistant starch, a gut-health booster that helps fill you up without making your blood sugar go crazy.

½ cup avocado oil

2 green plantains, peeled and cut into 1-inch-thick slices

Fine sea salt and freshly ground black pepper

1. Heat the avocado oil in a large cast-iron skillet over medium-high heat. Working in batches if needed to avoid overcrowding the pan, carefully place the plantain slices in the oil and cook until they begin to brown and soften, 3 to 4 minutes. Using tongs, flip them over and fry until the other side is browned, about 2 minutes.

2. Transfer the plantains to a platter lined with paper towels to drain. Turn off the heat under the skillet but leave the oil in the pan.

3. Lay a piece of parchment paper on a cutting board. Place the plantain pieces on the parchment paper, lay another piece of parchment on top, and flatten the plantains with a rolling pin to a ½-inch thickness. (Alternatively, you can flatten them one at a time with the bottom of a glass.)

4. Rewarm the oil over medium heat. Working in batches, fry the plantains a second time until they are crunchy but still tender inside, 1 to 2 minutes total. Transfer to another plate lined with paper towels to absorb the excess oil. Season to taste with salt and pepper and serve hot.

NOTE:

Tostones are best eaten right away. They lose their crispness if they sit around.

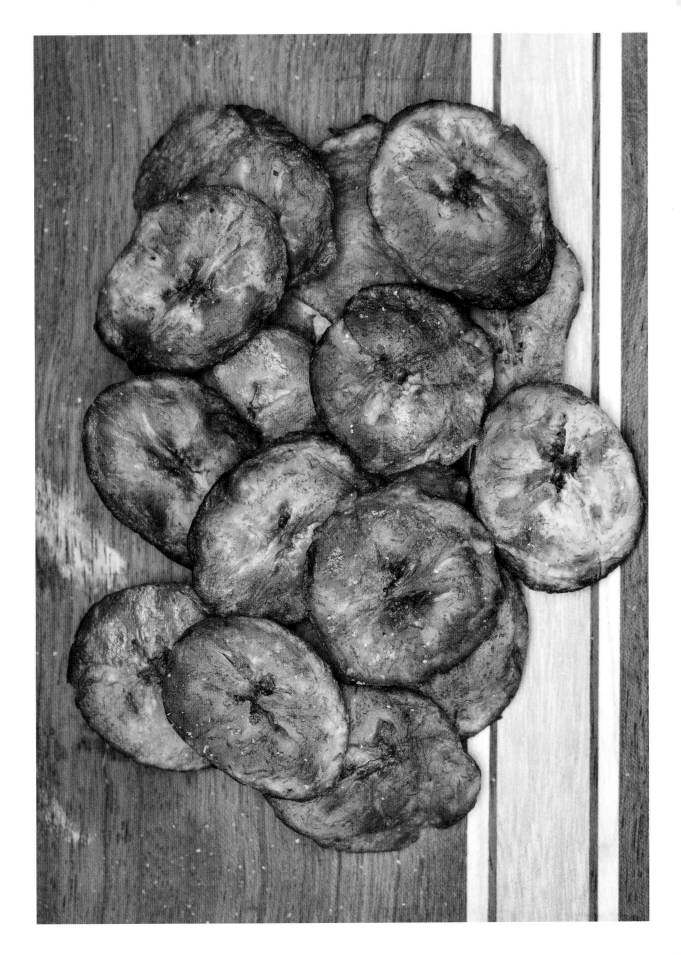

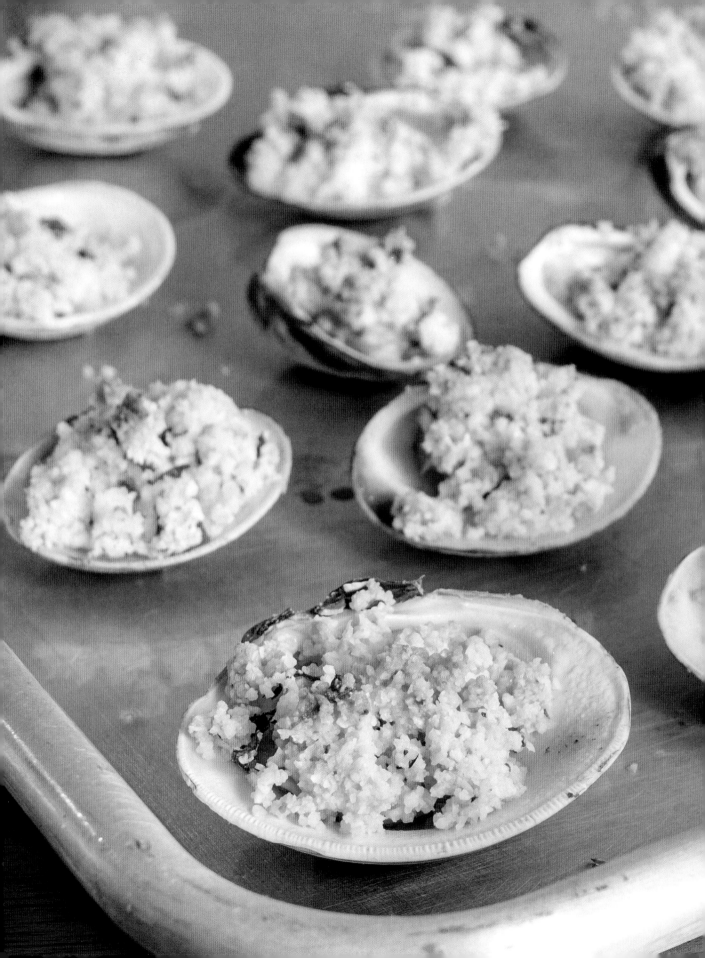

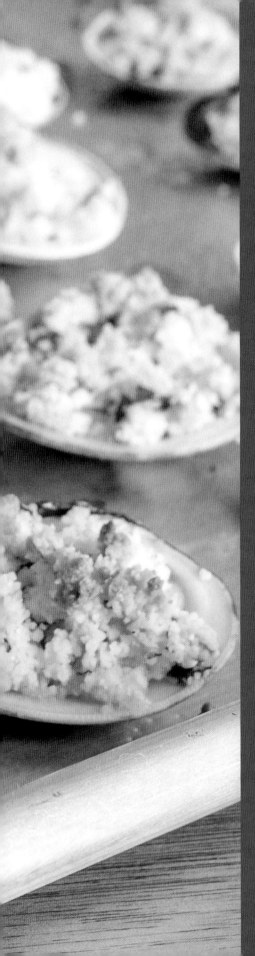

CHAPTER 11:

APPETIZERS & SNACKS

STUFFED MUSHROOMS

SERVES: 4 | **PREP TIME:** 15 minutes | **COOK TIME:** 36 minutes

Cheese and pancetta–Italian bacon–are all you need to make beautiful, luscious stuffed mushrooms. If you serve these at a party, they are guaranteed to go fast.

8 large white mushrooms

1 tablespoon (½ ounce) unsalted butter

½ white onion, finely chopped (about 1 cup)

2 cloves garlic, minced (about 2 teaspoons)

4 thin slices pancetta, shredded

¾ cup shredded mozzarella cheese (about 3 ounces)

1. Preheat the oven to 400°F. Line a rimmed baking sheet with parchment paper.

2. Clean the mushrooms; trim the bottoms of the stems. Cut off the stems and set aside, then cut around the inner rims of the mushroom caps to make space for the filling.

3. Melt the butter in a large skillet over medium heat. Add the mushroom stems and onion and cook, stirring often, until softened, about 5 minutes. Add the garlic and cook, stirring, until fragrant, about 1 minute longer. Remove from the heat.

4. In a medium bowl, combine the mushroom and onion mixture with the pancetta and cheese. Scoop the mixture into the mushroom caps and place on the lined baking sheet.

5. Bake until the cheese has melted, the filling is golden, and the mushrooms are browned, about 30 minutes. Serve hot.

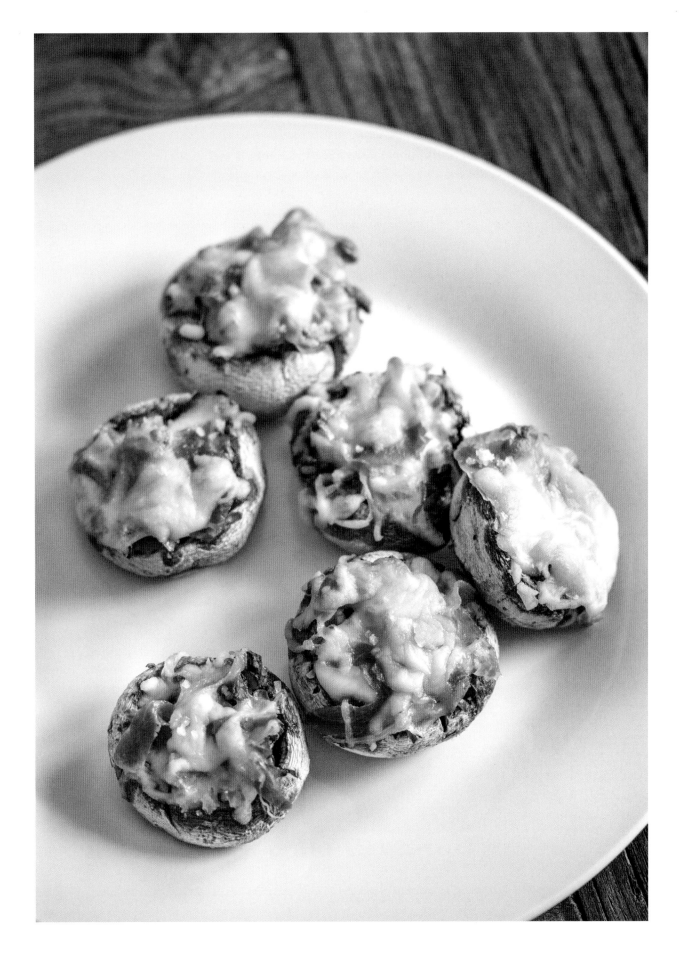

BAKED STUFFED CLAMS

SERVES: 8 | **PREP TIME:** 30 minutes | **COOK TIME:** 30 minutes

Beth's mom, Tama, made the world's best baked stuffed clams. It was one of Beth's favorite dishes of hers. Sadly, Tama is gone now, and Beth never did get that recipe. But here's ours: it's free of grains but full of flavor and our own brand of mama love. It's fancy enough to serve at a dinner party but easy and budget-friendly enough to make anytime. We like to think Tama would have loved them.

CLAMS:

1 tablespoon (½ ounce) unsalted butter

1 tablespoon extra-virgin olive oil

3 cloves garlic, minced (about 1 tablespoon)

40 Little Neck clams, scrubbed

½ cup dry white wine

TOPPING:

1 lemon, scrubbed and dried

2 tablespoons (1 ounce) unsalted butter

2 tablespoons extra-virgin olive oil

2 cloves garlic, grated (about 2 teaspoons)

1 cup blanched almond flour

¼ cup freshly grated Parmesan or Pecorino Romano cheese (about ¾ ounce)

2 tablespoons chopped fresh flat-leaf parsley

½ teaspoon dried oregano leaves

Fine sea salt and freshly ground black pepper

1. Preheat the oven to 450°F. Oil a rimmed baking sheet.

2. Make the clams: Put the butter, olive oil, and garlic in a large unheated saucepan or Dutch oven. Place over medium-low heat; cook gently until the butter melts and the mixture begins to sizzle, 2 to 3 minutes. Allow to sizzle for 30 seconds more. Add the clams in a single layer (or mostly so), working in batches if needed to avoid overcrowding the pan, which would make it hard for the clams to open. Stir to coat the clams with the butter mixture, then pour in the wine and ¼ cup water. Raise the heat to medium, cover, and allow the clams to cook until the shells open, 5 to 7 minutes. After 5 minutes, begin to check and remove opened clams one at a time, pouring any liquid in them back into the pan. After 7 minutes, discard any clams that haven't opened. Strain the cooking liquid through a fine-mesh sieve into a small bowl.

3. Using tongs, transfer the clams to the prepared baking sheet; let cool until you can handle them. Pull off and discard the top shells.

4. Make the topping: Grate 1 teaspoon zest from the lemon, then cut the fruit into wedges for serving. In a small unheated skillet, combine the butter, olive oil, and garlic. Place over low heat and cook until the butter melts and the mixture begins to sizzle, 4 to 5 minutes. Let it sizzle for 30 seconds more, then transfer to a medium bowl. Add the almond flour, Parmesan, parsley, lemon zest, and oregano and stir well. The texture should be like wet sand; if the mixture is dry, add the reserved clam juice 1 teaspoon at a time to moisten. Taste and season with salt and pepper.

5. Top each clam with about ½ teaspoon of the topping mixture. Mist with cooking spray. Bake until the filling is golden and crisp, 8 to 10 minutes. Serve hot with the lemon wedges on the side.

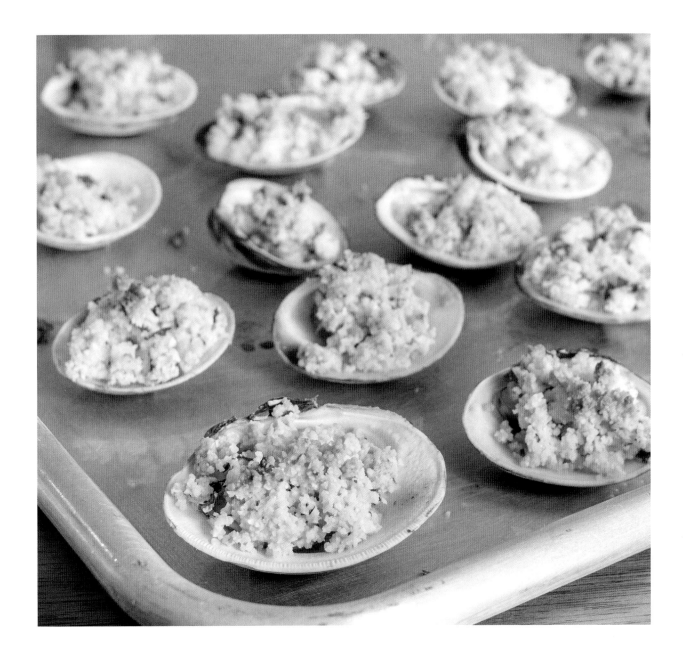

NOTES:

Clams vary in size; use more or less filling as needed.

If you're making these for a party, you can prep them up to 8 hours ahead, but wait to bake them. Top the clams with the filling on the baking sheet, cover, and refrigerate. Uncover and bake when you're ready to serve (you'll need to bake them a few minutes longer if they're right out of the fridge).

If you have topping left over, you can freeze it and use it for more clams later, or spread it on fish before baking.

WARM BACON JALAPEÑO POPPER DIP

SERVES: 4 to 6 | **PREP TIME:** 20 minutes | **COOK TIME:** 40 minutes

Jalapeño poppers are awesome—spicy, crunchy, and cheesy. But they can be a little bit of a hassle to make, especially if you're having people over. We thought, why not deconstruct them into a dip that you can make in advance? This dip is much easier to serve at a party because you're not stuck in the kitchen frying peppers while everyone else is socializing. Pro tip: If you have any dip left over (unlikely, but...), keep it covered in the fridge and add a spoonful to scrambled eggs.

2 ounces bacon (about 2 slices)

3 large jalapeño peppers, seeds and ribs removed, finely diced (about ¾ cup)

3 scallions, sliced on a diagonal (about ⅓ cup; reserve dark green parts for garnish if desired)

Pinch of fine sea salt

2 (8-ounce) packages cream cheese, at room temperature

¾ cup avocado oil mayonnaise

½ cup shredded sharp cheddar cheese (about 2 ounces)

½ cup freshly grated Parmesan cheese (about 1 ounce), divided

1 (7-ounce) can pickled jalapeño slices, drained and chopped

½ cup pork panko

Grain-free crackers, homemade (page 308) or store-bought, and/or sliced vegetables, for serving

1. Preheat the oven to 350°F.

2. Put the bacon in a medium unheated cast-iron or other ovenproof skillet; place over medium-low heat. (*Note:* If your skillet isn't ovenproof, have an 8-inch baking dish ready.) Cook the bacon until it is crisp and the fat has rendered, turning it a few times, about 10 minutes. Transfer the bacon to a cutting board and set aside.

3. Raise the heat to medium and add the diced jalapeños and white and light green parts of the scallions to the fat in the skillet. Sprinkle with the salt and cook, stirring occasionally, until tender, 3 to 4 minutes. Transfer to a small bowl to cool slightly. Chop the bacon.

4. In a large bowl, using an electric mixer, beat the cream cheese, mayonnaise, cheddar, and ¼ cup of the Parmesan until well blended. Scrape down the sides of the bowl, add the jalapeño mixture, pickled jalapeños, and bacon; beat again just to mix. Spread in the skillet or baking dish. Combine the remaining ¼ cup of Parmesan and panko, then sprinkle over the jalapeño mixture. Mist the top with cooking spray.

5. Bake until the dip is heated through and golden on top, 20 to 25 minutes. Sprinkle with the sliced dark green parts of the scallions, if desired, and serve with crackers and/or vegetables.

NOTE:

Broil the finished dip for a minute or two to crisp the topping if you like. Watch it carefully to prevent burning.

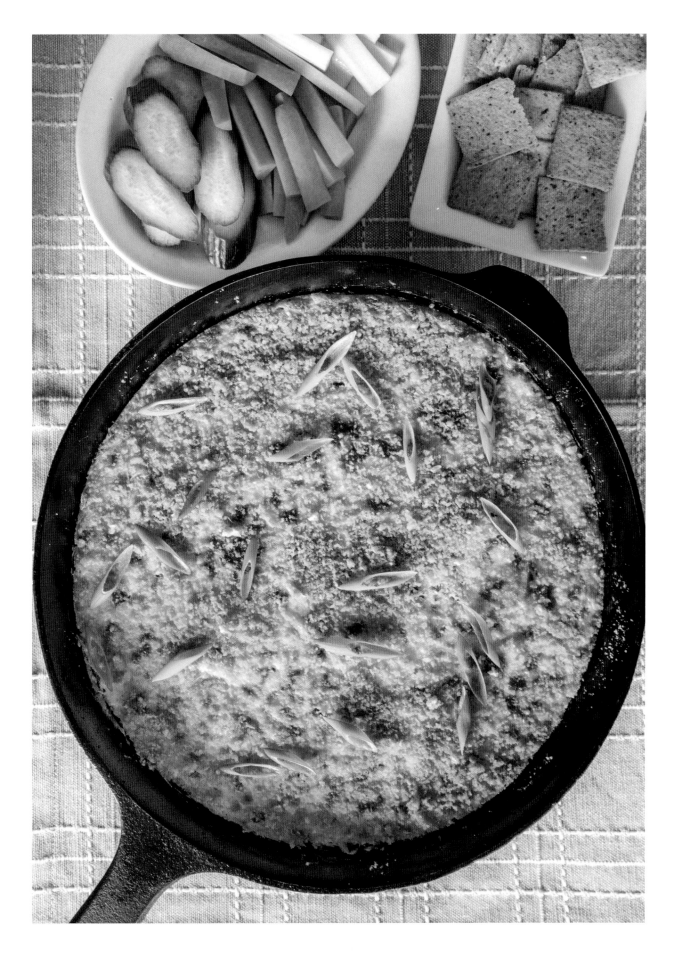

AIR FRYER MOZZARELLA STICKS

MAKES: 12 pieces (4 servings) | **PREP TIME:** 30 minutes, plus 1 hour to freeze | **COOK TIME:** 5 minutes

Isn't it fantastic when you can take food you love that isn't so great for you, make it healthier, and have it taste every bit as good (or even better)? These mozzarella sticks are grain-free and air-fried, so you get all that crisp cheesy goodness *and* get to feel like a champ afterward. Bread extras to keep in the freezer and air-fry at will; your future self will thank you. Do not skip the second round of dipping: the sticks fall apart in the air fryer without the extra layer of breading.

¼ cup (35 grams) cassava flour

½ teaspoon garlic powder

¼ teaspoon onion powder

¼ teaspoon dried oregano leaves

⅛ teaspoon fine sea salt

⅛ teaspoon freshly ground black pepper

2 large eggs

1 cup pork panko, divided

6 part-skim mozzarella sticks, cut in half crosswise

Chopped fresh flat-leaf parsley, for garnish (optional)

Warmed marinara sauce, for dipping (optional)

1. In a shallow bowl, combine the cassava flour, garlic powder, onion powder, oregano, salt, and pepper. In a separate shallow bowl, beat the eggs. Put half of the panko in a third shallow bowl. Line a plate or rimmed baking sheet with parchment or waxed paper.

2. Working one at a time, dredge a mozzarella stick in the flour mixture. Tap off the excess. Dip in the egg, shaking off the excess, then dredge in the panko. Place on the lined plate. Repeat until all of the sticks are coated.

3. Add the remaining panko to the bowl with the panko. Repeat dipping, first in the cassava flour mixture, then the egg, then the panko. Freeze for at least 1 hour. (Once they're frozen, you can transfer the sticks to a resealable bag and freeze them for up to 3 months.)

4. Preheat an air fryer to 380°F for 5 minutes. Mist the air fryer basket with cooking spray. Place the frozen mozzarella sticks in a single layer in the basket (work in batches if necessary, keeping the remaining sticks in the freezer). Mist the tops with cooking spray. Air-fry for 5 minutes, until golden brown and crisp. Serve warm, sprinkled with parsley and with marinara sauce alongside for dipping, if desired.

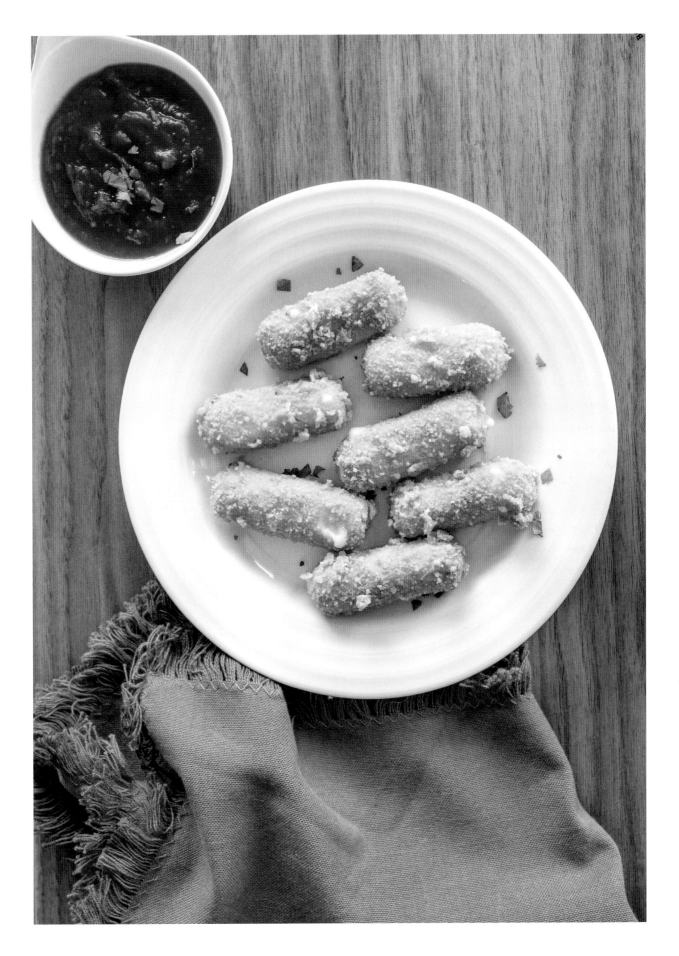

PAFFLE

MAKES: 1 paffle | **PREP TIME:** 5 minutes | **COOK TIME:** 4 minutes

Cheese, egg, and pork rinds—it's no surprise that this combo, when waffle-ized, makes a really satisfying quick meal or base for eggs, a BLT, avocado toast, or cold cuts. What *is* surprising is that this carb-free food feels carb-y when you eat it. It's rich, meaty, and hearty, the savory cousin to the sweet Cinnamon Bun Chaffles (page 210). Feel free to double or triple this recipe; it multiplies easily.

1 large egg

½ cup pork panko

⅓ cup shredded mozzarella cheese (about 1.3 ounces)

¼ teaspoon garlic powder

Pinch of fine sea salt

Pinch of cayenne pepper (optional)

Pinch of freshly ground black pepper

1. Preheat a waffle iron to high.

2. In a medium bowl, beat the egg. Stir in the panko, mozzarella, garlic powder, salt, and cayenne, if using. Season with the pepper. The mixture will be very thick, like cookie dough.

3. Mist the waffle iron lightly with cooking spray. Scoop the mixture into the center of the iron, close, and cook until golden brown and crisp, 3 to 4 minutes (or as the manufacturer instructs). Serve hot.

NOTE:

To ensure your waffles don't stick, a nonstick waffle iron is ideal; if you're using a waffle iron without a nonstick surface, use a brush to grease it with oil or melted ghee or butter. If using a nonstick waffle iron, remember to use a nonmetal tool to remove the paffle, such as a silicone spatula, to avoid scratching the finish.

How to change up your paffle

Use ¼ cup mozzarella and 1 tablespoon grated Parmesan, and add diced pepperoni and ¼ teaspoon dried oregano or basil leaves to the batter. Serve with marinara sauce for dipping.

Use shredded cheddar instead of mozzarella. Some chopped fresh chives go nicely in here, too.

Add different spices—try a blend like za'atar or curry powder, or a mix of chili powder and cumin.

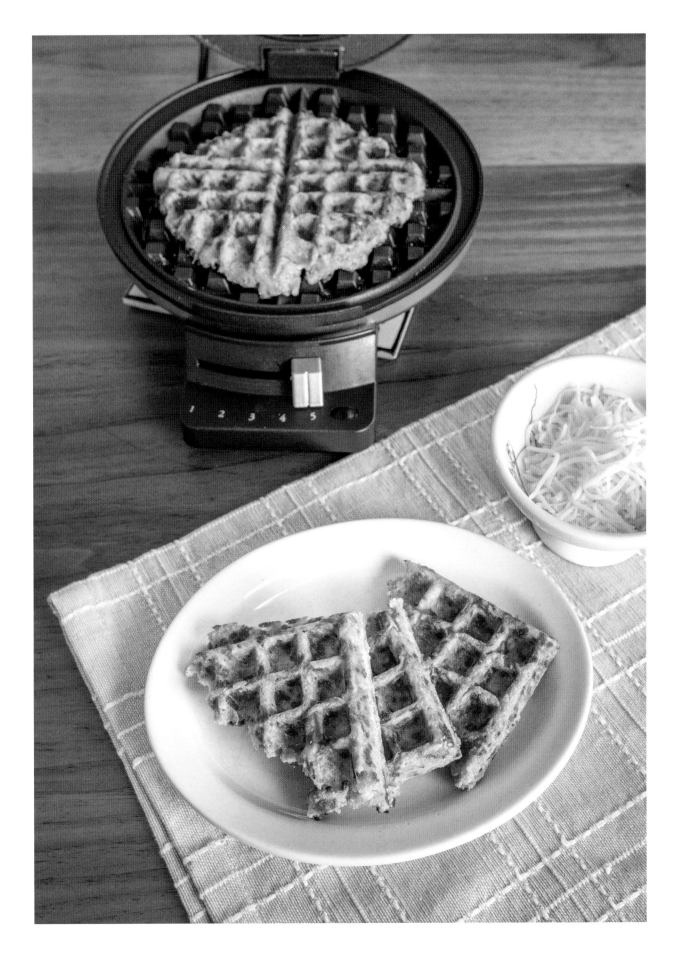

ELVIS BANANA BREAD

MAKES: One 9-inch loaf (10 slices) | **PREP TIME:** 15 minutes | **COOK TIME:** 1 hour

We don't know if it's true that Elvis ate fried peanut butter, banana, and bacon sandwiches, but that flavor combo is forever associated with the King. Here, it's every bit as indulgent but also good for you in banana bread form. Use crunchy or smooth peanut butter; either one works.

4 ounces bacon (about 4 slices)

1½ cups (156 grams) blanched almond flour

¼ cup (36 grams) arrowroot powder

3 tablespoons (18 grams) unflavored grass-fed collagen peptides

1 teaspoon baking soda

¼ teaspoon fine sea salt

3 medium ripe bananas, mashed (about 1¼ cups)

⅓ cup unsweetened, salted peanut butter (see Notes)

¼ cup maple syrup

2 large eggs

1 teaspoon vanilla extract

2 ounces dark chocolate (at least 70% cacao), finely chopped (optional)

¼ cup chopped roasted salted peanuts (optional)

1. Preheat the oven to 350°F. Line a 9 by 5-inch loaf pan with parchment paper.

2. Put the bacon in a medium unheated skillet over medium-low heat; cook until crisp, flipping once or twice, about 10 minutes. Transfer to a cutting board to cool, then finely chop or crumble.

3. In a large bowl, whisk together the almond flour, arrowroot, collagen, baking soda, and salt. Put the bananas, peanut butter, maple syrup, eggs, and vanilla in a medium bowl and whisk well. Add the banana mixture to the flour mixture and stir until well combined. If using the chocolate and peanuts, set aside 1 tablespoon of each for garnish, then fold the remaining chocolate and peanuts and the chopped bacon into the batter.

4. Spread the batter evenly in the lined loaf pan. Sprinkle the reserved chocolate and peanuts on top, if using. Bake until a toothpick inserted in the center comes out clean, 45 to 50 minutes. Cover loosely with foil while baking if the top is browning too quickly.

5. Put the pan on a rack to cool for 10 minutes, then turn the bread out onto the rack to cool completely. Store leftovers covered in the fridge for up to 4 days, or wrap tightly and freeze for up to 3 months.

NOTES:

Peanut butters vary in saltiness. This recipe was developed using lightly salted peanut butter. Taste the brand you're using to see how salty it is and adjust the salt in the recipe accordingly. (A little extra saltiness in a peanut butter–banana bread isn't necessarily a bad thing.) If using unsalted peanut butter, consider adding an extra pinch or two of salt to the dry mixture.

Feel free to swap in an equal amount of almond or cashew butter or tahini if peanut butter isn't your thing.

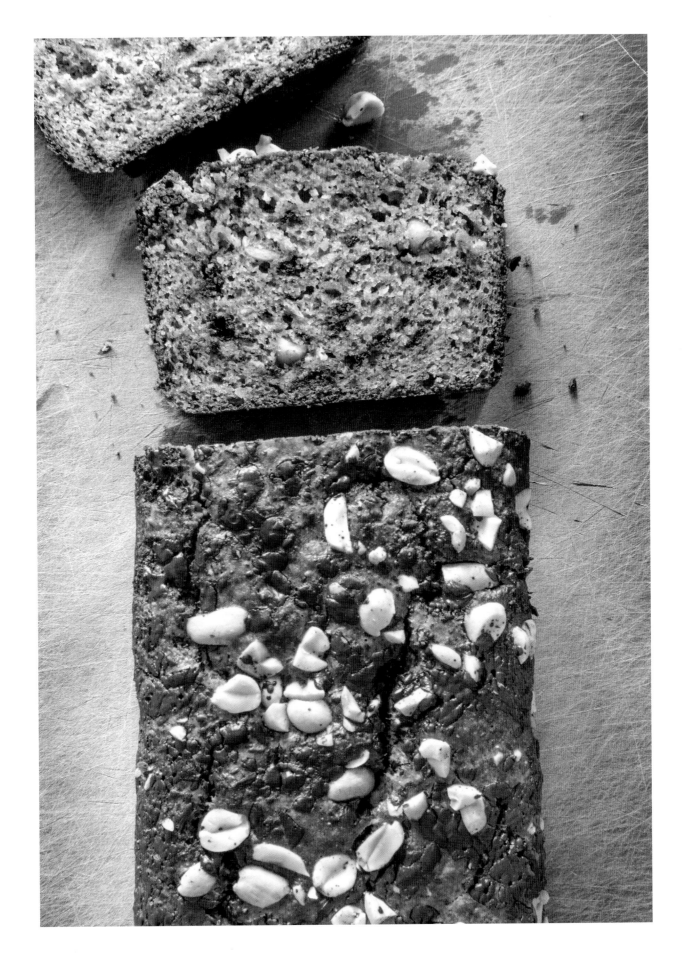

DARK CHOCOLATE-COCONUT GRANOLA CLUSTERS

MAKES: About 7 cups (14 to 18 servings) | **PREP TIME:** 15 minutes | **COOK TIME:** 35 minutes

Is it a snack, breakfast, or dessert? The answer is yes. This grain-free granola is super rich and indulgent thanks to cacao powder and dark chocolate. But it isn't super sweet, so you can have it with yogurt for breakfast, grab a handful as a snack, or try it crumbled on a hot fudge sundae to add something extra to a special dessert (see the recipe on page 320).

½ cup unsweetened almond butter

½ cup maple syrup

⅓ cup bacon fat

1 teaspoon vanilla extract

½ teaspoon fine sea salt

1 cup sliced almonds

½ cup chopped raw pecans or walnuts

¼ cup hemp hearts

1 cup unsweetened shredded coconut

¼ cup (24 grams) raw cacao powder

¼ cup (26 grams) blanched almond flour

2 ounces dark chocolate (at least 70%), finely chopped

1. Preheat the oven to 325°F. Line a rimmed baking sheet with parchment paper.

2. Put the almond butter, maple syrup, and bacon fat in a medium saucepan. Set over low heat and cook, stirring often, until smooth and well combined. Remove the pan from the heat; stir in the vanilla and salt.

3. In a large bowl, combine the almonds, pecans, hemp hearts, coconut, cacao, and almond flour. Add the almond butter mixture and fold together until the ingredients are well combined. Spread in a thin, even layer on the lined baking sheet. (If it's too thick, it won't crisp up.)

4. Bake until the granola is golden and beginning to get crisp (it will crisp up further as it cools), 25 to 30 minutes. Place the baking sheet on a wire rack; sprinkle the top with the chopped chocolate (it will melt; this is what you want). Let cool completely before breaking the granola into clusters. Store in an airtight container in the fridge for up to a week.

NOTE: —————————————————————

If you don't have bacon fat (why not?), you can swap in unrefined coconut oil or olive oil.

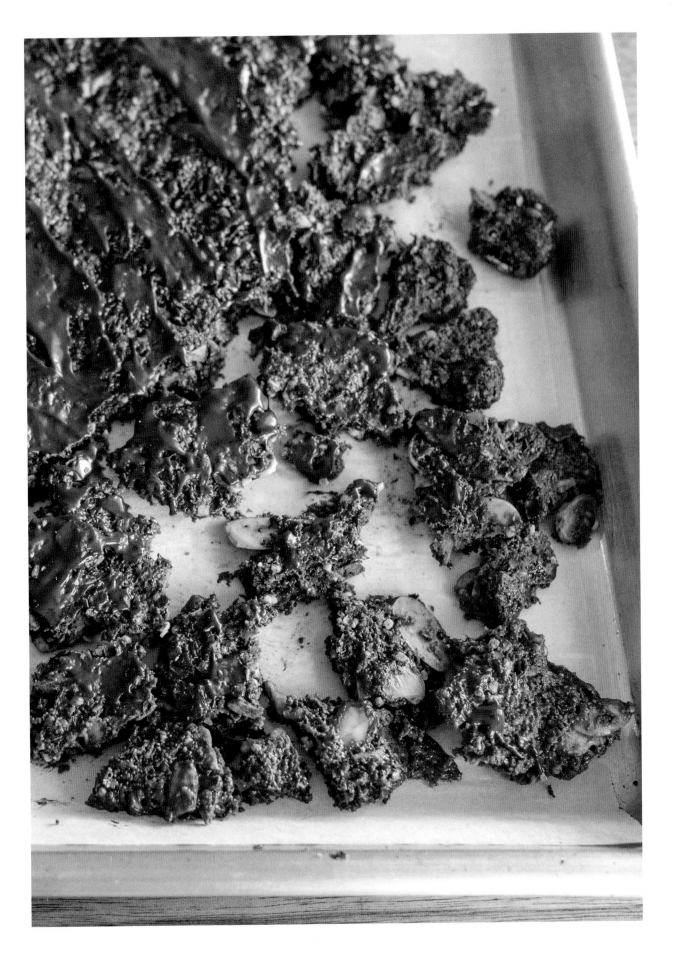

KETO EGG BREADS

SERVES: 6 | **PREP TIME:** 10 minutes | **COOK TIME:** 23 minutes

Going grain-free can have a lot of advantages, but missing bread is definitely a downside. No wonder people found a workaround with keto egg bread, a spongy, remarkably carblike low-carb swap. These single-serving breads are great on their own as a snack, with soup, or cut in half and used for sandwiches or sloppy joe (see the recipe on page 182). As with the chaffles (see page 210), eggs and cheese come together and are magically transformed into a fluffy revelation. We like to use mascarpone, the Italian double for cream cheese best known for its use in tiramisu, because it's more neutrally flavored than the more common, tangier cream cheese, but you can substitute cream cheese if mascarpone isn't readily available.

3 large eggs, separated

⅛ teaspoon cream of tartar

¼ cup mascarpone, at room temperature

⅛ teaspoon fine sea salt

1. Preheat the oven to 300°F. Line a rimmed baking sheet with parchment paper.

2. In a large bowl, using an electric mixer, beat the egg whites on high speed until foamy. Add the cream of tartar and continue beating until stiff peaks form, about 2 minutes.

3. In a second large bowl, use the mixer or a whisk to beat the mascarpone, egg yolks, and salt until smooth, about 1 minute.

4. Carefully and gradually fold the egg whites into the mascarpone mixture with a silicone spatula until just combined; don't overmix or you'll break down the air bubbles in the egg whites.

5. Scoop the mixture onto the lined baking sheet in six circles, about 1 inch thick, spaced a few inches apart. Bake until they set and begin to turn golden, 20 to 23 minutes.

NOTES:

You can store the breads in an airtight container in the fridge for 2 to 3 days, but the texture is best if eaten the same day.

Feel free to add spices of your choosing to impart some flavor—try ¼ to ½ teaspoon cinnamon for a sweet option or the same amount of garlic powder for savory, for example.

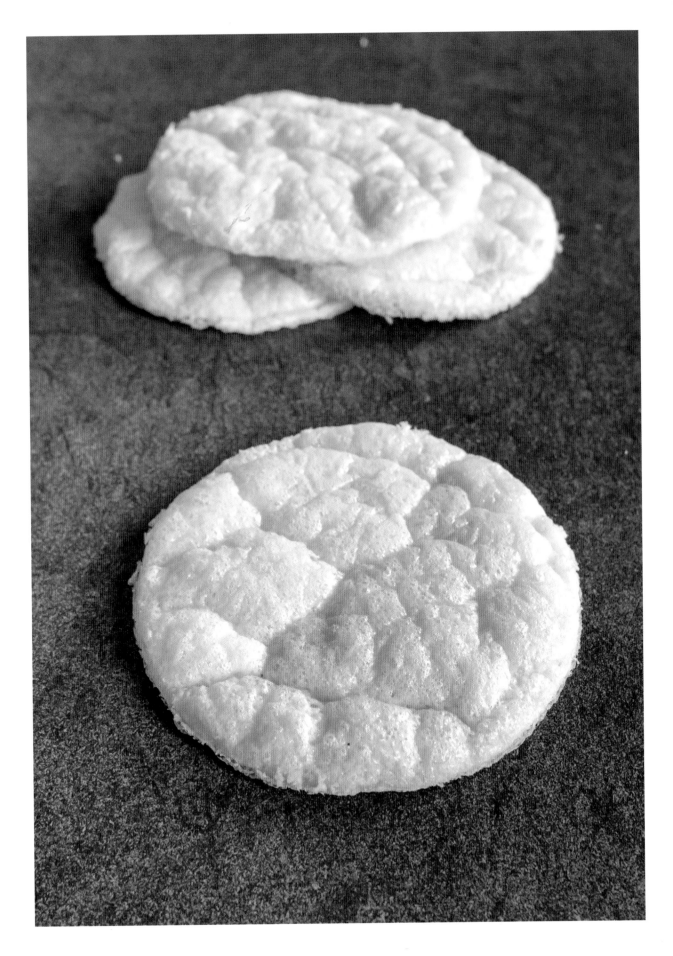

TURKEY JERKY

SERVES: 6 | **PREP TIME:** 10 minutes, plus 1 hour to freeze and 12 hours to marinate | **COOK TIME:** 8 hours

Come on, it's just plain fun to say "turkey jerky." This version is super tasty and not overly salty or sweet, as some packaged jerky can be.

1 pound boneless, skinless turkey breast, patted dry

¼ cup coconut aminos

¼ cup apple cider vinegar

2 tablespoons raw honey

2 tablespoons Cholula chili garlic hot sauce or mild- to medium-hot hot sauce of choice

½ teaspoon garlic powder

½ teaspoon onion powder

½ teaspoon fine sea salt

½ teaspoon freshly ground black pepper

Special equipment:
Food dehydrator (optional but recommended; see Notes for oven method)

1. Arrange the turkey breast flat on a plate or rimmed baking sheet, cover, and freeze until firm but not frozen solid, about 1 hour.

2. While the turkey is in the freezer, combine the coconut aminos, vinegar, honey, hot sauce, garlic powder, onion powder, salt, and pepper in a large baking dish or gallon-sized resealable bag.

3. When the turkey is firm, place it on a cutting board, trim any visible fat and membranes, and slice along the grain into ¼-inch-thick strips. Make the strips as uniform as possible to ensure even drying. Put the turkey in the dish or bag with the marinade and mix until well coated. Cover and refrigerate for 12 hours.

4. Remove the turkey strips and pat dry with a paper towel (discard the marinade). Place the strips in a single layer on the dehydrator tray and set to the dehydrator to160°F.

5. Remove the jerky from the dehydrator when it is fully dried and has the consistency of beef jerky, about 8 hours. If you prefer a chewier or more dry jerky, adjust the drying time accordingly; the longer it dehydrates, the drier and tougher it will get. If you prefer chewier jerky, taste-test it at about 7 hours to determine if it has reached your desired texture.

NOTES:

If you don't have a dehydrator, you can use the oven. Preheat it to its lowest setting (usually 200°F). Place the strips on a wire rack set inside a rimmed baking sheet and bake for about 10 hours. (Because ovens don't circulate air as well as dehydrators do, the process of removing moisture from the meat takes a little longer.) Check the jerky every few hours and crack the oven door every couple of hours to let moisture escape.

Store the jerky in an airtight glass container in the fridge for up to a week.

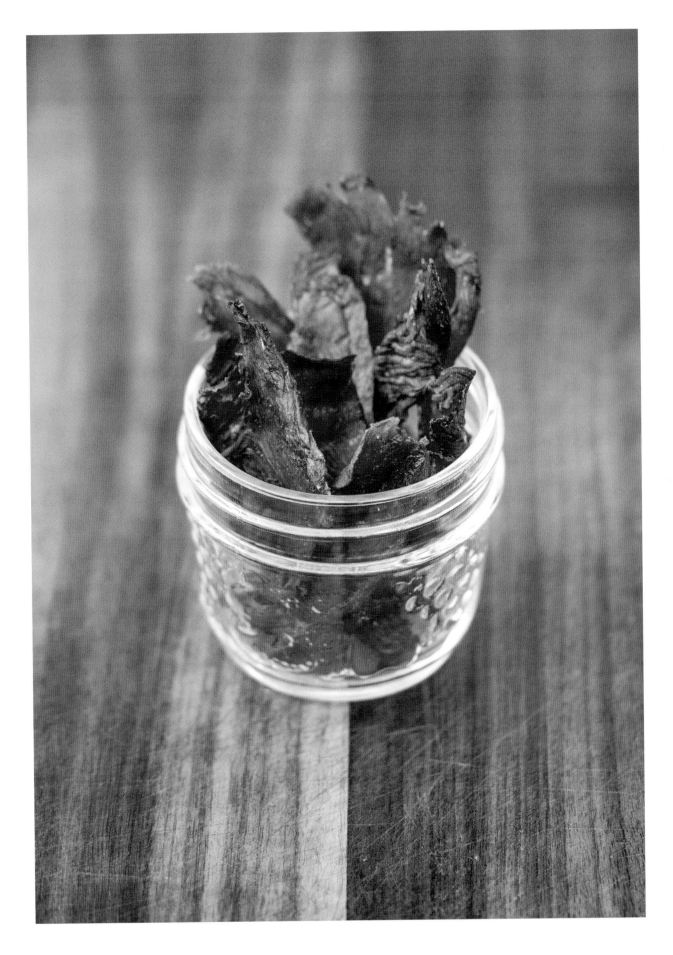

PORK RIND NACHOS

SERVES: 4 | **PREP TIME:** 5 minutes | **COOK TIME:** 10 minutes

These nachos have the same salty, crunchy decadence of your favorite plate of nachos but far fewer carbs. Make them your own by adding the toppings, cheese, and shredded meat of your choice.

1 (2.5-ounce) bag pork rinds

½ cup chopped bell pepper (any color)

¼ cup chopped white or red onion

½ cup shredded cheddar cheese or cheese of choice (about 2 ounces)

¼ teaspoon cayenne pepper or smoked paprika, for finishing (optional)

1. Preheat the oven to 350°F. Line a rimmed baking sheet with parchment paper.

2. Spread the pork rinds in a single layer on the lined baking sheet. Layer on the bell pepper, onion, and cheese. (Add a second layer of pork rinds and toppings if there are any left over.)

3. Bake until the cheese is melted and beginning to brown, 8 to 10 minutes (alternatively, you can broil the nachos on low for 5 to 6 minutes).

4. Sprinkle the nachos with cayenne or smoked paprika, if desired, and serve immediately.

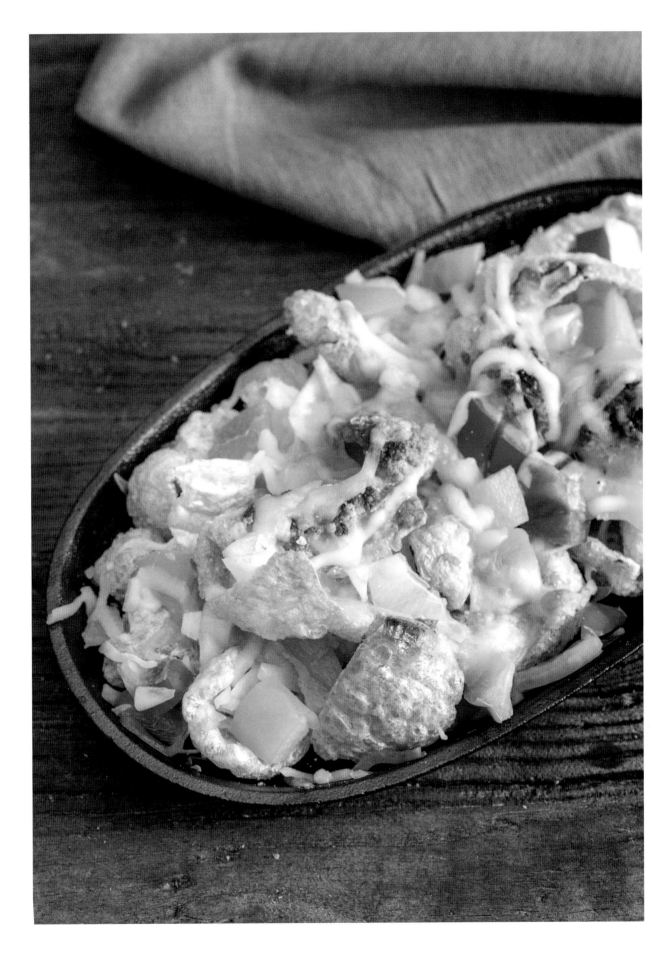

FORAGER TRAIL MIX

MAKES: About 3 cups (6 servings) | **PREP TIME:** 10 minutes |
COOK TIME: 20 minutes

We admit it: we're snackers. Creating trail mixes with new combinations of flavors and textures keeps things fun on road trips and hikes, and this stuff makes a great treat for little ones, too. As with many of our recipes, the beauty of this one is that you can customize it to your preferences. You can skip the dried fruit or include it if you want more carbs (freeze-dried fruit tends to be high in flavor and texture and very low in carbs and fiber). Use whichever nuts and seeds you want, experiment with different cheeses and spices—no matter what combination you come up with, it will make a delicious and savory treat.

1 cup mixed raw cashews, almonds, and shelled sunflower seeds or nuts and seeds of choice

¾ cup freshly grated Parmesan cheese (about 2¼ ounces)

¾ cup shredded mozzarella or cheddar cheese (about 6 ounces)

½ to ¾ teaspoon spice(s) or seasoning blend of choice (optional; see Notes)

1 cup pork rinds

1 cup freeze-dried berries of choice

1. Place the oven racks in the top and bottom third positions and preheat the oven to 400°F. Line two rimmed baking sheets with parchment paper.

2. Toss the nuts and seeds on one of the lined baking sheets and bake on the top rack until toasted and turning golden, about 20 minutes, stirring halfway through. Transfer to a medium bowl.

3. While nuts and seeds are baking, make the cheese crisps: In a small bowl, combine the Parmesan and mozzarella. Place 1-tablespoon heaps on the other lined baking sheet, spaced about 2 inches apart (they will spread during baking). Sprinkle with the spices, if using. Bake on the bottom rack until the edges are browned, 6 to 8 minutes. Check frequently and remove the pan promptly to prevent burning. Allow to cool for about 5 minutes, then transfer the crisps to paper towels to drain.

4. Break apart the cheese crisps and add them to the bowl of nuts/seeds, along with the pork rinds and freeze-dried berries. Toss, taste, and add more spices, if desired.

NOTES:

We like to use ¼ teaspoon each of cayenne pepper, chili powder, and/or garlic powder, but almost anything goes here. Since Parmesan is salty, we recommend using a seasoning blend without salt, but it's up to you.

Because of the different ingredients, this mix will keep in an airtight container for only a day or two. Best to eat it fresh.

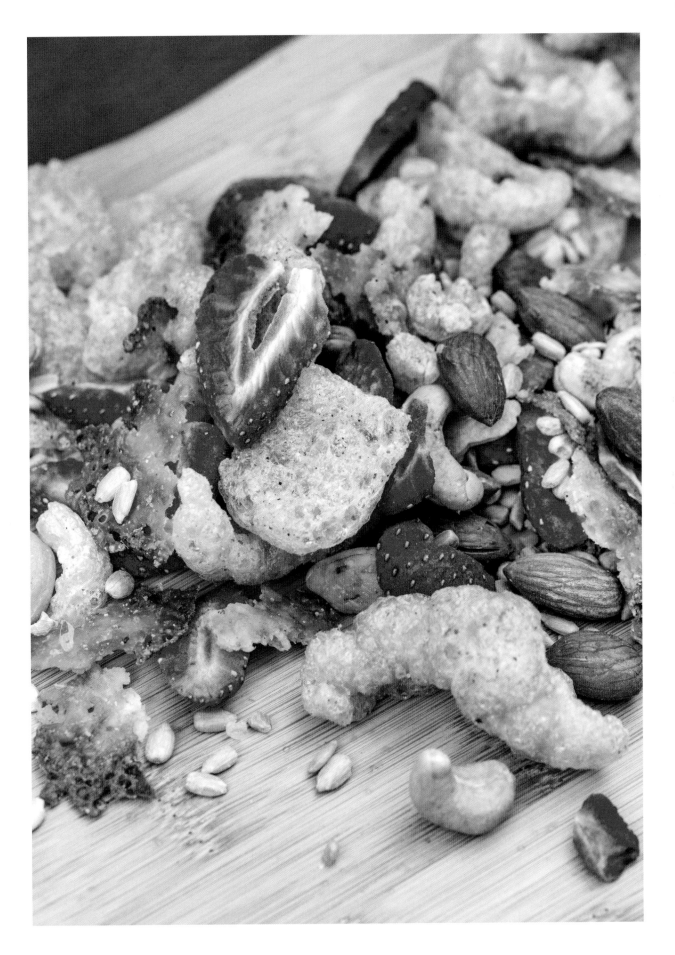

"ANIMAL" CRACKERS

SERVES: 6 | **PREP TIME:** 10 minutes | **COOK TIME:** 10 minutes

These grain-free crackers are named for the subtle addition of desiccated organ meat and collagen rather than fun shapes (though you can try that if you want). They make great snacks (kids love them too) and work well on our Savory Dessert Plate (page 332) or alongside Smoked Salmon Pâté (page 310) or Lemon-Tarragon Lobster Salad (page 228).

1¼ cups (160 grams) blanched almond flour, plus more for rolling

¼ cup (32 grams) flaxseed meal

¼ cup (32 grams) unflavored grass-fed collagen peptides

1 tablespoon desiccated beef liver powder

1 tablespoon sesame seeds

½ teaspoon fine sea salt

½ teaspoon freshly ground black pepper, plus more for finishing, if desired

2 tablespoons extra-virgin olive oil

1 large egg

Flaky sea salt, for finishing

1. Place the oven racks in the top and bottom third positions; preheat the oven to 450°F.

2. In a large bowl, combine the almond flour, flaxseed meal, collagen, liver powder, sesame seeds, salt, and pepper.

3. In a small bowl, whisk together the olive oil and egg.

4. Slowly add the egg mixture to the flour mixture, using moistened hands to mix them together. The mixture may be sticky, and that's OK; just make sure it's mixed well and not clumpy. Divide the dough into two equal portions.

5. Generously sprinkle more almond flour across a large piece of parchment paper; place one of the pieces of dough on the parchment and sprinkle more flour across the top of the dough to prevent sticking. Put another large piece of parchment on top and roll out with a rolling pin to a ¼-inch thickness.

6. Remove the top layer of parchment and, using a pizza cutter or chef's knife, cut the dough into 2-inch crackers; don't separate (they'll break apart easily once baked). Sprinkle generously with flaky salt and ground pepper, if desired. Slide the bottom sheet of parchment with the crackers onto a cookie sheet. Repeat with the second half of the dough, using a second cookie sheet.

7. Bake until the crackers just turn golden brown, about 10 minutes. Watch them carefully; they can burn easily. Let cool completely on the pans, about 10 minutes, before breaking apart.

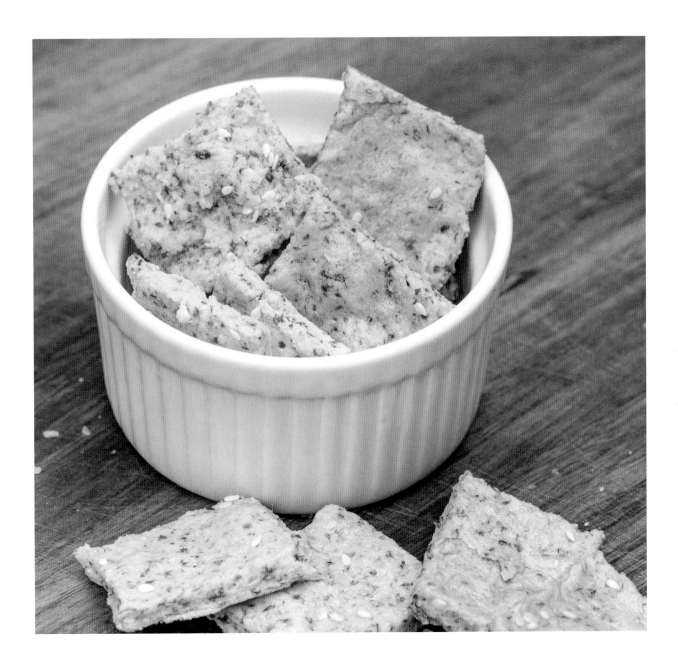

NOTES:

You can buy liver powder online and in some health food stores. Be sure to buy 100% grass-fed, grass-finished (it will say so on the label) for the most nutrient density.

We like to use cookie sheets here because it's much easier to slide the sheet of parchment paper with the cut-out crackers onto flat pans than ones with rims, but you can use rimmed baking sheets if you don't have cookie sheets.

These crackers will keep in an airtight container on the counter for up to 5 days.

SMOKED SALMON PÂTÉ

MAKES: 1 cup (6 to 8 servings) | **PREP TIME:** 5 minutes, plus 30 minutes to chill

This is essentially a dressed-up version of smoked salmon cream cheese spread—but please, call it "pâté" so it sounds fancy. You can change up the flavor with different spices if you like. A spoonful of beet horseradish would be nice, or try chives along with (or in place of) the dill.

4 ounces cream cheese, at room temperature

2 tablespoons (1 ounce) unsalted butter, at room temperature

3 ounces cold-smoked salmon, such as Nova lox, coarsely chopped

1 teaspoon fresh lemon juice

¼ teaspoon chopped fresh dill, plus more for garnish if desired

½ teaspoon fine sea salt

¼ teaspoon freshly ground black pepper

Lettuce wraps, endive spears, or grain-free crackers, homemade (page 308) or store-bought, for serving

1. In a food processor, blend the cream cheese and butter until smooth, about 1 minute, stopping to scrape down the sides of the bowl at least once.

2. Add the salmon, lemon juice, dill, salt, and pepper. Process until smooth, about 1 minute longer.

3. Spoon the pâté into a small bowl and sprinkle with more dill, if desired. Cover and chill until firm, about 30 minutes. Serve on lettuce wraps, endive spears, or crackers.

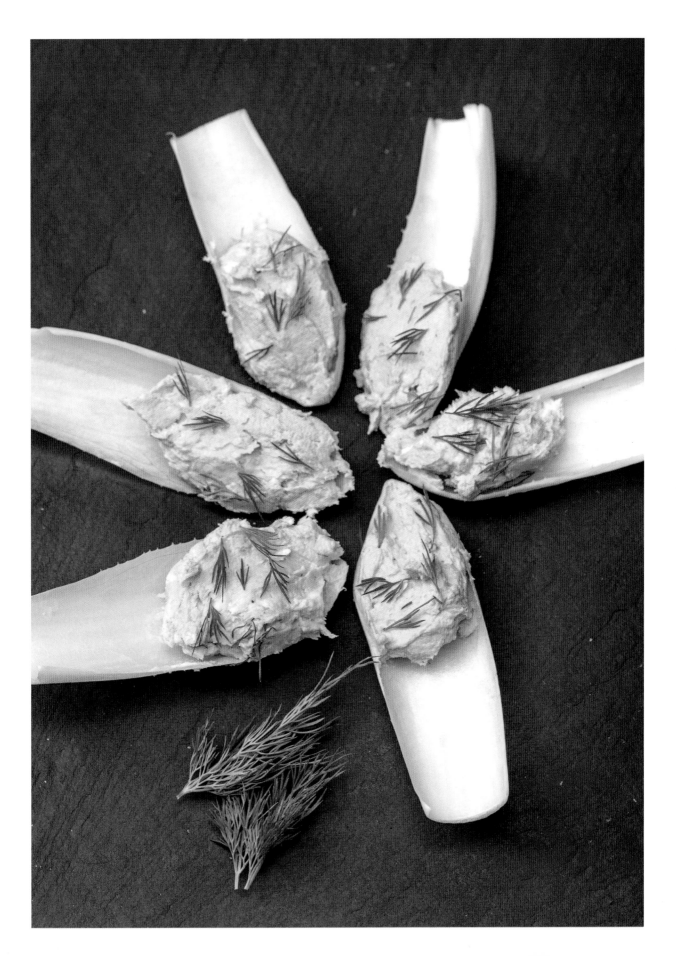

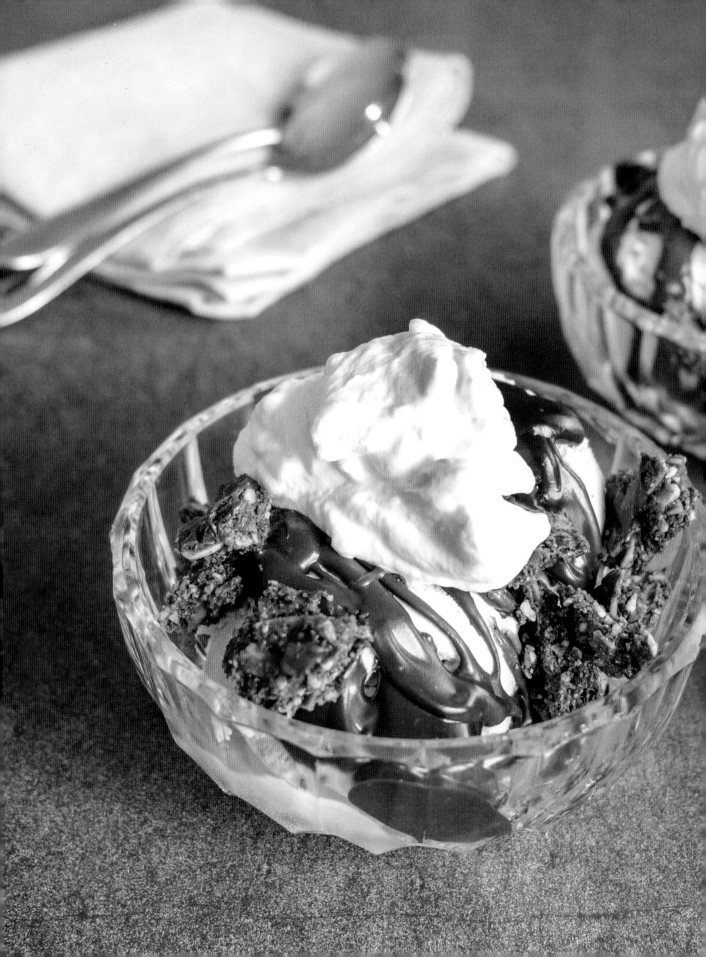

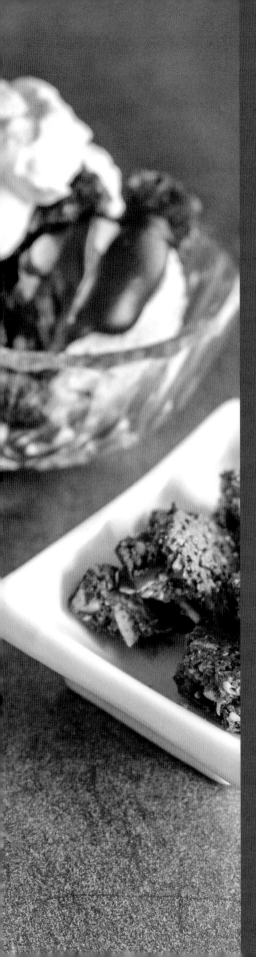

CHAPTER 12:

DESSERTS & BEVERAGES

VANILLA BEAN ICE CREAM

MAKES: 1 quart | **PREP TIME:** 30 minutes, plus 6½ hours to chill, churn, and freeze | **COOK TIME:** 10 minutes

Carnivore-ish ice cream? Well, yes—it has egg yolks, heavy cream, and whole milk. Our version is not as sweet as typical ice cream; we kept the sugar on the lighter side. But it's rich and satisfying thanks to all of the fat and the pronounced vanilla flavor from real vanilla bean. You can use a tablespoon of pure vanilla extract instead of the bean, but we recommend using a bean if you can get one; with so few ingredients and less sweetness, that strong vanilla flavor really shines.

1½ cups whole milk

¼ teaspoon fine sea salt

1 vanilla bean, split lengthwise

4 large egg yolks

½ cup (64 grams) coconut sugar

1½ cups heavy cream

Special equipment:
Ice cream maker

1. At least 12 hours in advance, place the bowl of an ice cream maker in the freezer.

2. Put the milk and salt in a medium saucepan. Scrape the seeds out of the vanilla bean. Add the seeds and the pod to the milk. Place over medium heat and bring just to a simmer, then reduce the heat to low.

3. Meanwhile, combine the egg yolks and sugar in a mixing bowl. Whisk until well combined and slightly thickened. Whisking constantly and vigorously, slowly drizzle a few ladles of the warm milk into the egg mixture. Slowly drizzle the egg mixture into the pan with the warm milk, whisking constantly and vigorously.

4. Raise the heat to medium-low. Cook the mixture, stirring the bottom and sides of the pan constantly, until it thickens enough to coat the back of a spoon, 3 to 5 minutes. Pour it through a fine-mesh sieve into a large bowl. Stir in the cream. Cover the bowl and refrigerate for at least 4 hours or overnight.

5. Pour the mixture into the bowl of the ice cream maker and churn it according to the manufacturer's instructions. Place in a freezer-safe container, cover, and freeze until firm, at least 2 hours.

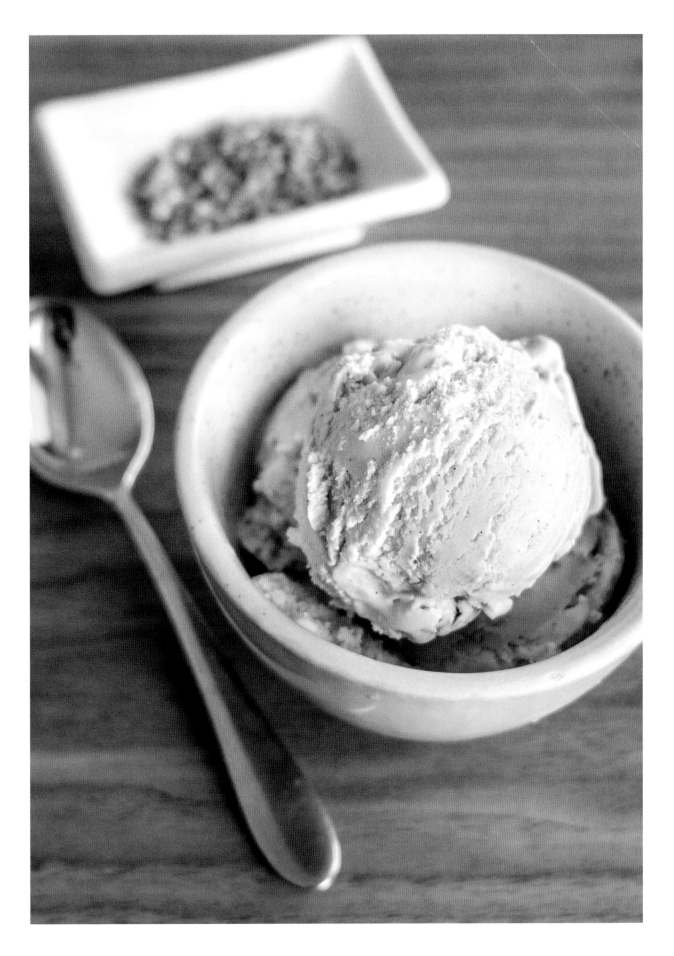

FRUIT JELLIES

MAKES: 15 to 20 pieces | **PREP TIME:** 5 minutes, plus 1 hour to chill |
COOK TIME: 5 minutes

Jellies, also known as gummies, are so much fun for kids and adults alike. It's deceptively easy to make them healthier with grass-fed gelatin and just a touch of natural sweetener instead of a pile of white sugar. You can use silicone candy molds in different shapes and sizes, or, if you have tiny molds like you'd use for gummy bears, use those (a dropper is handy to get the liquid into them). Eat these jellies within a day or two; beyond that, they become a bit rubbery and lose some of their flavor.

¾ cup unsweetened fruit juice, such as pomegranate, apple, green juice, or a combination

2 tablespoons fresh orange, lemon, or lime juice

Pinch of fine sea salt

1 tablespoon raw honey or maple syrup

1½ tablespoons unflavored grass-fed gelatin

Special equipment:
Gummy bear mold (50 cavities) (optional)

1. In a small saucepan, combine the fruit juice, citrus juice, and salt. Heat over medium heat until hot but not boiling; you should just see steam start to rise. Reduce the heat to low, then whisk in the honey. Sprinkle in the gelatin a little at a time, whisking until it dissolves.

2. Strain the mixture through a fine-mesh sieve into a small heatproof pitcher or liquid measuring cup. Pour or spoon the mixture into silicone molds; if your molds are quite small, use a small spoon or even an eye dropper. Alternatively, you can pour it into a loaf pan. Refrigerate until firm, at least 1 hour.

3. Push each section of the mold inside out to release the jellies. If you used a loaf pan, cut out shapes with a cookie cutter, or simply cut into squares, then use a small flexible or offset spatula to tease them out of the pan. Keep leftovers covered in the fridge for up to 2 days.

NOTE:

> *A green juice—often made with kale or spinach and sometimes cucumber, kiwi, or apple—is a good option for these because it's a fun way to get your kids (or yourself) to take in a few extra nutrients.*

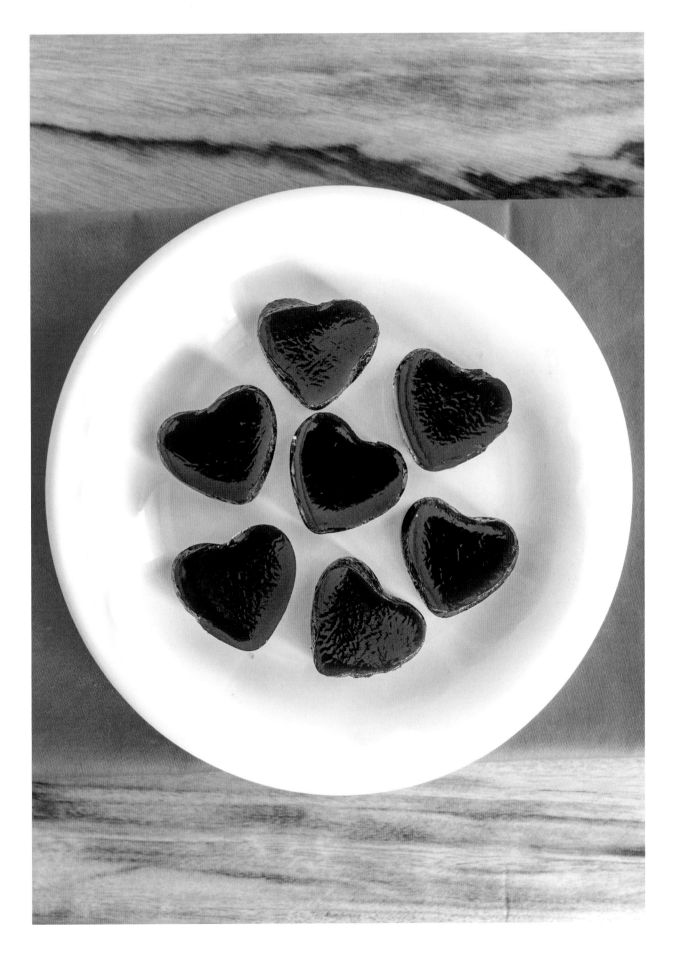

SECRET-INGREDIENT COOKIE DOUGH TRUFFLES

MAKES: About 24 truffles | **PREP TIME:** 30 minutes, plus 1 hour 45 minutes to freeze and chill | **COOK TIME:** 5 minutes

Naturally sweet cashew butter has a magical cookie dough quality in both flavor and texture. Adding cacao nibs and pork panko to these little truffles and dipping them in melted dark chocolate makes them a sweet-crunchy celebration in your mouth. Bring them to a party and watch them disappear, or make them for yourself and keep them in the freezer for chocolate "emergencies" (it's totally a thing).

1 cup unsweetened smooth cashew butter

½ cup pork panko

½ cup cacao nibs

¼ cup maple syrup

1 teaspoon vanilla extract

Pinch of fine sea salt (if your cashew butter is unsalted)

Coconut flour, if needed

1 cup dark chocolate chips, or 5 ounces dark chocolate, chopped (at least 70% cacao)

1 teaspoon coconut oil

Flaky sea salt, for finishing

1. In a large bowl, combine the cashew butter, panko, nibs, maple syrup, vanilla, and salt, if using. The mixture should be firm enough to hold together. If it isn't, stir in a tablespoon of coconut flour (or more, if needed).

2. Divide the mixture into 1-tablespoon portions (a small ice cream scoop is useful here). Freeze for 15 minutes, then roll into balls in your palms. Place on a plate and freeze for another 30 minutes.

3. Put the chocolate chips and coconut oil in a metal bowl set over a pan of simmering water. Heat, stirring often, until melted and smooth, about 5 minutes. Remove the bowl from the pan.

4. Line a rimmed baking sheet with parchment paper. One at a time, dip each ball into the chocolate, turning to coat it. Use a fork to lift it out; shake the excess chocolate back into the bowl. Place the coated balls on the lined baking sheet; sprinkle with a pinch of flaky salt. (If you have chocolate left over, you can drizzle it over the truffles for decoration, as shown.)

5. Refrigerate until the chocolate is firm, at least 1 hour. Serve cold. Store leftovers covered in the fridge for up to a week or in the freezer for up to 2 months.

> **NOTE:**
>
> *Keep the pan of water on the stove after you take the bowl of chocolate off. If the frozen truffles cause the chocolate to harden, place the bowl back over the simmering water for a few minutes to melt it again.*

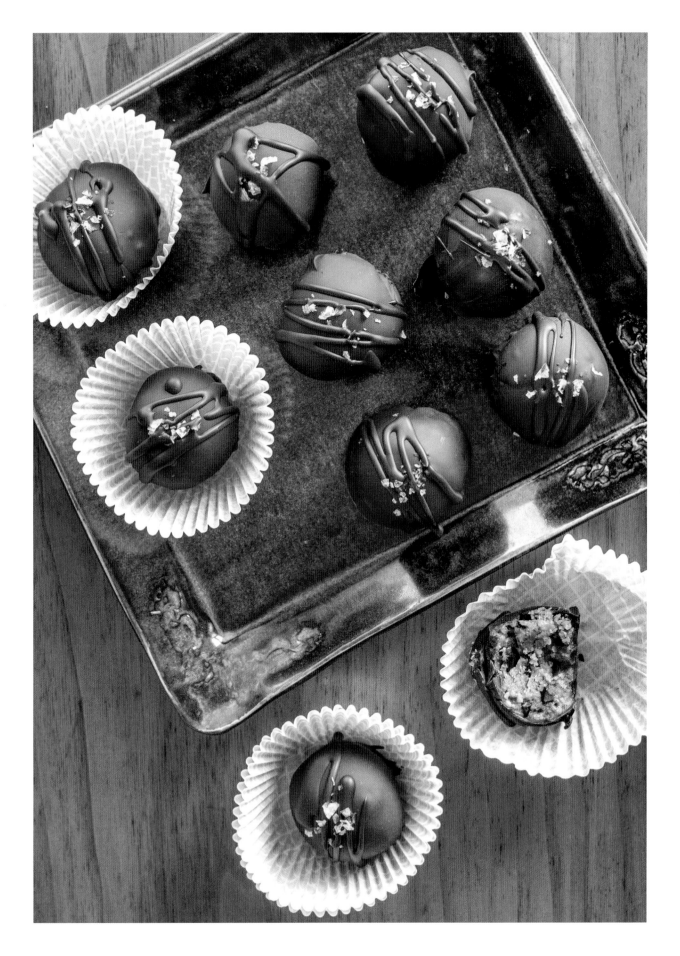

HOT FUDGE SUNDAES

SERVES: 4 | **PREP TIME:** 20 minutes | **COOK TIME:** 5 minutes

All right, no, a hot fudge sundae isn't the healthiest thing to eat—but we firmly believe that part of good health is balance, and life is made better when you enjoy the occasional sundae. Plus, when you make it yourself, you can be assured that the ingredients are of high quality. We add a sprinkle of our Dark Chocolate-Coconut Granola Clusters for a little crunch; you can leave it off or add a sprinkle of toasted nuts if you prefer. You'll definitely have hot fudge left over; keep it covered in the fridge for up to 2 weeks (though it never lasts that long for us). Rewarm it gently over low heat, and drizzle it on ice cream or berries.

HOT FUDGE *(MAKES 1¾ CUPS)*:

8 ounces dark chocolate (at least 70% cacao), chopped

¾ cup heavy cream

4 tablespoons (2 ounces) unsalted butter, cut into pieces

2 tablespoons raw honey

2 tablespoons coconut sugar

2 tablespoons raw cacao powder

⅛ teaspoon fine sea salt

Pinch of instant coffee (optional)

1 teaspoon vanilla extract

WHIPPED CREAM:

½ cup heavy cream

SUNDAES:

4 to 8 scoops Vanilla Bean Ice Cream (page 314) or store-bought ice cream of choice

½ cup Dark Chocolate-Coconut Granola Clusters (page 298)

1. Place a medium metal bowl and the beaters from an electric mixer in the freezer.

2. Make the hot fudge: Combine the chocolate, cream, butter, honey, sugar, cacao, salt, and coffee, if using, in a medium saucepan. Place over medium-low heat and cook, stirring often, until the chocolate is melted and smooth and the sugar has dissolved, 4 to 5 minutes. Remove from the heat and stir in the vanilla. Let cool slightly.

3. Make the whipped cream: Remove the bowl and beaters from the freezer. Pour in the cream and beat on medium-high speed until soft peaks form.

4. To serve, divide the ice cream among four bowls. Drizzle each bowl with 1 to 2 tablespoons of hot fudge. Sprinkle with 1 to 2 tablespoons of the granola clusters. Top with a dollop of whipped cream and serve.

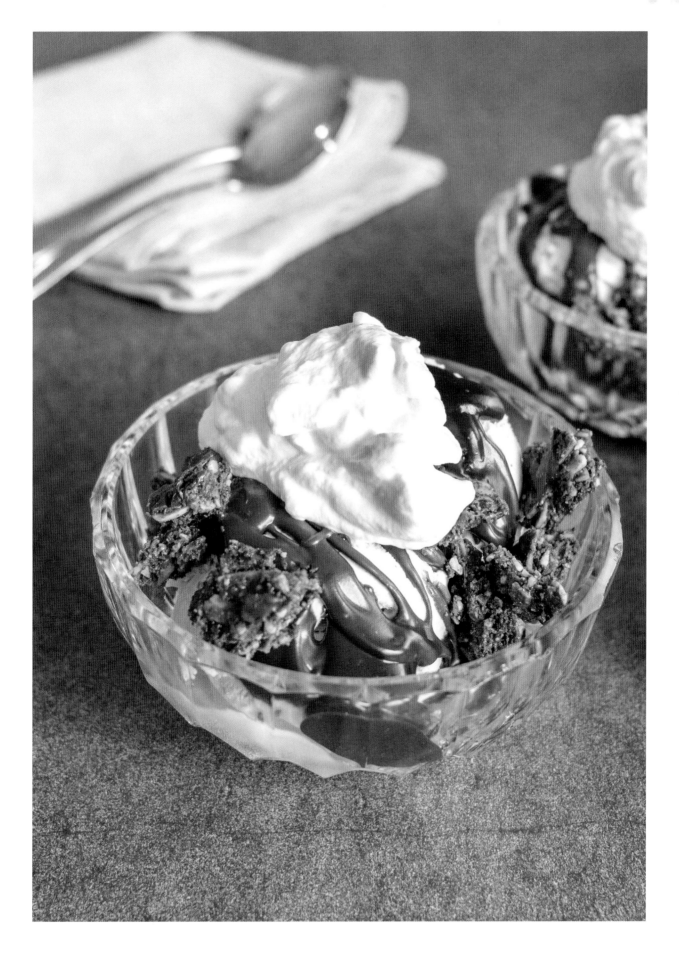

FRENCH TOAST EGG CUSTARD

SERVES: 6 | **PREP TIME:** 10 minutes | **COOK TIME:** 50 minutes

If you're a fan of crème brûlée, you'll love this carnivore-ish take: it's lightly sweet, creamy, and a touch eggy. Full of healthy fats and bolstered with beneficial collagen, this custard is a decadent and satisfying treat that won't weigh you down after dinner.

4 large egg yolks, at room temperature

½ cup maple syrup

2 cups unsweetened full-fat coconut cream or heavy cream

¼ cup (32 grams) unflavored grass-fed collagen peptides

1 teaspoon vanilla extract

1 teaspoon ground nutmeg

1 teaspoon ground cinnamon, plus extra for sprinkling if desired

½ teaspoon ground cardamom

⅛ teaspoon fine sea salt

1. Preheat the oven to 325°F.

2. In a large bowl, blend the egg yolks and maple syrup with an electric mixer or whisk until combined (don't overmix). Drizzle in the coconut cream, whisking as you pour, until all of the ingredients are combined. Whisk in the collagen, vanilla, nutmeg, cinnamon, and cardamom until just combined.

3. Divide the mixture among six 6-ounce ramekins. Sprinkle a little extra cinnamon on top, if desired. Place the ramekins in a roasting pan or large glass baking dish (minimum height 2 inches). Fill the pan or dish with enough warm water to reach halfway up the sides of the ramekins.

4. Bake the custards until they are just set but still jiggle slightly when lightly shaken, and a toothpick goes through a custard cleanly, about 50 minutes. (Do not overcook, or the custards will get rubbery.) Carefully remove the custards from the water bath. Serve warm, or let cool, cover, and refrigerate to serve cold. Cover leftovers with plastic wrap and keep in the fridge for up to 2 days.

NOTE:

You can use an instant-read thermometer to make sure the custard is cooked to the right doneness. The thermometer should read 170°F to 175°F when stuck in the center.

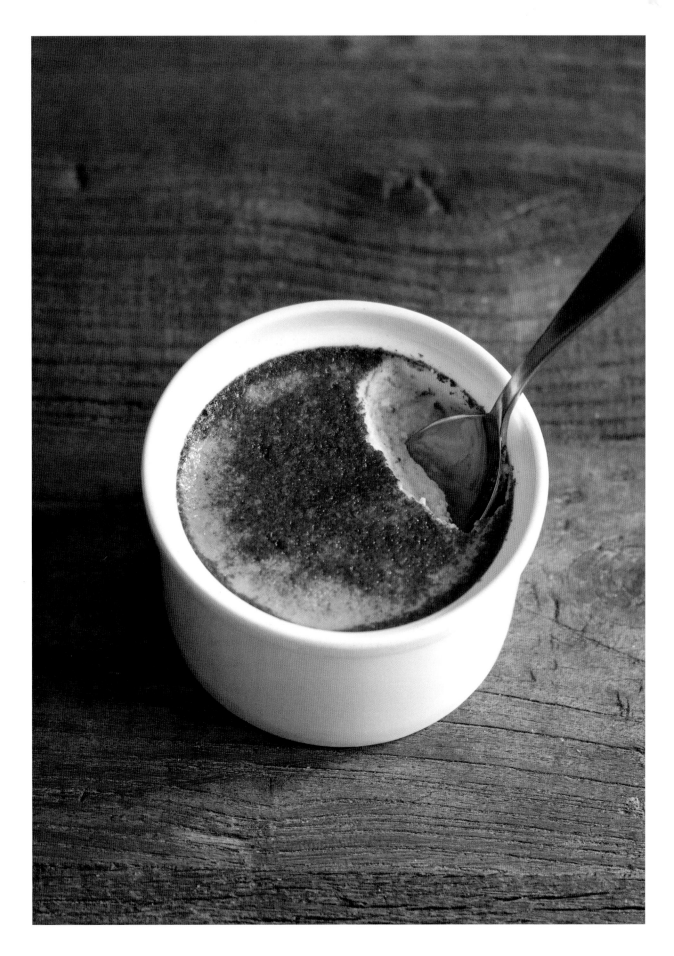

MAPLE BACON MERINGUES

MAKES: About 20 meringues | **PREP TIME:** 20 minutes, plus 1 hour to dry in oven |
COOK TIME: 1 hour

Just because you may prefer a high-protein, whole-foods diet doesn't mean you won't crave classic sweets now and then. These meringues are a relatively sweet treat, but the bacon adds a savory chewiness that's addictive. They're so light and crunchy, and just a few usually quell the craving.

¼ cup (32 grams) coconut sugar

5 ounces bacon (about 5 slices)

¼ cup maple syrup

2 large egg whites

¼ teaspoon cream of tartar

½ teaspoon vanilla extract (optional)

1. Preheat the oven to 350°F. Line two rimmed baking sheets with parchment paper, then place a cooling rack inside one of the lined baking sheets.

2. Rub the sugar into both sides of the bacon slices. Lay the bacon on the wire rack. Bake until brown, caramelized, and beginning to crisp, about 20 minutes. Place between pieces of paper towel to soak up the excess grease. Chop the bacon into small pieces and set aside. Lower the oven temperature to 225°F.

3. In a small saucepan, cook the maple syrup over medium heat just until it starts to boil.

4. Using a stand mixer, beat the egg whites and cream of tartar on high speed until stiff peaks form, about 5 minutes. With the mixer running, slowly drizzle the hot maple syrup into the bowl with the egg whites, pouring it down the side of the bowl. Add the vanilla, if using. Continue to beat until the mixture is thick and glossy, 3 to 4 minutes longer.

5. Attach a small round or star-shaped tip to a piping bag and fill it with the meringue mixture. Pipe 1-inch-wide, 1-inch-tall circles of meringue on the second lined baking sheet (you don't have to leave extra space between them; they won't spread). Sprinkle the bacon bits on top.

6. Bake the meringues until crisp but not browned, about 1 hour, keeping the oven door closed at all times so the meringues don't deflate. Turn off the oven and leave the meringues inside to dry for another hour.

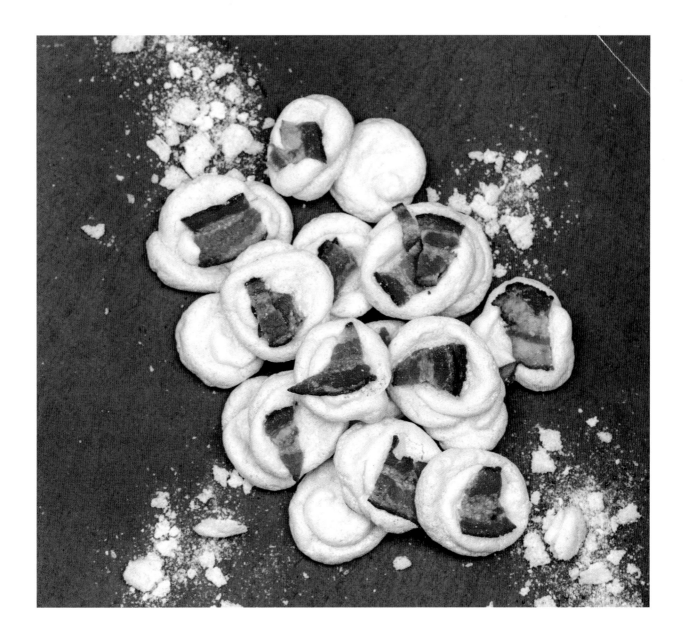

NOTES:

Meringues can be finicky—you don't want to under- or overbeat the egg whites, and humidity can leave you with soggy, chewy meringues. Make sure that all of your bowls and utensils are perfectly dry, and don't try this recipe on an overly humid day.

Enjoy the meringues within a day for the best texture; store leftovers in an airtight container at room temperature.

If you don't have a stand mixer, you can use a hand mixer; it's just a bit more work as you'll need both hands to hold the mixer and steady the bowl. The timing should be about the same.

JAPANESE-STYLE CHEESECAKE

SERVES: 12 | **PREP TIME:** 15 minutes | **COOK TIME:** 1 hour 10 minutes

This recipe is inspired by a Japanese cheesecake shop in Ashleigh's neighborhood that makes the best light, fluffy, barely sweet cakes. It is a bit labor-intensive for a cake, but the light, creamy decadence is absolutely worth it. It's cheesy and rich like a traditional American cheesecake but not as heavy or dense (which does mean it's easy to eat more of it; you've been warned...).

Unsalted butter, for greasing

6 large eggs

⅛ teaspoon cream of tartar

2 (8-ounce) packages cream cheese, at room temperature

2 tablespoons fresh lemon juice

1 teaspoon vanilla extract

¾ cup (96 grams) coconut sugar

1 cup (128 grams) blanched almond flour

1 teaspoon baking powder

1. Preheat the oven to 325°F. Cut a 9-inch circle out of parchment paper, as well as a strip to line the side of the pan. Grease both sides of the paper with butter. Line the bottom and side of a 9-inch springform pan with the greased parchment. Wrap aluminum foil across the bottom and up the side of the pan to make it watertight.

2. Separate the eggs, placing the yolks and whites in separate large mixing bowls. Add the cream of tartar to the whites and, using an electric mixer, beat on medium speed until soft peaks form, about 3 minutes. Set aside. Rinse and dry the beaters.

3. Put the cream cheese in the bowl with the egg yolks and beat on medium-high speed until smooth, creamy, and free of lumps, about 2 minutes (scrape down the sides of the bowl as you go to ensure even mixing). Add the lemon juice, vanilla, and sugar and beat until smooth, about 1 minute longer. Add the almond flour and baking powder and beat until fully combined, another minute or so.

4. Using a silicone spatula, gently fold about one-third of the egg whites into the cream cheese mixture until just incorporated (do not overmix, or the egg whites will deflate). Repeat with the remaining two-thirds. Pour the batter into the prepared pan, smoothing the top with the spatula.

5. Carefully place the pan in the center of a large baking pan that's at least 2½ inches deep. Pour water into the baking pan until it reaches about one-third of the way up the side of the springform pan (about 1½ inches of water). Bake until a skewer inserted in the center of the cake comes out clean and the cake jiggles slightly in the center when lightly shaken, about 1 hour 10 minutes.

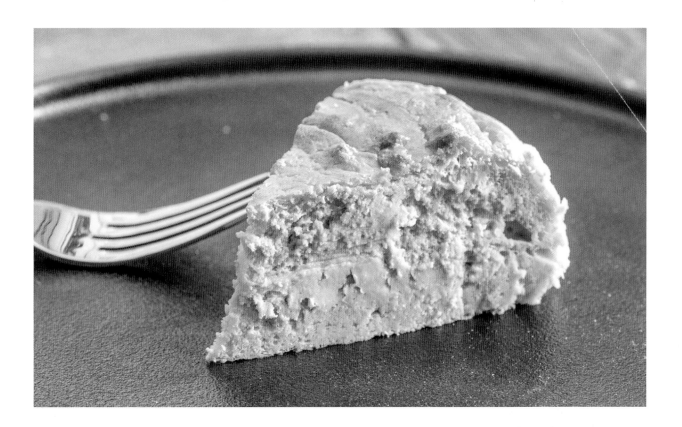

6. Carefully lift the springform pan from the water bath and remove the foil. Let the cake cool in the oven with the door open for about 20 minutes, then on a wire rack on the counter until room temperature. Remove from the pan by carefully running a knife all around the side to loosen the cake, then unhinge the clasp on the pan and carefully transfer the cake to a cake plate, discarding the parchment paper. Serve at room temperature or let cool, cover, and refrigerate to serve cold (we think it's best after it's been chilled for at least 2 hours). The cake will keep in an airtight container in the fridge for up to 1 week or in the freezer for up to 2 months.

NOTES:

When folding in the whipped egg whites in Step 4, it's crucial not to overmix; doing so will reduce the air bubbles in the whites, which are what give the finished cake its awesome texture.

The cake may deflate an inch or so after baking, which is normal; letting it cool slowly in the oven and then on the counter before refrigerating helps set the cake and prevent too much deflation as a result of significant temperature change.

ORANGE WHITE CHOCOLATE-DIPPED DUCK FAT SUGAR COOKIES

MAKES: 12 cookies | **PREP TIME:** 15 minutes, plus 45 minutes to chill | **COOK TIME:** 12 minutes

The name is a mouthful, and so are the cookies. Orange-infused white chocolate is a delicious sweet balance to rich sugar cookies; duck fat imparts a serious depth of flavor (but they don't taste like duck, we promise). Feel free to play with different spices or to use dark chocolate instead of white.

2 cups Paleo or gluten-free baking flour blend

½ teaspoon baking powder

¼ teaspoon fine sea salt

1 cup (128 grams) coconut sugar

4 tablespoons (2 ounces) unsalted butter, at room temperature

¼ cup duck fat, at room temperature

1 large egg

1 teaspoon vanilla extract

WHITE CHOCOLATE DIP:

⅓ cup white chocolate chips

1 tablespoon coconut oil

½ teaspoon orange extract

Grated zest of 1 orange, for finishing

1. Preheat the oven to 325°F. Line a rimmed baking sheet with parchment paper.

2. In a large bowl, whisk together the flour, baking powder, and salt.

3. In another large bowl, using an electric mixer on medium speed, cream the sugar, butter, and duck fat until fluffy and fully combined, about 3 minutes. Beat in the egg and vanilla. Slowly add the flour mixture to the butter mixture, beating until just combined (don't overmix). Cover and refrigerate the dough until firm, about 15 minutes.

4. Form the dough into 12 balls about 2 inches in diameter, then flatten with the palm of your hand until they're about 1 inch thick. Place on the lined baking sheet, spaced about 2 inches apart.

5. Bake until the cookies are lightly browned around the edges, about 12 minutes. Transfer the cookies to a wire rack to cool.

6. When the cookies have cooled completely, make the dip: Melt the white chocolate and coconut oil in a microwave-safe bowl in 30-second intervals until smooth, stirring after each interval. Stir in the orange extract.

7. Dip the cookies in the chocolate mixture, lay them back on the parchment, and sprinkle with the orange zest. Refrigerate for 30 minutes to set the chocolate before serving. The cookies will keep in an airtight container for up to 5 days; they don't need to be refrigerated unless your house is very warm.

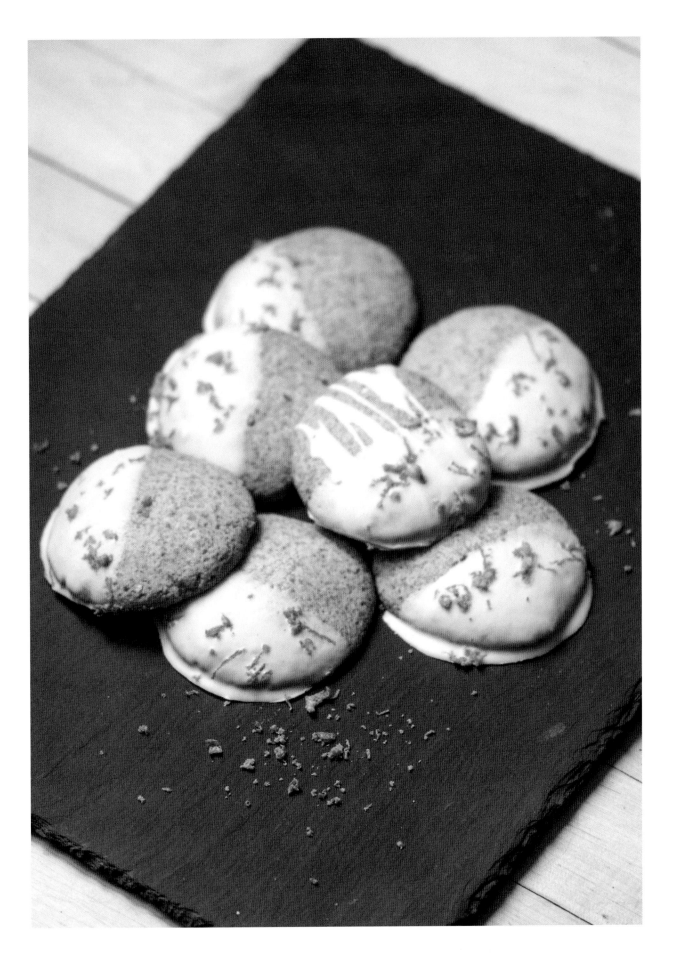

SNEAKY CHOCOLATE CHIP CARNIVORE PROTEIN BARS

MAKES: 12 bars | **PREP TIME:** 10 minutes, plus 1 hour to chill

These rich, chewy bars may remind you of a popular refrigerated protein bar you can find at your local grocery store, but with these, you can control the amount of sugar, and you get the added bonus of some powdered (and tasteless) organ meats to boost the nutrient profile. This is a great way to get more nutrient density into your kids' snacks, and adults will love these bars, too.

1 cup (128 grams) oat flour or Paleo/gluten-free flour blend

¼ cup (32 grams) vanilla-flavored whey protein powder

¼ cup (32 grams) unflavored grass-fed collagen peptides

1 tablespoon powdered beef organs

¼ teaspoon fine sea salt

½ cup unsweetened, unsalted natural peanut butter or nut butter of choice

⅓ cup raw honey

1 teaspoon vanilla extract

1 to 2 tablespoons coconut oil

½ cup mini chocolate chips, plus more for garnish if desired

1. Grease an 8 by 4-inch loaf pan. In a large bowl, whisk together the oat flour, protein powder, collagen, powdered organs, and salt. Add the peanut butter, honey, vanilla, and 1 tablespoon of coconut oil. Mix with moistened hands. The mixture should be thick and have the consistency of play dough; add up to 1 tablespoon more coconut oil if it's crumbly or dry. Mix in the chocolate chips.

2. Press the mixture into the greased loaf pan and press more chocolate chips into the top, if desired. Cover and refrigerate for at least 1 hour before cutting into bars. Store covered in the fridge for up to 1 week.

NOTE:

Oats are naturally gluten-free but sometimes end up containing gluten because of cross contamination with wheat, rye, or other grains on neighboring fields or during processing. If you have celiac disease or you're gluten sensitive, be sure to seek out certified gluten-free oats and oat flour, which are carefully grown, harvested, and processed to prevent cross-contamination.

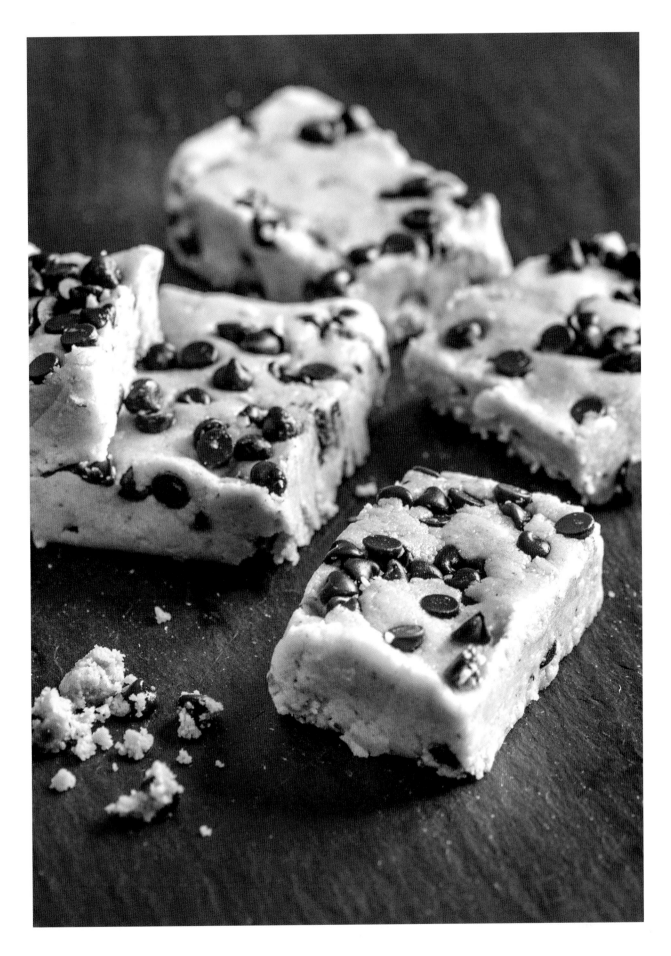

SAVORY DESSERT PLATE

SERVES: 4 to 8 | **PREP TIME:** 10 minutes

For those who prefer a more savory after-dinner treat (you know who you are: you always go for the cheese plate for dessert in restaurants), it's easy to take some of our snack recipes, throw them together on a cheese plate or charcuterie board, and impress your friends with some tasty animal-based delicacies.

1 batch Forager Trail Mix (page 306)

1 batch Turkey Jerky (page 302)

1 batch each of "Animal" Crackers (page 308) and compound butter(s) of choice (see pages 348 to 351)

1 batch Dark Chocolate-Coconut Granola Clusters (page 298)

1 batch Air Fryer Mixed Sweet Potato Chips (page 276)

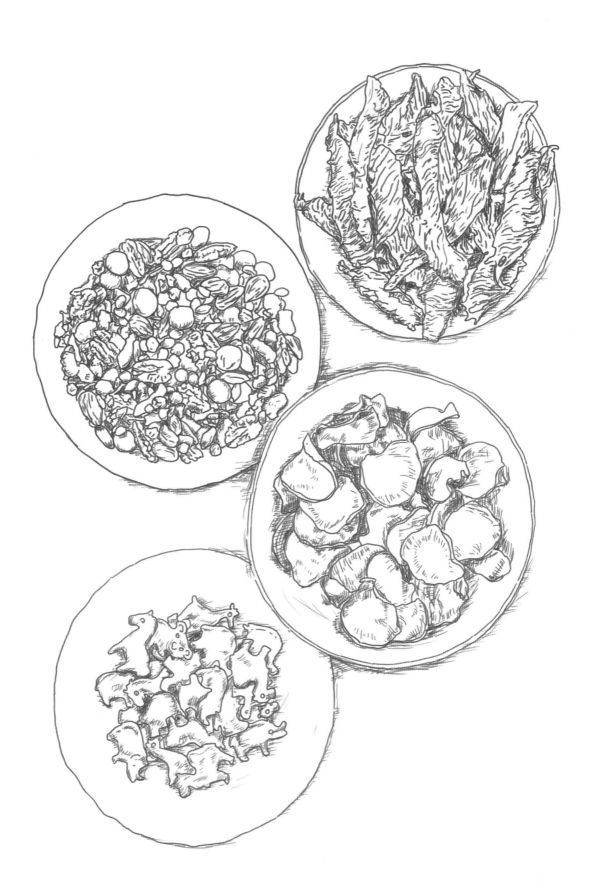

BLOOD ORANGE GIN FIZZ

SERVES: 1 | **PREP TIME:** 10 minutes

An egg white in this classic gin-based cocktail makes it frothy, and shaking it without ice first (called "dry shaking") whips in air and makes it even frothier. We love the sweet-tart flavor and beautiful color of blood oranges, but you can swap in traditional lemon juice if you prefer.

2 ounces gin

1 ounce fresh blood orange juice

1½ teaspoons raw honey

1 large egg white

Ice cubes

Club soda, for topping

1. Put the gin, blood orange juice, honey, and egg white in a cocktail shaker. Shake well for 15 seconds, until the mixture is beginning to get frothy.

2. Add a few ice cubes to the shaker; shake again until the ingredients are chilled and frothier.

3. Strain into a martini or daiquiri glass, top with club soda, and serve.

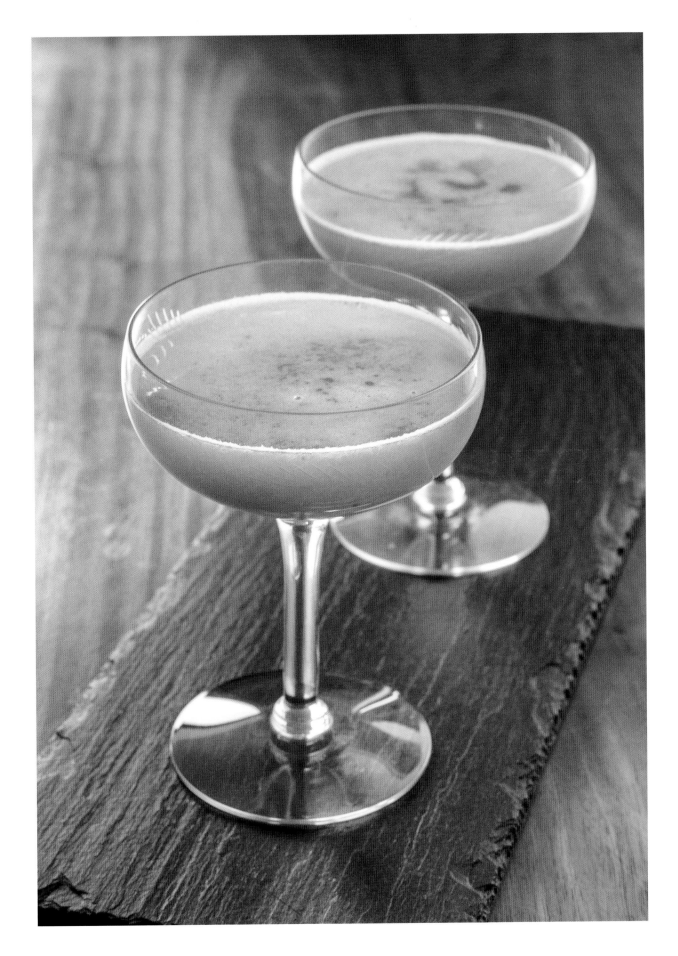

SPICY TORO SHOT

SERVES: 1 | **PREP TIME:** 10 minutes, plus 24 hours to infuse

Beth first encountered the Bull Shot cocktail while working as a waitress in an NYC restaurant decades ago. It was made with canned beef broth, and back then it sounded...well, weird. Now that we know all of the benefits of bone broth, we decided to give it a second look. This version incorporates spicy jalapeño-infused tequila and lime juice instead of the traditional vodka and lemon for a unique cocktail that will wake you right up at brunch time.

JALAPEÑO-INFUSED TEQUILA *(MAKES ENOUGH FOR 4 SHOTS)*:

8 ounces silver (aka white) tequila

½ jalapeño, sliced in half lengthwise, seeds and ribs removed

FOR 1 TORO SHOT:

Ice

2 ounces jalapeño-infused tequila (from above)

¾ cup beef bone broth

2 teaspoons fresh lime juice

¼ teaspoon Worcestershire sauce

¼ teaspoon fine sea salt

¼ teaspoon freshly ground black pepper

⅛ teaspoon ground celery seed (see Note, page 158)

Hot sauce (optional)

1. Infuse the tequila: Pour the tequila into a jar with a lid. Add the jalapeño. Cover and let stand at room temperature for 24 hours. Strain the tequila; discard the jalapeño.

2. To make one toro shot, fill a large rocks glass with ice. Fill a cocktail shaker with ice. To the shaker, add 2 ounces of the infused tequila along with the broth, lime juice, Worcestershire, salt, pepper, and ground celery seed; shake well. Strain into the ice-filled glass. Top with a few shakes of hot sauce, if you like, and serve.

NOTES:

If you like a glass with a salted rim, run a lime wedge around the rim of the glass and then dip it in coarse salt before filling the glass with ice.

Use the remaining infused tequila for more toro shots or other cocktails.

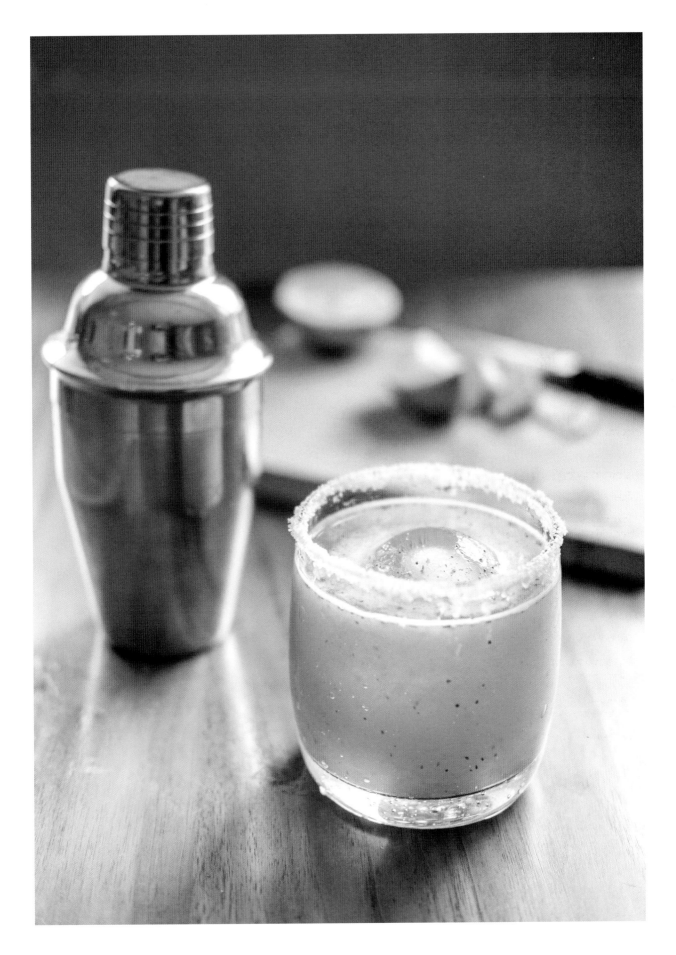

ANTIOXIDANT-RICH SIPPING BROTH

SERVES: 3 (8 ounces per serving) | **PREP TIME:** 10 minutes, plus 30 minutes to soak |
COOK TIME: 16 to 24 hours

Bone broth is enjoying a renaissance, though it's an ancient food. Adding spices to the broth while it simmers infuses it with deep flavor and makes it truly sippable. Enjoy some on a cold winter's afternoon, or have it instead of coffee if you do one of those caffeine cleanses we've heard about.

1 pound beef bones

3 cups filtered water, plus more as needed

3 tablespoons apple cider vinegar

2 cinnamon sticks, plus more for garnish if desired

1 teaspoon turmeric powder

1 teaspoon fine sea salt

1 teaspoon freshly ground black pepper

½ teaspoon cayenne pepper

½ teaspoon whole cloves

1. Put the beef bones, filtered water, and vinegar in a 6-quart slow cooker, making sure the bones are covered by about 1 inch of water. Allow the mixture to sit without turning on the heat for 30 minutes.

2. Stir in the cinnamon sticks, turmeric, salt, black pepper, cayenne, and cloves. Cover and cook on low for 16 to 24 hours, checking the water level about every 3 hours and adding more filtered water as needed to keep the bones covered.

3. Remove the bones and cinnamon sticks with tongs or a slotted spoon. Strain the broth through a fine-mesh sieve into a 1-quart mason jar. When no longer piping hot, taste and season with salt and pepper to your liking. Pour into 8-ounce cups and enjoy while still hot, garnished with a cinnamon stick or two if desired, or let cool completely before covering and refrigerating; the broth will keep in an airtight container in the fridge for up to 1 week.

NOTES: ───────────────────────

Ashleigh often includes vegetables in her bone broth for more depth of flavor and nutrients, but since this one is meant to be enjoyed as a sipping broth and is used to make the Spicy Bone Broth Hot Chocolate on page 340, we kept it simple, letting the beefiness and spices stand alone.

The taste of your water can impact the flavor of the broth. Filtered water is recommended but is not necessary; if you have great-tasting tap water, that's fine.

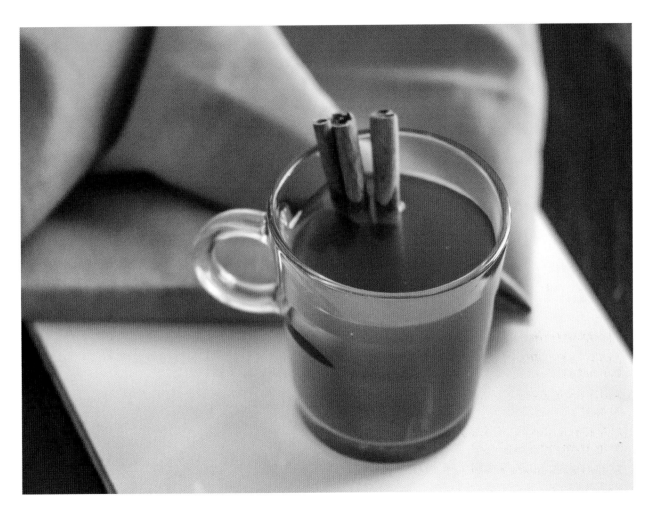

NOTES:

When you reheat the broth, don't let it come to a boil, which would break down the healthy fats and collagen. Bring it just to a simmer over low heat.

You can freeze broth in a freezer-safe container; it should keep for up to 6 months. Pro tip: For bone broths made with vegetables and savory herbs, the basis of so many good savory preparations, we recommend freezing the broth in cubes (using silicone trays for easy removal), then popping out the frozen cubes and storing them in airtight freezer bags.

We have a wide range of cooking time here, and it really depends on how much time you have. You'll want to simmer for at least 16 hours to let the bones release their collagen; the longer you simmer, the more nutrients will be released. Twenty-four hours is generally the maximum you want to cook broth; if the bones start to get really soft, dissolve, or crumble, then you know you've gone a little too far.

SPICY BONE BROTH HOT CHOCOLATE

SERVES: 2 (10 ounces per serving) | **PREP TIME:** 5 minutes

Meat and chocolate are basically our two favorite food groups, and it turns out there are many ways to combine them with delicious results. For those chilly days when a cup of hot chocolate hits the spot, why not supercharge it with some spicy collagen-rich bone broth? It won't make your hot chocolate taste beefy, but it may cut the sweetness a little bit, which isn't a bad thing.

1 cup unsweetened full-fat coconut cream or heavy cream

2 ounces dark chocolate (at least 85% cacao), chopped

½ cup Antioxidant-Rich Sipping Broth (page 338)

½ teaspoon vanilla extract

Stevia or monk fruit (powdered or extract/liquid), or maple syrup (optional)

Coconut or dairy whipped cream, for serving (optional)

Special equipment:
Small handheld frother (optional)

1. Put the cream and chocolate in a small saucepan over low heat. Bring to a simmer, whisking until the chocolate is fully melted and incorporated, 4 to 5 minutes.

2. Stir in the broth and heat until warmed through, about 1 minute longer. Remove from the heat and stir in the vanilla.

3. Pour the mixture into two 10-ounce mugs and add sweetener to taste, if desired. If you have a small handheld frother, use it to create some bubbles on top, about 15 seconds each. Top with whipped cream, if desired, and serve.

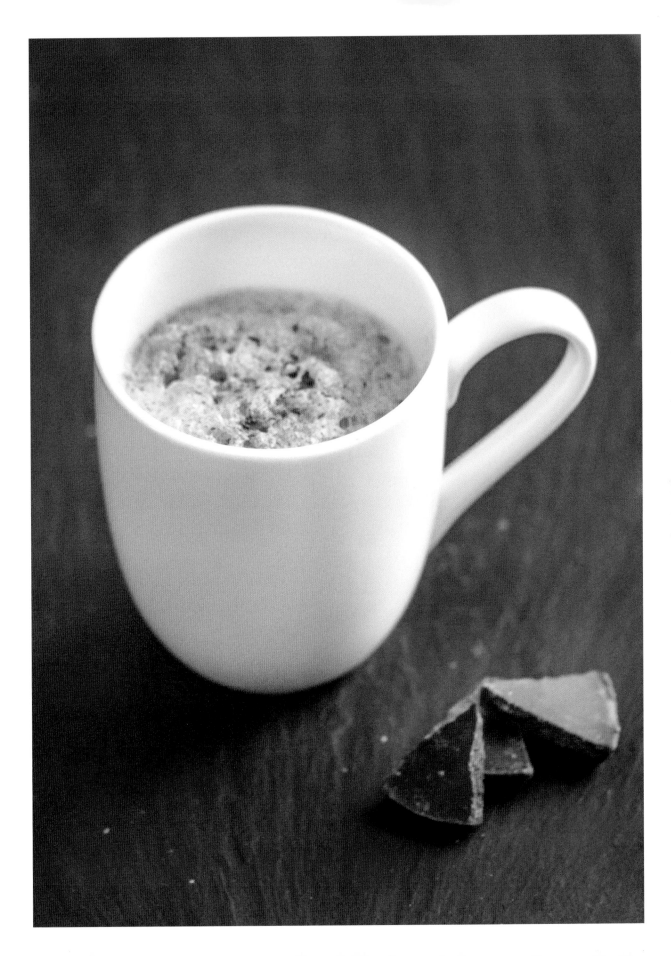

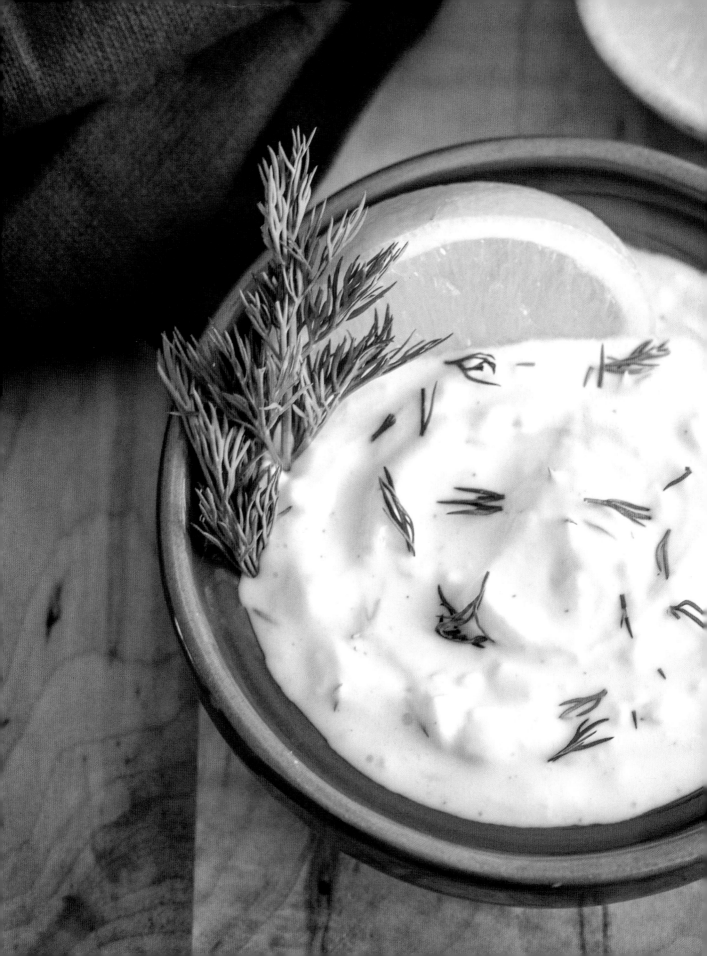

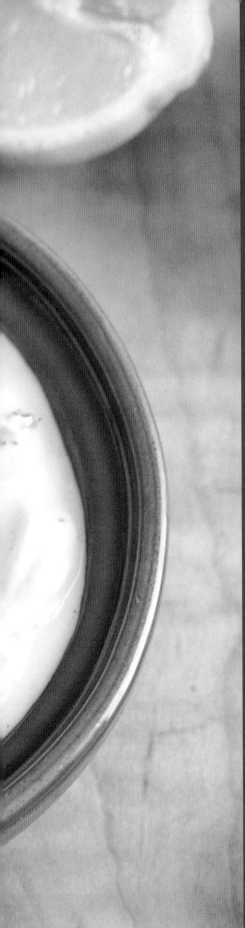

CHAPTER 13:

SAUCES & CONDIMENTS

BACON RANCH DIP

MAKES: ⅔ cup | **PREP TIME:** 20 minutes | **COOK TIME:** 9 minutes

This dip is a real crowd-pleaser: bacon and ranch, what's not to like? It's especially good with Air Fryer Buffalo Chicken Nuggets (page 118). A lot of ranch recipes call for dried herbs, but we really like the fresh parsley and dill in here. They punch up the flavor so much that it's worth the extra effort. Want to use this as a dressing? See the variation below.

3 ounces bacon (about 3 slices)

2 cloves garlic, minced (about 2 teaspoons)

¼ cup avocado oil mayonnaise

¼ cup sour cream

½ teaspoon mustard powder

1 teaspoon grated lemon zest

1 tablespoon fresh lemon juice

3 tablespoons chopped fresh flat-leaf parsley

2 teaspoons minced fresh dill

¼ teaspoon raw honey

Fine sea salt and freshly ground black pepper

1. Put the bacon in a large unheated skillet. Turn the heat to medium-low and cook until the bacon is crisp but not overly browned, turning the slices over a few times, about 10 minutes. Transfer the bacon to a cutting board. Pour off all but 1 tablespoon of the bacon fat (reserve the extra fat for another use).

2. Reduce the heat to low, then add the garlic to the skillet and cook until fragrant, about 1 minute. Transfer to a blender or small food processor. Add the mayonnaise, sour cream, mustard powder, lemon zest and juice, parsley, dill, and honey; blend until smooth. (Alternatively, you can whisk the ingredients together in a medium bowl.)

3. Finely chop the bacon and fold it into the dip. Taste and season with salt and pepper. Serve, or cover and refrigerate to serve later; it will keep for up to 5 days. The dip will thicken in the refrigerator.

BONUS: Bacon Ranch Dressing. This dip can double as a salad dressing. Just whisk in a little olive oil, milk, or even water to thin it to the consistency you want. Taste and add more seasoning, if needed.

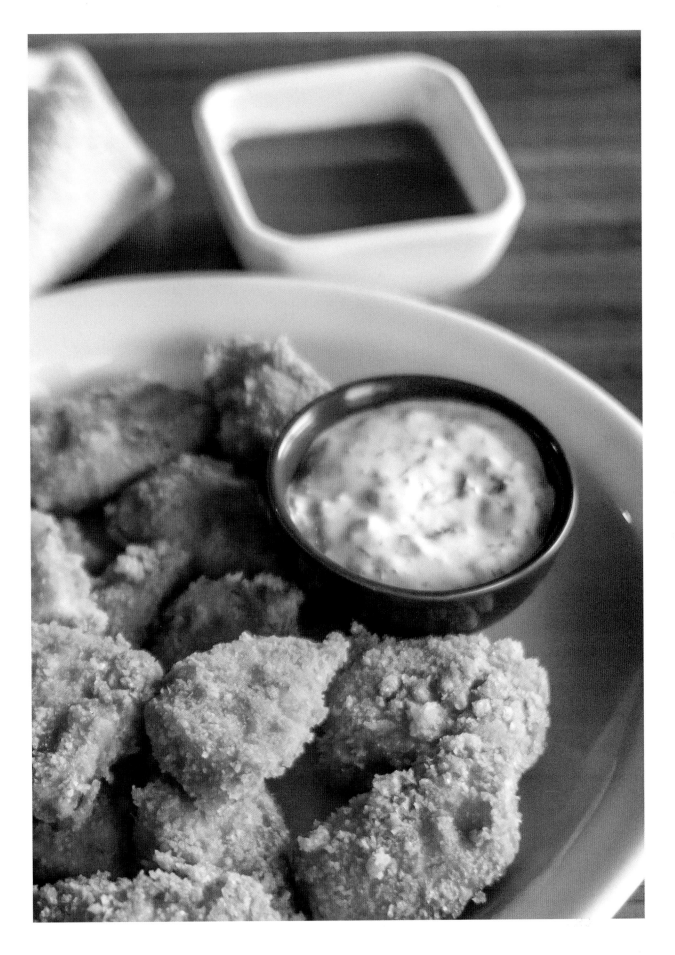

LEMON-CAPER AIOLI

MAKES: 1 cup | **PREP TIME:** 15 minutes | **COOK TIME:** 2 minutes

Technically, aioli isn't supposed to have mayo in it, and it isn't the same thing as mayo. Mayonnaise is an emulsion of egg yolks and oil, and aioli is supposed to be an emulsion of garlic and olive oil. You can take some poetic license as we did and call this aioli, or you can be more correct and call it lemon-caper mayo. Whatever you want to call it, *make it.* Slather it on our Roasted Whole Red Snapper (page 236), or enjoy it with any fish or shellfish.

2 tablespoons extra-virgin olive oil

3 scallions, white and light green parts, thinly sliced (about ¼ cup)

1 clove garlic, minced (about 1 teaspoon)

2 tablespoons drained capers

1 tablespoon chopped fresh flat-leaf parsley, plus more for garnish if desired

½ teaspoon grated lemon zest

2 tablespoons fresh lemon juice

¼ teaspoon raw honey

¼ teaspoon hot sauce

½ cup avocado oil mayonnaise

Fine sea salt and freshly ground black pepper

1. Combine the olive oil, scallions, and garlic in a small unheated skillet. Place over low heat and cook undisturbed until the mixture begins to sizzle. Allow it to sizzle for 1 minute more, then transfer to a small food processor.

2. Add the capers, parsley, lemon zest and juice, honey, hot sauce, and mayonnaise; blend until smooth. Taste and season with salt and pepper. (You can make the aioli up to 2 days ahead; keep it covered and refrigerated.)

NOTE:

If you don't have a small food processor, or you just prefer the sauce with more texture, mince the scallions, capers, and parsley and, in Step 2, whisk all of the ingredients together.

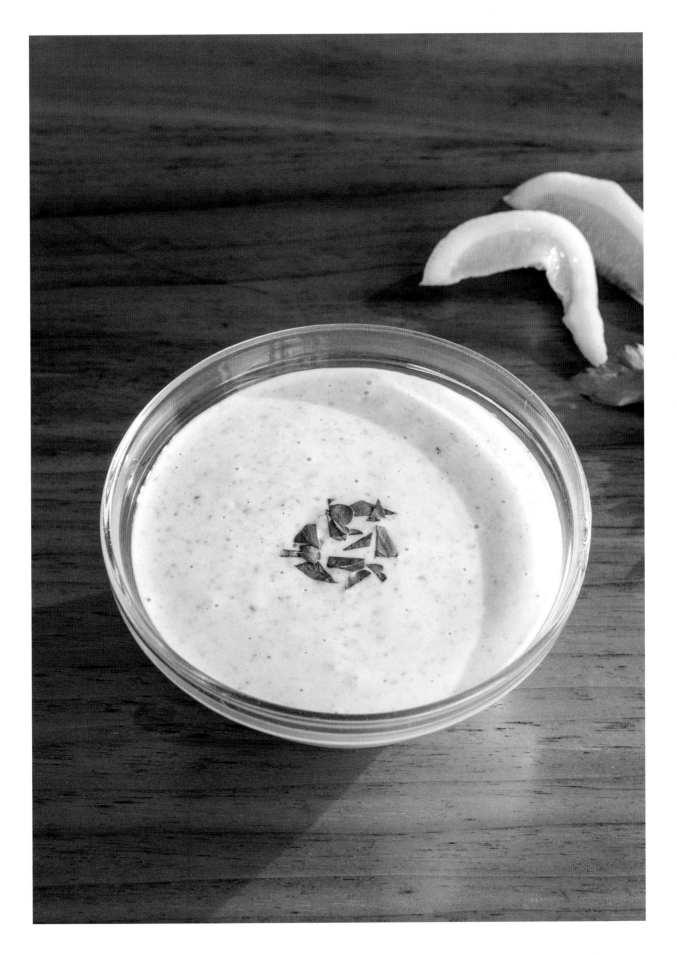

COMPOUND BUTTER THREE WAYS

Compound butter is a fantastic culinary trick. Just combine unsalted butter with a few simple ingredients and you have a sexy spread for grain-free bread or a shortcut sauce for steak, fish, chicken, or vegetables. You can also make a sweet compound butter to dress up pancakes, waffles, or muffins. Here are three butters we love—plus a bonus: the blue cheese butter on page 82 is a fourth one.

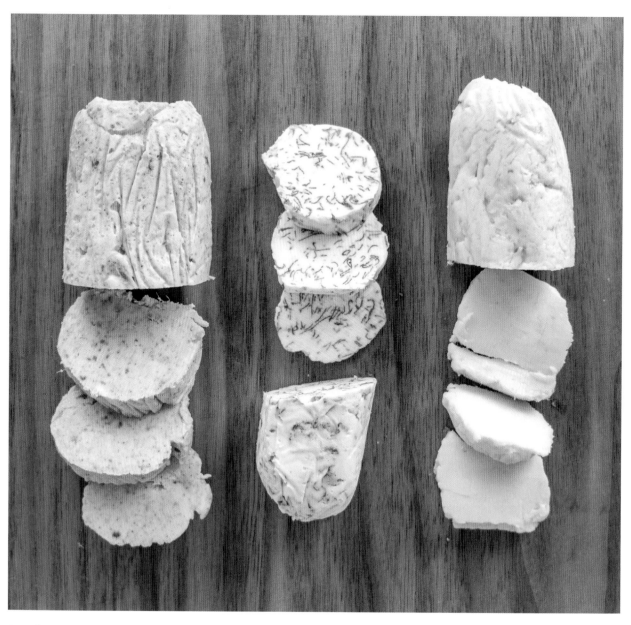

Anchovy Butter

MAKES: About 5 tablespoons | **PREP TIME:** 10 minutes, plus 30 minutes to chill

This butter is rich and luscious, with just a touch of heat from the paprika. It's not fishy; the anchovies add saltiness and umami to the butter. And it's so versatile: it can elevate steak, chicken, fish, or vegetables.

4 tablespoons (2 ounces) unsalted butter, at room temperature

4 jarred or tinned olive oil-packed anchovy fillets

½ teaspoon fresh lemon juice

¼ teaspoon garlic powder

⅛ teaspoon hot paprika

Fine sea salt and freshly ground black pepper, to taste

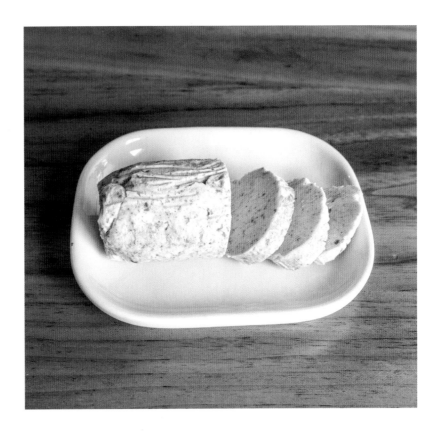

To make compound butter

Simply mash the butter with the other ingredients in a bowl until everything is well incorporated. Alternatively, if you have a small food processor, you can blend the butter with the other ingredients. Roll the compound butter into a log, wrap in plastic wrap, and refrigerate for at least 30 minutes before slicing; it will keep for up to a week. Or place the wrapped butter in a resealable bag and freeze it for up to 2 months. This method applies to all of the flavor variations that follow.

Parsley-Chive Butter

MAKES: About 5 tablespoons | **PREP TIME:** 10 minutes, plus 30 minutes to chill

Try this herby butter on seafood (like the Grilled Mussels on page 238), or melt a slice on top of mashed root vegetables, such as our Parsnip Mash (page 272).

4 tablespoons (2 ounces) unsalted butter, at room temperature

2 tablespoons chopped fresh flat-leaf parsley

2 teaspoons minced fresh chives

½ teaspoon grated lemon zest

Fine sea salt and freshly ground black pepper, to taste

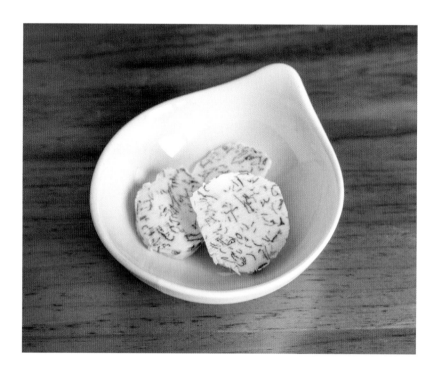

Honey-Lemon-Ginger Butter

MAKES: About 5 tablespoons | **PREP TIME:** 10 minutes, plus 30 minutes to chill

Sweet and spicy, this butter would be outrageously good on grain-free toast, muffins, pancakes, or waffles. You can also lick it right off a spoon—we won't judge.

4 tablespoons (2 ounces) unsalted butter, at room temperature

2 teaspoons raw honey

1 teaspoon fresh lemon juice

1 teaspoon grated fresh ginger

Pinch of fine sea salt

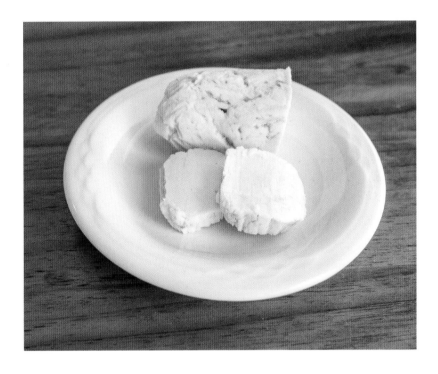

TZATZIKI

MAKES: About 1¼ cups | **PREP TIME:** 15 minutes | **COOK TIME:** 2 minutes

Cucumber, fresh mint, lemon, garlic, thick yogurt—this classic sauce hits all of the notes. Use sheep's milk yogurt if it's available to you; it's higher in both protein and fat than cow's milk yogurt, so it's ultra-rich and creamy. Like goat's milk yogurt, it's also easy on the gut for the lactose sensitive, but it's more mildly flavored than goat. (We're not knocking goat—we love it—but the milder sheep's milk is better for this sauce.) If you opt for cow's milk yogurt, you can use regular or Greek, depending on how thick you like your tzatziki.

½ English cucumber

Fine sea salt

1 tablespoon extra-virgin olive oil

1 clove garlic, minced (about 1 teaspoon)

¾ cup full-fat plain yogurt (preferably sheep's milk)

2 teaspoons chopped fresh mint leaves

½ teaspoon grated lemon zest

¼ teaspoon raw honey

Freshly ground black pepper

Pinch of red pepper flakes, for garnish (optional)

1. Grate the cucumber on the large holes of a box grater. Put the cucumber in a fine-mesh sieve, sprinkle with salt, and gently toss. Let stand for 10 minutes.

2. Meanwhile, combine the olive oil and garlic in a small unheated skillet. Place over low heat and cook until the mixture begins to sizzle. Allow to sizzle for 30 seconds more, then transfer to a medium bowl.

3. Press down on the cucumber in the sieve to squeeze out some of the water. Wrap the cucumber in a clean kitchen towel and squeeze hard to remove as much water as possible. Transfer the cucumber to the bowl with the garlic mixture. Stir in the yogurt, mint, lemon zest, and honey until well combined. Taste and season with salt and pepper. (You can make the tzatziki up to 3 days ahead; cover and refrigerate. Stir before serving.)

4. Spoon into a serving dish and garnish with red pepper flakes, if desired.

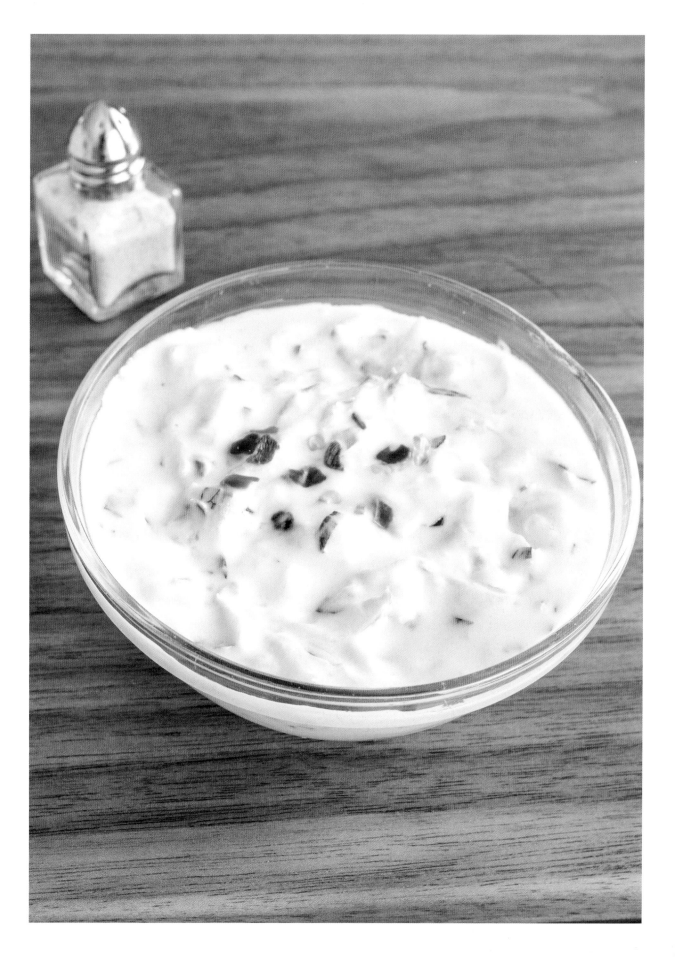

GARLIC AND DILL YOGURT DIP

MAKES: About 1 cup | **PREP TIME:** 10 minutes, plus 1 hour to chill

We love this recipe because it's easy, delicious, and packed with protein, which is kind of our thing. This dip is a great accompaniment to any protein dish, but we especially love it with chicken and lamb, like the Spicy Air Fryer Chicken Thighs on page 134 and the Lamb Kefta on page 88. Just make it and keep it in the fridge—you'll find yourself putting it on everything.

1 cup full-fat plain Greek yogurt

2 cloves garlic, crushed to a paste

1 tablespoon fresh lemon juice

½ teaspoon chopped fresh dill, plus more for garnish if desired

½ teaspoon fine sea salt

½ teaspoon freshly ground black pepper

In a small bowl, combine all of the ingredients. Cover and chill for at least 1 hour before serving. Garnish with fresh dill, if desired. Store leftovers in an airtight container in the fridge for up to 4 days.

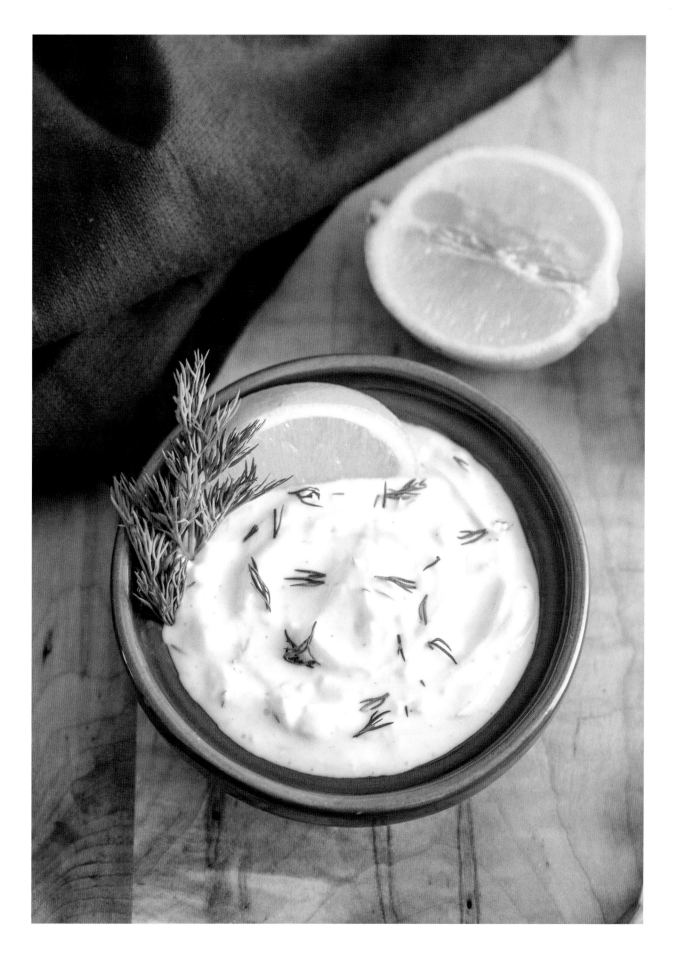

WARM BACON VINAIGRETTE

MAKES: About ½ cup | **PREP TIME:** 10 minutes | **COOK TIME:** 13 minutes

If you love bacon as much as we do, you want it in basically everything…including salad. Make it happen by using bacon fat as the base for this vinaigrette. Add the bacon bits to the dressing or scatter them on top of the salad (or eat the bacon while you make the salad, we're just saying).

4 ounces bacon (about 4 slices), diced

3 tablespoons stone-ground mustard

2 tablespoons raw honey

3 cloves garlic, minced (about 1 tablespoon)

½ teaspoon fine sea salt

½ teaspoon freshly ground black pepper

¼ cup apple cider vinegar

1. Put the diced bacon in a medium unheated skillet. Turn the heat to medium-low and cook until crisp, about 10 minutes. Using a slotted spoon, transfer the bacon to a bowl lined with paper towels. Remove the skillet from the heat.

2. Add the mustard, honey, garlic, salt, and pepper to the skillet with the bacon fat. Whisk until well combined.

3. While whisking, drizzle the vinegar into the skillet. Continue to whisk until the vinaigrette has emulsified and thickened slightly, about 3 minutes. Add the bacon bits to the vinaigrette, if desired.

4. Serve warm, or pour into a glass jar, cover, and refrigerate to serve later. It's best warm, so if you've refrigerated it, pour it into a skillet or saucepan and rewarm over low heat, whisking. The dressing will keep, covered and refrigerated, for up to 4 days.

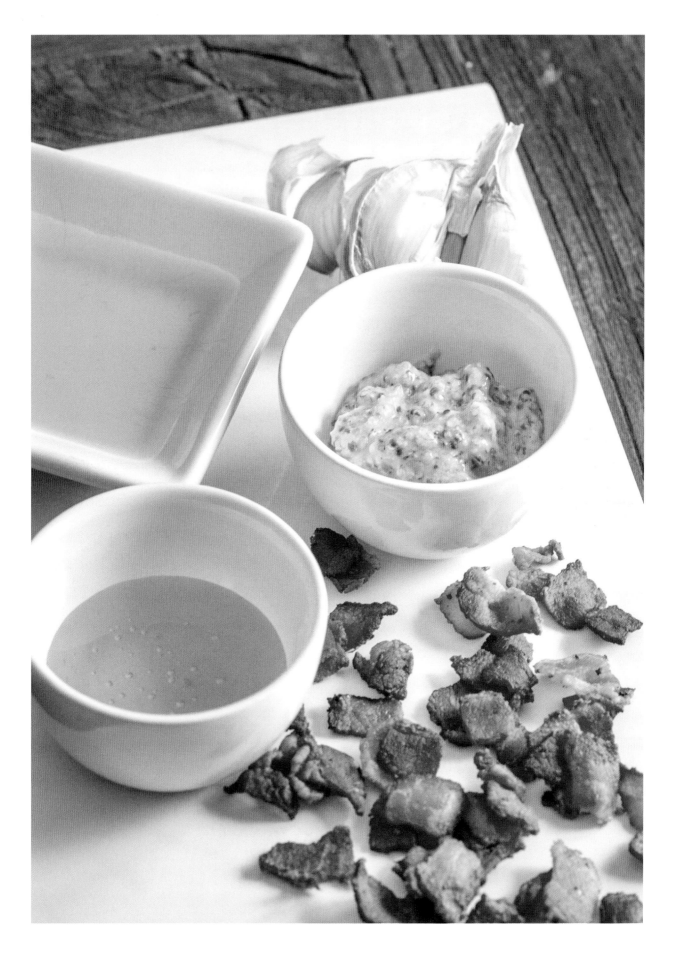

CINNAMON AND VANILLA-INFUSED GHEE

MAKES: 1 cup | **PREP TIME:** 5 minutes | **COOK TIME:** 5 minutes

Ghee is a rich, delicious, über-buttery fat that works well for many people who have issues with dairy; since the butter is clarified, the milk solids are removed, making ghee easier to digest. You can make this recipe savory by replacing the vanilla bean and cinnamon sticks with spices like turmeric or thyme, and you can use infused ghee anywhere you'd use butter: on bread, vegetables, or maybe some tasty chaffles (see the recipe on page 210).

1 vanilla bean

1 cup ghee

2 cinnamon sticks, or ½ teaspoon ground cinnamon

⅛ teaspoon fine sea salt

1. Slice open the vanilla bean lengthwise and carefully scrape out the seeds.

2. Put the ghee, vanilla pod and seeds, cinnamon sticks, and salt in a small saucepan; place over medium heat. Cook, stirring continuously, until the ghee has melted and become fragrant, about 5 minutes.

3. Remove the pan from the heat. Remove the cinnamon sticks and vanilla pod and pour the infused ghee into a heatproof glass container. Let cool at room temperature for about 1 hour or, once no longer hot, in the fridge for about 30 minutes before using. The ghee will firm back up to a soft spreadable consistency as it cools. Store in an airtight glass container at room temperature for up to 3 months.

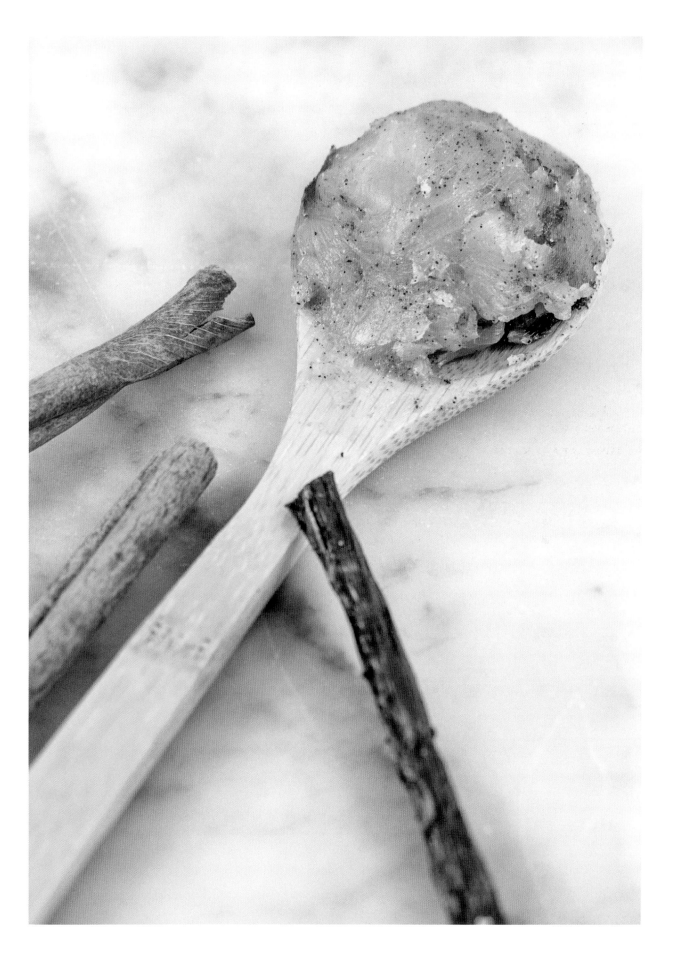

SPICY FRUIT SALSA

MAKES: 4 cups | **PREP TIME:** 15 minutes

This perfectly sweet and spicy summer salsa tastes great with grilled chicken or pork chops (page 174) or with sweet potato chips (page 276). Swap peaches for the pineapple if they're in season, include cilantro if you like it, and add some finely diced jalapeño if you'd like your salsa even spicier.

1 cup diced fresh pineapple

1 cup diced mango

½ medium red onion, finely diced (about ½ cup)

½ red bell pepper, seeded and finely diced (about ½ cup)

¼ cup fresh lime juice (from 2 to 3 limes)

¼ teaspoon fine sea salt

¼ teaspoon cayenne pepper or chipotle powder

In a medium bowl, combine the pineapple, mango, onion, and bell pepper. Add the lime juice, salt, and cayenne; toss to combine. Taste and season with additional salt, if needed. Store leftovers in an airtight container in the fridge for up to 3 days.

NOTE:

Feel free to make this salsa the day before serving it; the flavors will come together beautifully.

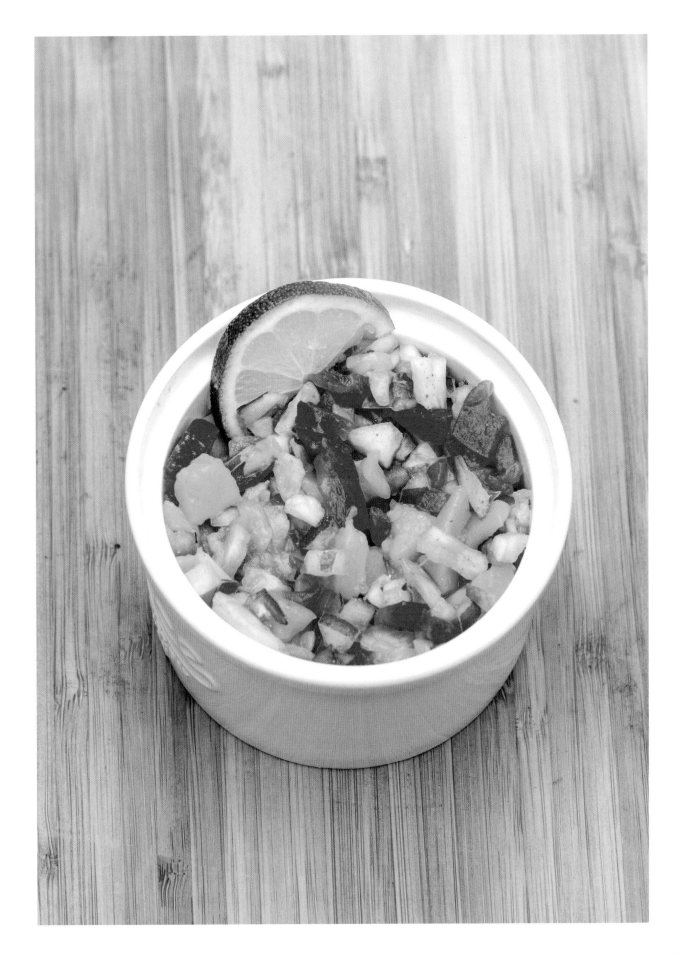

ACKNOWLEDGMENTS

From Beth: Big, big thanks to Ashleigh, my dear friend and partner on this book, truly a labor of love in every way. You teach me so much and inspire me every day. To my love and my partner, Mark. Everything is better because of you (including some of the photos in this book, taken with your camera and often with or by you). To my daughter, Dylan, who encouraged me and helped me laugh at myself, and who teaches me every day by example what it means to be an amazing human. To my biggest cheerleader, my mom, Tama: I miss you every day. To my agent, Joy Tutela, for your wisdom and generosity. To my dedicated taster and photo consultant, Ella d'Aulaire, thank you. To family and friends too abundant to name, but all of whom helped with this book with their enthusiasm and love—I am so grateful for each one of you.

From Ashleigh: First, thank you to my partner-in-crime, Beth. Ever since we met, we've talked excitedly about doing a project together, and it was Beth's genius that brought forth the idea of a healthy, protein-forward cookbook. I can't think of anyone else I'd rather work with on such a noble—and delicious—project. Thank you to my favorite person on the planet, my husband, Alex. He is my biggest source of support and positivity, and his enthusiasm (and willingness to barbecue) never wavers. Thank you to my talented and dear friend Heather, who did food photography for this and my first book—sharing exciting projects with people you love makes the process that much more rewarding, and I'll always cherish our adventure-filled weekend shoots. And to everyone who supported this project and shares in our love of good, nourishing food: this is for you.

Special thanks to the experts who shared their abundant wisdom about animal proteins:

- John Addis, owner of Fish Tales

- Jess Coslow, livestock manager for Stone Barns Center for Food and Agriculture

- Ariane Daguin, founder of D'Artagnan

- Ryan Farr, founder of 4505 Meats

- Jennifer Gregg, VP of operations for Vital Farms

- Mike Salguero, CEO of ButcherBox

- Heather Marold Thomason, founder of Primal Supply Meats

- Bri Van Scotter, author of *Complete Wild Game Cookbook*

Shout-out to the local butcher shops in Brooklyn that answered many questions, accommodated special requests with a smile, and encouraged us:

- Fleishers

- Paisanos

- Staubitz Market

We'd also like to extend a big thanks to the whole staff at Victory Belt. You are incredible partners. We are so grateful for your excitement about this book, all of your hard work and dedication in creating it with us, and how fun and fulfilling you made the entire process.

And of course, thanks to you, our readers and supporters. Thank you for opening these pages, being willing to learn and try new things, and sharing in our passion for nourishing, delicious food. You were in our minds throughout this whole process.

RESOURCES

Farming/Agriculture

Certified Humane: certifiedhumane.org

Organic livestock requirements: www.ams.usda.gov/sites/default/files/media/Organic%20Livestock%20Requirements.pdf

Cooking Basics

Food52: food52.com

Kitchn: www.thekitchn.com

Serious Eats: www.seriouseats.com

The Spruce Eats: www.thespruceeats.com

Purveyors of Quality Proteins

This is by no means all of them; we're lucky to have a wealth of online sources for high-quality proteins. These are some that we love and have used extensively.

ButcherBox: www.butcherbox.com

Crowd Cow: www.crowdcow.com

D'Artagnan: www.dartagnan.com

Holy Grail Steak Co.: holygrailsteak.com

Porter Road: porterroad.com

Thrive Market: thrivemarket.com

US Wellness Meats: grasslandbeef.com

Vital Choice: www.vitalchoice.com/

Walden Local Meat (Northeastern U.S. only): waldenlocalmeat.com

RECOMMENDED READING

Badger, Mike. "The Nutrition of Pasture-Raised Chicken and Meats." Accessed May 20, 2021. https://apppa.org/The-Nutrition-of-Pasture-Raised-Chicken-and-Meats.

Clover Meadows Beef. "What Everyone Ought to Know About Beef Cuts." Accessed May 20, 2021. https://www.clovermeadowsbeef.com/beef-cuts/.

Cofnas, Nathan. "Is Vegetarianism Healthy for Children?" *Critical Reviews in Food Science and Nutrition* 59, no. 13 (2019): 2052–60.

Ede, Georgia. "The History of All-Meat Diets." Accessed April 6, 2021. https://www.diagnosisdiet.com/full-article/all-meat-diets.

Edwards, Rebekah. "Paprika: The Antioxidant-Rich Spice That Fights Disease." Accessed June 13, 2021. https://draxe.com/nutrition/paprika/.

Encyclopedia of Food Sciences and Nutrition, 2nd ed. "Carcass and Meat Characteristics." Accessed April 7, 2021. https://www.sciencedirect.com/topics/agricultural-and-biological-sciences/game-animals.

Institute of Agriculture and Natural Resources, University of Nebraska-Lincoln. "Pork Meat Identification." Accessed May 20, 2021. https://animalscience.unl.edu/pork-meat-identification.

Kresser, Chris. "RHR: How Protein Supports Your Muscle Health, with Dr. Gabrielle Lyon." Accessed April 6, 2021. https://chriskresser.com/how-protein-supports-your-muscle-health-with-dr-gabrielle-lyon/#Why_Protein_Quality_Matters_for_Muscles.

Nourish by WebMD. "Health Benefits of Coriander." Accessed June 13, 2021. https://www.webmd.com/diet/health-benefits-coriander#1.

Oregon Health Authority. "Safe Eating of Shellfish." Accessed June 13, 2021. https://www.oregon.gov/oha/PH/HealthyEnvironments/Recreation/Documents/Shellfish-safety.pdf.

Penn State News. "Research Shows Eggs from Pastured Chickens May Be More Nutritious." Accessed May 20, 2021. https://www.psu.edu/news/agricultural-sciences/story/research-shows-eggs-pastured-chickens-may-be-more-nutritious/.

Plataforma SINC. "How to Remove Environmental Pollutants from Raw Meat." Accessed June 2, 2021. https://www.sciencedaily.com/releases/2016/05/160506100202.htm.

Rodgers, Diana. "Amazing Grazing: Why Grass-Fed Beef Isn't to Blame in the Climate Change Debate." Accessed April 10, 2021. https://sustainabledish.com/beef-isnt-to-blame/.

Rodgers, Diana. "Eat Meat. Improve Your Mood." Accessed April 7, 2021. https://sustainabledish.com/eat-meat-improve-your-mood/.

Rodgers, Diana. "Meat Is Magnificent." Accessed April 7, 2021. https://sustainabledish.com/meat-is-magnificent/.

Rodgers, Diana. "More Protein, Better Protein." Accessed April 7, 2021. https://sustainabledish.com/protein-better-protein/.

Rodgers, Diana. "Why Is It Necessary to Eat Animals?" Accessed April 10, 2021. https://robbwolf.com/2016/08/03/why-is-it-necessary-to-eat-animals/.

Rodgers, Diana. "Women and Meat." Accessed April 10, 2021. https://sustainabledish.com/women-and-meat/.

VanHouten, Ashleigh. *It Takes Guts: A Meat-Eater's Guide to Eating Offal with Over 75 Healthy and Delicious Nose-to-Tail Recipes.* Las Vegas, Nev.: Victory Belt Publishing, 2020.

RECIPE INDEX

Beef, Lamb & Goat

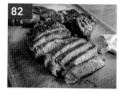
Rib Eye with
Blue Cheese Butter

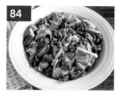
Cheeseburger Salad

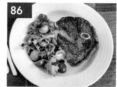
Za'atar Lamb
Shoulder Chops

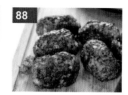
Lamb Kefta

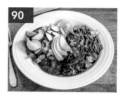
Chipotle
Shredded Beef

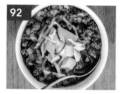
Super Meaty Chili

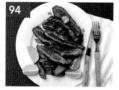
Carne Asada

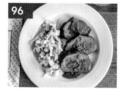
Beef Tenderloin
Roast with Bourbon
Pan Sauce

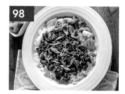
Korean-Style
Ground Beef

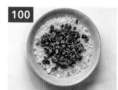
Beef Confit

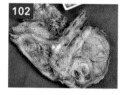
Garlic-Herb
Lamb Chops with
Applesauce

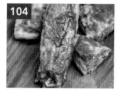
Stuffed Cabbage
Rolls

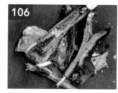
Spice-Rubbed
Goat Ribs

Poultry

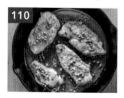
Chicken Piccata

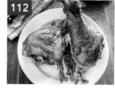
Turkey Legs Confit

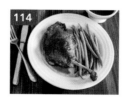
Red Wine–Braised
Duck Legs

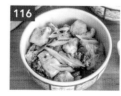
Stir-Fried Chicken
and Vegetables

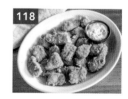
Air Fryer Buffalo
Chicken Nuggets

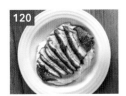
120
Five-Spice Duck Breast with Orange and Red Wine Jus

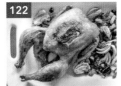
122
Roast Chicken with Vegetables

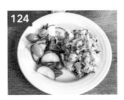
124
Creamy Chicken, Bacon, and Broccoli Casserole

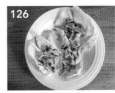
126
Vietnamese Chicken Meatball Lettuce Wraps

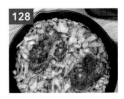
128
Skillet Chicken Thighs with Cabbage

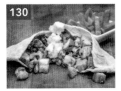
130
Chicken Shawarma

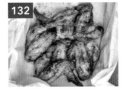
132
Hot Honey Chicken Wings

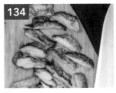
134
Spicy Air Fryer Chicken Thighs

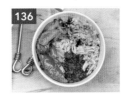
136
Mexican-Style Shredded Chicken Bowl

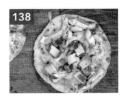
138
Shredded Chicken Tostadas

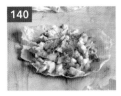
140
Chicken Salad with Fennel and Asian Pear

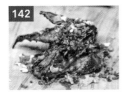
142
Sweet Chili and Orange Duck Wings

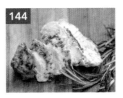
144
Air Fryer Herbed Butter Turkey Breast

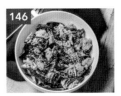
146
Turkey and Cabbage Bowl

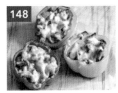
148
Stuffed Peppers

Pork

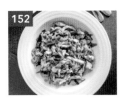
152
Mu Shu Pork Bowls

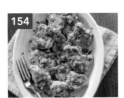
154
Pork Medallions with Mustard Pan Sauce

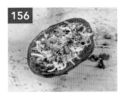
156
Loaded Sweet Potatoes

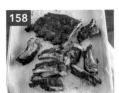
158
Slow-Baked Ribs

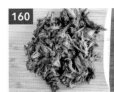
160
Pulled Pork

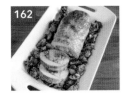
162
Sausage and Apple–Stuffed Pork Loin Roast

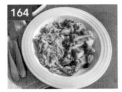
164
Air Fryer Pork Katsu

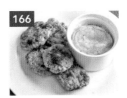
166
Pork Breakfast Sausage Patties

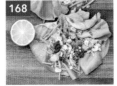
168
Vietnamese-Style Roast Pork Lettuce Wraps

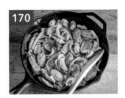
170
Sausage and Peppers

Pork (continued)

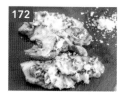
172

Breadless Croque Monsieur

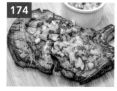
174

Grilled Pork Chops with Spicy Fruit Salsa

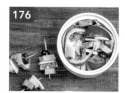
176

Italian Sub Salad

Game

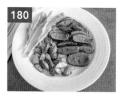
180

Coffee-Rubbed Venison Denver Leg

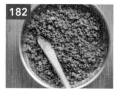
182

Bison Sloppy Joe

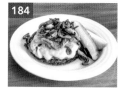
184

Open-Faced Bison Patty Melts

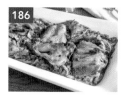
186

Braised Rabbit with Mushrooms and Mustard

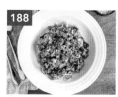
188

Sausage and Ostrich Bolognese

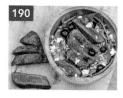
190

Elk Steak Salad

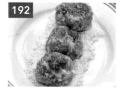
192

Wild Boar Meatballs

Eggs

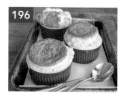
196

Cheddar-Chive Soufflés

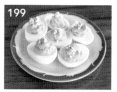
199

Buffalo Deviled Eggs

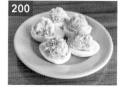
200

Crab Cake Deviled Eggs

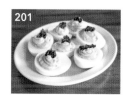
201

Ginger-Wasabi Deviled Eggs

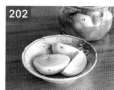
202

Spicy Kimchi Pickled Eggs

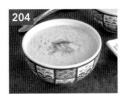

204

Egg Drop Soup

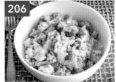

206

Denver Scramble

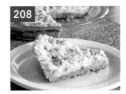

208

Quiche Lorraine

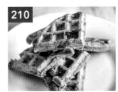

210

Cinnamon Bun Chaffles

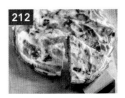

212

Caramelized Onion and Leek Frittata with Prosciutto

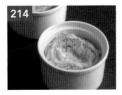

214

Easy Ham and Egg Mug Omelets

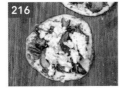

216

Cauliflower-Cheese Breakfast Wraps

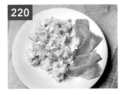

220

Creamy Scrambled Eggs with Smoked Salmon

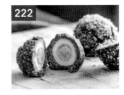

222

Carnivore Baked Scotch Eggs

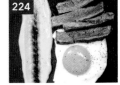

224

Steak and Eggs with Lemon "Hollandaise" Sauce

Seafood

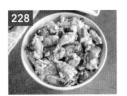

228

Lemon-Tarragon Lobster Salad

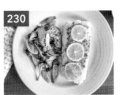

230

Lemon-Garlic Butter Roasted Cod

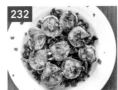

232

Seared Scallops with Bacon, Fried Capers, and Shallot Butter

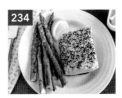

234

Everything Bagel Salmon

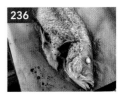

236

Roasted Whole Red Snapper

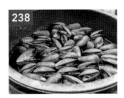

238

Grilled Mussels

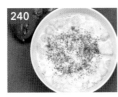

240

Traditional Nova Scotia Chowder

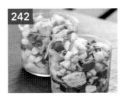

242

Trout Ceviche

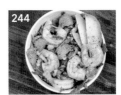

244

Shrimp, Avocado, and Citrus Salad

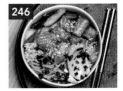

246

Salmon Poke Bowl

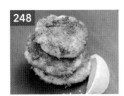

248

Bermuda-Style Codfish Cakes

Offal

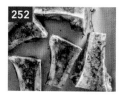
Roasted Marrow Bones

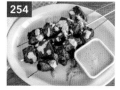
Peruvian-Style Grilled Beef Heart

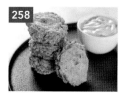
Savory Meat "Muffins"

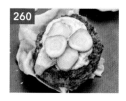
Bone Marrow Burgers

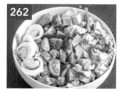
Grilled Chicken Heart Cobb Salad

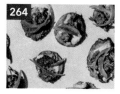
Tongue Sliders

Sides

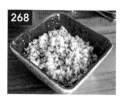
Cauliflower Rice (That Doesn't Suck)

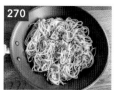
Zucchini Noodles (That Don't Suck)

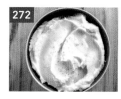
Parsnip Mash

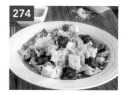
Caesar Salad with Pork Belly "Croutons"

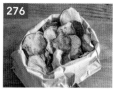
Air Fryer Mixed Sweet Potato Chips

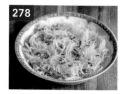
Garlicky Spaghetti Squash

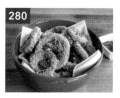
Pork Panko Onion Rings

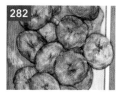
Tostones

Appetizers & Snacks

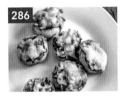
286

Stuffed Mushrooms

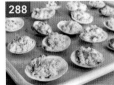
288

Baked Stuffed Clams

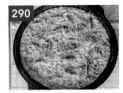
290

Warm Bacon
Jalapeño Popper Dip

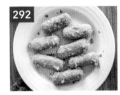
292

Air Fryer
Mozzarella Sticks

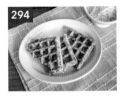
294

Paffle

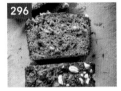
296

Elvis Banana Bread

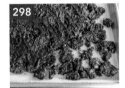
298

Dark Chocolate-
Coconut Granola
Clusters

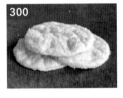
300

Keto Egg Breads

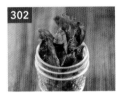
302

Turkey Jerky

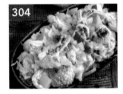
304

Pork Rind Nachos

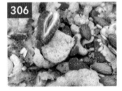
306

Forager Trail Mix

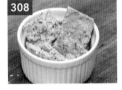
308

"Animal" Crackers

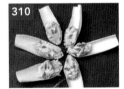
310

Smoked Salmon Pâté

Desserts & Beverages

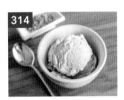
314

Vanilla Bean
Ice Cream

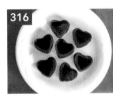
316

Fruit Jellies

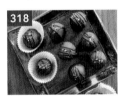
318

Secret-Ingredient
Cookie Dough
Truffles

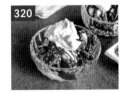
320

Hot Fudge Sundaes

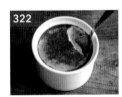
322

French Toast
Egg Custard

Desserts & Beverages (continued)

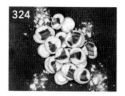
Maple Bacon Meringues

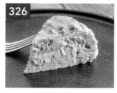
Japanese-Style Cheesecake

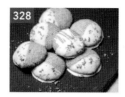
Orange White Chocolate-Dipped Duck Fat Sugar Cookies

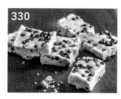
Sneaky Chocolate Chip Carnivore Protein Bars

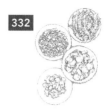
Savory Dessert Plate

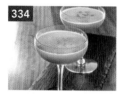
Blood Orange Gin Fizz

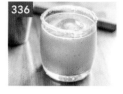
Spicy Toro Shot

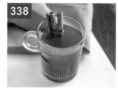
Antioxidant-Rich Sipping Broth

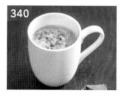
Spicy Bone Broth Hot Chocolate

Sauces & Condiments

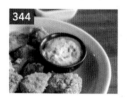
Bacon Ranch Dip

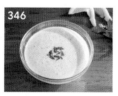
Lemon-Caper Aioli

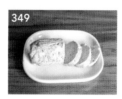
Anchovy Butter

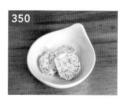
Parsley-Chive Butter

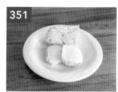
Honey-Lemon-Ginger Butter

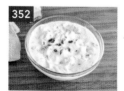
Tzatziki

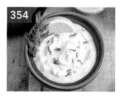
Garlic and Dill Yogurt Dip

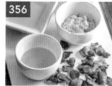
Warm Bacon Vinaigrette

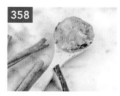
Cinnamon and Vanilla-Infused Ghee

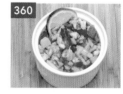
Spicy Fruit Salsa

GENERAL INDEX